Lecture Notes in Computer Science 14976

Founding Editors

Gerhard Goos
Juris Hartmanis

The series Lecture Notes in Computer Science (LNCS), including its subseries Lecture Notes in Artificial Intelligence (LNAI) and Lecture Notes in Bioinformatics (LNBI), has established itself as a medium for the publication of new developments in computer science and information technology research, teaching, and education.

LNCS enjoys close cooperation with the computer science R & D community, the series counts many renowned academics among its volume editors and paper authors, and collaborates with prestigious societies. Its mission is to serve this international community by providing an invaluable service, mainly focused on the publication of conference and workshop proceedings and postproceedings. LNCS commenced publication in 1973.

Xianghua Xie · Iain Styles · Gibin Powathil ·
Marco Ceccarelli
Editors

Artificial Intelligence in Healthcare

First International Conference, AIiH 2024
Swansea, UK, September 4–6, 2024
Proceedings, Part II

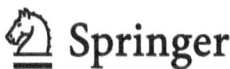 Springer

Editors
Xianghua Xie ⓘ
Swansea University
Swansea, UK

Iain Styles ⓘ
Queen's University
Belfast, UK

Gibin Powathil ⓘ
Swansea University
Swansea, UK

Marco Ceccarelli ⓘ
University of Rome Tor Vergata
Rome, Italy

ISSN 0302-9743 ISSN 1611-3349 (electronic)
Lecture Notes in Computer Science
ISBN 978-3-031-67284-2 ISBN 978-3-031-67285-9 (eBook)
https://doi.org/10.1007/978-3-031-67285-9

This Springer imprint is published by the registered company Springer Nature Switzerland AG
The registered company address is: Gewerbestrasse 11, 6330 Cham, Switzerland

If disposing of this product, please recycle the paper.

Preface

This LNCS volume contains the papers presented at the inaugural edition of the International Conference on Artificial Intelligence on Healthcare (AIiH 2024), which was organized in September 2024 in the beautiful city of Swansea, UK.

AIiH aims to provide a prominent platform for researchers and practitioners who are devoted to improving healthcare using modern artificial intelligence. We recognize that healthcare applications present complex and sometimes unique challenges across a wide spectrum, from ethics to technical developments, and that generic AI methods are often inadequate. By creating this dedicated forum, we encourage discussion and dissemination of efficient and effective AI solutions and technologies for healthcare, and in turn we hope to influence research, technology adoption, and decision making in healthcare.

The papers submitted to AIiH 2024 were thoroughly double-blindly reviewed by up to four referees per paper and 47 papers were selected as full papers for the conference proceedings from 70 submissions (excluding late-breaking abstracts). A total of 25 papers were accepted for oral presentation at the conference. Contributing authors were from 17 countries, which reflected the international nature of the conference. The best paper prize was selected and awarded at the conference. AIiH 2024 also offered 5 full bursaries to students in order to encourage participation, particularly where financial support was needed.

We would like to thank all reviewers for their diligent work and prompt responses. In particular, we would like to highlight the following outstanding reviewers for their hard work in providing detailed, insightful and high-quality reviews for all the papers assigned to them: Frederick W. B. Li from University of Durham, Betsy Dayana Marcela Chaparro Rico from Swansea University, John Chiverton from University of Portsmouth, Jingjing Deng from University of Durham, Hanchi Ren from Swansea University, Ioannis Ivrissimtzis from University of Durham, Gani Balbayev from Eurasian National University, Temitayo Olugbade from University of Sussex, and Matteo Russo from University of Rome Tor Vergata. AIiH 2024 offered a 50% discount on the registration fee to all reviewers who fully engaged in the review process.

We were honored to have 9 distinguished scholars as invited speakers. Amir Atapour-Abarghouei from University of Durham delivered the conference tutorial on Deep Generative Neural Networks. The 5 keynotes were given by Hao Ni from University College London, Timothy Rittman from University of Cambridge, Konstantinos Kamnitsas from University of Oxford, Jacques Fleuriot from University of Edinburgh, and Eiichiro Tanaka from Waseda University. AIiH 2024 also featured a 3-speaker Panel Session on Translating AI Research into Practice by Alba Di Pardo from IRCCS Istituto Neurologico Mediterraneo Neuromed, Noura Al Moubayed from Durham University & Evergreen Life, and Mark Penney from AstraZeneca. We are grateful for their inspiring contributions.

We are indebted to a number of people who contributed generously to the organization of the conference: Daniele Cafolla, Jiaxiang Zhang, Raoul Van Loon, Jiaxiang Zhang, Lu Zhang, Jingjing Deng, Hanchi Ren, Beiyu Lin, Rex Ying, and many student volunteers. The conference received generous support from several companies and institutions. We would like to thank Springer for extending their support to publish the proceedings in LNCS. Finally, we thank all the presenting authors and attendees who made the first edition of this new conference series intellectually stimulating and enjoyable.

July 2024

Xianghua Xie
Iain Styles
Gibin Powathil
Marco Ceccarelli

Organization

General Co-chairs

Xianghua Xie   Swansea University, UK
Iain Styles   Queen's University Belfast, UK

Program Co-chairs

Gibin Powathil   Swansea University, UK
Marco Ceccarelli   University of Rome Tor Vergata, Italy

Special Session Co-chairs

Jiaxiang Zhang   Swansea University, UK
Rex Ying   Yale University, USA

Sponsorship Co-chairs

Daniele Cafolla   Swansea University, UK
Raoul Van Loon   Swansea University, UK

Publicity Co-chairs

Lu Zhang   Swansea University, UK
Beiyu Lin   University of Nevada, USA

Publication Co-chairs

Jingjing Deng   Durham University, UK
Hanchi Ren   Swansea University, UK

International Program Committee

Mario Acevedo Alvarado	Panamerican University, Mexico
Gani Balbayev	Satbayev University, Kazakhstan
Barry Bentley	Cardiff Metropolitan University, UK
Yona Binti-Abd-Gaus	Durham University, UK
Neelanjan Bhowmik	Durham University, UK
Matteo Bottin	University of Padua, Italy
Sarah Brüningk	ETH Zürich, Switzerland
Fabio Caraffini	Swansea University, UK
Giuseppe Carbone	University of Calabria, Italy
Betsy D. M. Chaparro Rico	Swansea University, UK
Changrun Chen	University of Kent, UK
I-Ming Chen	NTU, Singapore
Xi Chen	University of Bath, UK
John Chiverton	University of Portsmouth, UK
Hassan Eshkiki	Swansea University, UK
Maria Garrosa Solana	University of Madrid "Carlos III", Spain
Kenji Hashimoto	Waseda University, Japan
Chen Hu	Swansea University, UK
Ioannis Ivrissimtzis	Durham University, UK
Richard Jiang	University of Lancaster, UK
Stamos Katsigiannis	Durham University, UK
Med Amine Laribi	University of Poitiers, France
Frederick Li	Durham University, UK
Siyu Li	University of Kent, UK
Hongying Liu	Tianjin University, China
Wei Liu	Xi'an UPT, China
Xuekang Liu	University of Kent, UK
Xiaoke Ma	Xidian University, China
Yingliang Ma	University of East Anglia, UK
Vicente Mata Amela	Universitat Politècnica de València, Spain
Temitayo Olugbade	University of Sussex, UK
Victor Petuya	University of the Basque Country, Spain
Long Qian	Queen Mary University of London, UK
Muhammad Raza	University of Edinburgh, UK
Suraj Ramchand	Swansea University, UK
Hanchi Ren	Swansea University, UK
Sa Ren	Sheffield University, UK
Matteo Russo	University of Rome "Tor Vergata", Italy
Sriram Sagi	NetApp, USA
Saber Sami	University of East Anglia, UK

Contents – Part II

Medical Signal and Image Processing

Assisted Living Technology

Digital Twinning, Virtual Pathology and Oncology

Patient Data, Privacy and Ethics

Contents – Part I

AI Driven Robotics for Healthcare

AI in Mental Health

AI in Proactive Care and Intervention

AI in Proactive Care and Intervention

Cluster and Trajectory Analysis of Multiple Long-Term Conditions in Adults with Learning Disabilities

Emeka Abakasanga[1] , Rania Kousovista[1], Georgina Cosma[1(✉)],
Gyuchan Thomas Jun[2], Reza Kiani[3], and Satheesh Gangadharan[3]

[1] Department of Computer Science, School of Science, Loughborough University,
Loughborough, UK
g.cosma@lboro.ac.uk
[2] School of Design and Creative Arts, Loughborough University, Loughborough, UK
[3] Leicestershire Partnership NHS Trust, Leicester, UK

Abstract. Individuals with learning disabilities (LD) are at a heightened risk of experiencing multiple long-term conditions (MLTCs) due to various factors, which can lead to increased premature mortality rates and compromised quality of life. Despite this, there is limited research employing cluster analysis to identify and categorise similar patterns of MLTCs in patients with learning disabilities. This study applies machine learning clustering algorithms to data from 13,069 adults with learning disabilities in Wales, using a 3-cluster Gaussian Mixture Model for 6,830 males and a 3-cluster BIRCH algorithm for 6,239 females. Cluster 3 for males and Cluster 1 for females represented 'relatively healthy' groups, characterised by predominantly younger patients with lower MLTC counts and lower hospitalization rates. However, these clusters exhibited the lowest age at mortality, 62 years for males and approximately 65 years for females, indicating a higher likelihood of preventable deaths. Subsequently, prevalent combinations of MLTCs and common disease trajectories were analysed within these clusters. Identifying distinct MLTC clusters, prevalent combinations, and trajectories provides crucial insights for optimizing care pathways, targeted interventions, and resource allocation tailored to the specific needs of individuals with learning disabilities. This ultimately aims to improve health outcomes and quality of life for this population.

Keywords: Cluster analysis · Trajectories · Learning disability · Multiple long-term conditions

1 Introduction

Clustering is a vital technique in healthcare research, enabling the grouping of similar patient data to identify patterns and structures within complex datasets. By identifying patient clusters with shared clinical profiles or combinations of

ⓒ The Author(s), under exclusive license to Springer Nature Switzerland AG 2024
X. Xie et al. (Eds.): AIiH 2024, LNCS 14976, pp. 3–16, 2024.
https://doi.org/10.1007/978-3-031-67285-9_1

diseases, researchers can inform disease stratification, personalised medicine, predictive modelling, and healthcare resource allocation. Moreover, clustering techniques facilitate the discovery of latent relationships and trajectories among patient data, enhancing targeted interventions, refining clinical decision-making, and ultimately improving patient outcomes.

Despite the broad application of clustering for patients with various Long Term Conditions (LTCs) [3,11,17,18,21,22], as well as in drug discovery and development for disease management [13], there is a noticeable gap in research on the co-occurrence patterns of Multiple Long Term Conditions (MLTC) among individuals with Learning Disabilities (LD) [10,14].

Individuals with learning disabilities exhibit a significantly higher prevalence of MLTC due to genetic, behavioural, and social factors, and shared aetiology among certain conditions [4,5,10]. This heightened MLTC prevalence, coupled with barriers to healthcare access, contributes to increased premature mortality rates and compromises the quality of life for this population [7]. Therefore, this study aims to explore potential clusters of MLTC in individuals with learning disabilities using machine learning and statistical approaches, offering crucial insights for devising individualised strategies based on patient characteristics.

In our initial analysis, six distinct machine learning and statistical clustering algorithms were applied to datasets of Welsh residents diagnosed with a learning disability between January 2000 and December 2021 [1]. The data was separately analysed for males and females to discern unique patient subgroups based on their distribution of LTC diagnoses at the study's end date. The algorithms employed were agglomerative clustering, Balanced Iterative Reducing and Clustering using Hierarchies (BIRCH) [23], KMeans [2], KModes [8], Gaussian Mixture Model (GMM) [15], and the Latent Class Analysis (LCA) model [16]. For each sex, the performances of all algorithms were compared, and the algorithm producing the most distinct clusters was selected. The Silhouette Coefficient (SC) index served as the metric to quantify cluster separability [20], with values ranging from -1 for strongly overlapping or misclassified clusters to 1 for well-defined/separated clusters. SC values near zero indicate overlapping clusters or a dataset lacking a clear structure. The 3-cluster GMM algorithm and the 3-cluster BIRCH demonstrated optimal performance in the male and female cohorts, respectively. This study further analyses the optimal algorithms to identify key characteristics of individuals across their respective clusters, prevalent co-occurring MLTC groups, and the most frequent trajectories of LTCs for both male and female cohorts within their predominant clusters. These findings provide valuable insights for enhancing patient outcomes and quality of life, facilitating the reduction of early mortality, optimizing healthcare resource allocation, tracking potential disease progression per patient, and providing pertinent data to advance clinical research and understand disease mechanisms, ultimately optimizing healthcare policies for this population.

2   Methods

2.1   Dataset

The clusters in this study were obtained for patients in Wales with learning disabilities, using Electronic Health Record (EHR) contained within the Secure Anonymised Information Linkage (SAIL) databank. SAIL is a Trusted Research Environment (TRE) for Wales, which enables the use of anonymised individual-level, population-scale, linked data sources [6,12,19]. All data from SAIL were accessed securely under strict conditions compliant with the General Data Protection Regulation (GDPR), and facilitated through a privacy-protective haven and remote access system known as the SAIL Gateway. Specifically, this study accessed primary care General Practice (GP) records from the Welsh Longitudinal General Practice (WLGP) data, secondary care inpatient hospitalisation records contained in the Patient Episode Database for Wales (PEDW), patients demographic, residency and registration records from the Welsh Demographic Service Dataset (WDSD) and mortality records from the Office for National statistics (ONS) contained in the Annual District Death Extract (ADDE) data.

2.2   Dataset Preparation

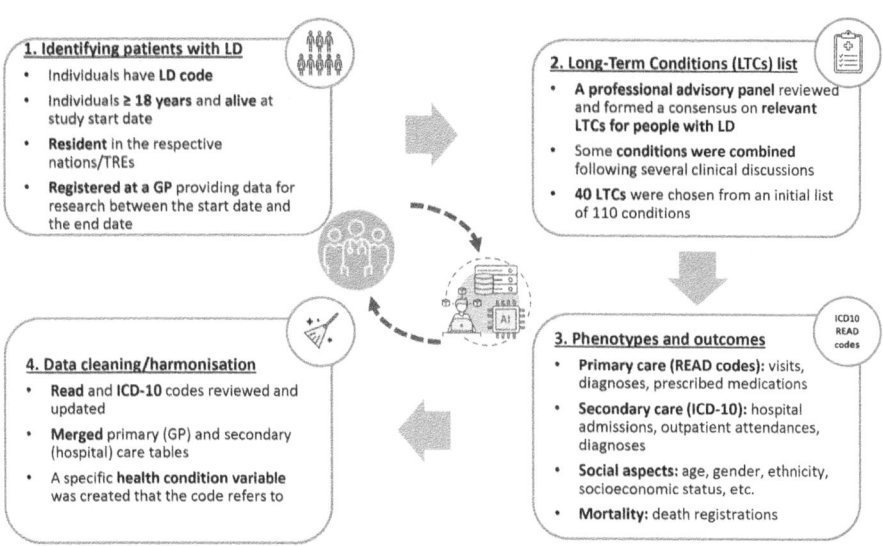

LD=Learning Disabilities; ICD-10= International Classification of Diseases version 10; TRE= Trusted Research Environment

Fig. 1. Data Preparation of cohort.

The data preparation was comprised of four steps as detailed in Fig. 1: Patient identification, reviewing the list of LTCs, data cleaning/harmonisation and phenotype/outcome extraction.

Patient Identification: This study was focused on adults, aged 18 and older, who are Welsh residents and identified as having a learning disability during the study period of January 1, 2000, to December 31, 2021, and registered with a SAIL GP at the study start date. A total of 14,323 unique patients were extracted.

List of LTCs: A professional advisory panel composed of clinicians and nurses from the National Health Service (NHS) reviewed and agreed upon relevant LTCs for people with learning disabilities. A final list was established consisting of 40 LTCs, some of which were combinations of similar conditions. The list includes Addison's disease, Anaemia, Barrett's oesophagus, Bronchiectasis, Cancer, Cardiac arrhythmias, Cerebral palsy, Chronic airway diseases, Chronic arthritis, Chronic constipation, Chronic diarrhoea, Chronic Kidney Disease (CKD), Chronic pain conditions, Chronic pneumonia, Cirrhosis, Coronary heart disease, Dementia, Diabetes, Dysphagia, Epilepsy, Hearing loss, Heart failure, Hypertension, Inflammatory Bowel Disease (IBD), Insomnia, Interstitial lung disease, Menopausal and perimenopausal conditions, Mental illness, Multiple Sclerosis (MS), Neuropathic pain, Osteoporosis, Parkinson's, Poly Cystic Ovaries (PCO), Psoriasis, Peripheral Vascular Disease (PVD), Reflux disorders, Stroke, Thyroid disorders, Tourette, Visual impairment. All 40 LTCs were associated with females, while all but Menopausal and perimenopausal conditions and PCO were associated with males.

Data cleaning and Harmonisation: Once the list of LTCs was concluded, all records of GP and hospital visits/consultations linked to the identified LTCs were extracted for each patient from birth; hence patients without any record linked to the 40 LTCs were excluded from the study. All primary care GP records were identified using read codes and the International Classification of Diseases version 10 (ICD-10) codes captured the secondary care hospital records. The resulting count after this process was 13,069 patients with 6,830 males and 6,239 females. The extracted GP and hospital data for all patients were harmonised to a single table for each sex (D_m for males and D_f for females); each row represents a unique patient and each unique variable column represents a binary indicator of the patient's diagnosis of one of the 40 LTCs at the study end date.

Characteristics and Outcome Extraction: For each patient in tables D_m and D_f additional variables were extracted indicating several patient outcomes and characteristics. The extracted outcomes included mortality information and the total number of unique hospitalisations for the patient at the study end date. Extracted patient characteristics include demographic information (age, sex and Welsh Index of Multiple Deprivation (WIMD))), patient's lifestyle and history (Body Mass Index (BMI), smoking history, alcohol consumption history, physical exercise), and presence of any prescribed antipsychotic, antidepressant, and mood stabilisers/anti-epileptic medications at the study end date. All information was obtained via read codes, for data collected at GP and ICD-10 codes for data collected at the hospital.

2.3   Cluster Analysis

A 3-cluster BIRCH algorithm was applied to the female dataset and a 3-cluster GMM was applied to the male dataset, to identify unique subgroups of patients based on the distribution of the LTC diagnosis. BIRCH is a hierarchical clustering algorithm suitable for large and non-uniformly distributed datasets. It aims to create compact and efficient clusters by organizing the feature space into non-overlapping regions called Clustering Feature (CF) entries, forming a CF Tree. In this study, BIRCH was implemented on the female dataset with a merging threshold value and branching factor set to 0.5 and 50, respectively. GMM is a probabilistic model-based clustering algorithm which assumes the data is generated from a mixture of Gaussian distributions and assigns probabilities to data points belonging to different clusters. It works effectively with both categorical and numerical data. In this study, GMM was implemented on the male dataset with a random state set to 1. Both BIRCH, and GMM were implemented using the scikit Learn library [9]. Following the identification of clusters for each sex, the characteristics of the patients within each cluster were analysed. In addition, the most common combinations of multiple coexisting long-term conditions were identified for the predominant clusters alongside their most frequent trajectories.

3   Results

3.1   Identifying Clusters of MLTC for Adults with Learning Difficulties

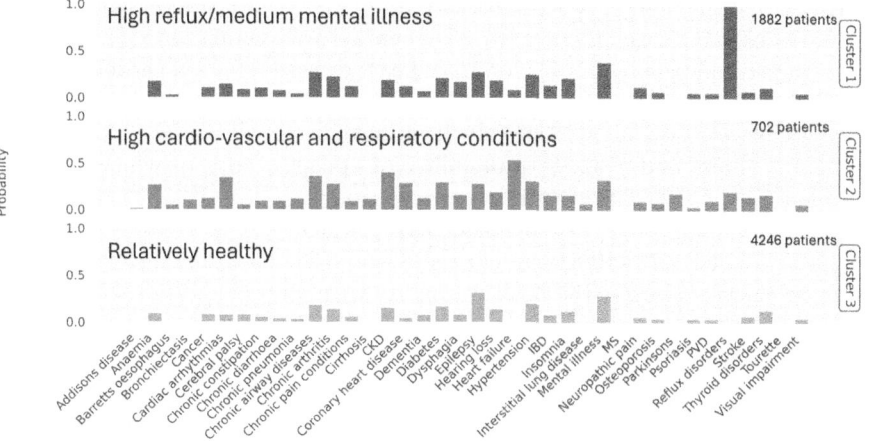

Fig. 2. Probability of LTCs across clusters for the 3-cluster GMM applied on male cohort.

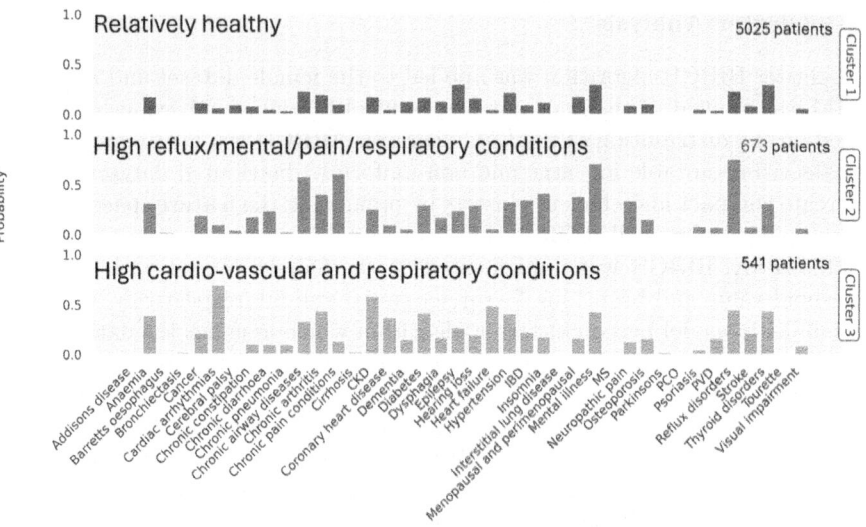

Fig. 3. Probability of LTCs across clusters for the 3-cluster BIRCH applied on female cohort.

The three identified clusters for the male and female cohorts were described based on the probability of their MLTC occurrence within each cluster (P_r) (See Figs. 2–3). For the male cohort, the GMM clustering identified 1882 (27.6%) patients in cluster 1, 702 (10.3%) in cluster 2, and 4246 (62.2%) in cluster 3. Cluster 1 was characterised by a 100% certainty of reflux disorders, a medium probability of mental illness (38.9%) (see Fig. 2), and ($P_r \leq 35\%$) for the other LTCs. Cluster 2 had the highest probabilities for developing heart failure (54.6%), CKD (41.6%), chronic airway diseases (37.3%), cardiac arrhythmia (35.8%), hypertension (31.8%), diabetes (30.3%), coronary heart disease (29.6%), chronic arthritis (28.8%), and anaemia (27.9%). Cluster 3, comprising the majority of the data, can be characterised as a 'relatively healthy' cluster with a 30 % probability of mental illness and a 32.7% probability of epilepsy, both of which are more prevalent in the population with learning disabilities.

For the female cohort, the 3-cluster BIRCH identified 5025 (80.5%) patients in cluster label 1, 673 (10.8%) in cluster 2, and 541 (8.7%) in cluster 3. Cluster 1 can be characterised as the healthy cluster, with all probabilities < 35%; however, it has the highest percentage of epilepsy at 29.2% compared to all other clusters. Cluster 2 had the highest probabilities for developing reflux disorders (74.6%), mental illness (70.6%), chronic pain conditions (60.3%), chronic airway diseases (57.5%), insomnia (41.2%), menopausal and perimenopausal conditions (37.9%), IBD (34%), neuropathic pain (33.7%), and hearing loss (28.5%). Cluster 3, with the smallest patient count, had the highest probabilities for developing cardiac arrhythmias (69.1%), CKD (57.9%), heart failure (47.9%), thyroid disorders (43.3%), diabetes (41.2%), hypertension (40.3%), anaemia (38.8%), coronary heart disease (36.6%), cancer (21.3%), stroke (21.3%), and dementia (15%).

3.2   What Were the Baseline Patient Characteristics Across the Identified Clusters?

Data from 6,830 males and 6,329 females with learning disabilities were analysed based on the most recent record for all patients, to characterise their respective cluster assignments as shown in Table @refTab:riskspsfactor.

For the male cohort, the mean (± Standard Deviation (std)) age of all men was 55.5 (13.9) years. Age distribution varied across clusters, as presented in Table @refTab:riskspsfactor. Notably, Cluster 3, representing 'relatively healthy' patients, had the youngest mean (± std) age of 53.8 (14) years, with a higher proportion of patients younger than 40 years compared to the other clusters.

Cluster 2 consisted of older patients, with a mean (± std) age of 64.8 (13.1) years. The 'relatively healthy' cluster 3 also exhibited a lower mean (± std) count of co-occurring MLTC at 3.2 (2.1) conditions per patient. In contrast, Cluster 2 had the highest mean number of MLTC per patient at 6.8 (3.2) LTCs. Overall, 84.2% of the male cohort had at least two LTCs. This rate was notably higher at 98.2% for patients in cluster 2, while the 'relatively healthy' cluster had 77.1% of its patients with at least two LTCs.

Regarding hospitalisation, Cluster 2 had the highest hospitalisation rate, with 56.8% of its members experiencing at least one hospital admission related to any of the considered LTCs. In contrast, the rate was lower in the 'relatively healthy' cluster, where 34.9% had at least one hospital admission. The mean (± std) count of admissions since birth for the considered LTCs was lowest in the 'relatively healthy' cluster at 3.7 (10.2) admissions per individual, while Cluster 2 had the highest at 8.9 (10.1) admissions per individual.

Regarding lifestyle factors, individuals with a history of smoking were predominantly in Cluster 2, and patient counts increased with deprivation (WIMD) across all clusters. Moreover, all clusters exhibited high obesity rates compared to other BMI classes. However, it's worth noting that BMI data was poorly coded, with approximately 85.9% of individuals missing BMI status for this cohort.

The mean (± std) age at mortality was observed to be lowest in the healthier cluster 3 at 62 (14) years and highest in cluster 2 at 66.7 (13.2) years. In summary, although several patients characterised in cluster 3 had a single LTC or relatively fewer MLTC counts and fewer hospitalisations compared to other clusters, 27% of its deceased individuals exhibited early mortality on average. This suggests that individuals in this cluster may be more susceptible to avoidable deaths compared to the other clusters.

For the female cohort, the 'relatively healthy' cluster (cluster 1) had the youngest mean (± std) age of 57 (14.8) years, with a higher proportion of patients aged below 40 years compared to clusters 2 and 3. Individuals in cluster 1 also had a lower mean (± std) count of co-occurring MLTC at 4.9 (3.1) conditions per individual, with 84.9% having at least 2 LTCs. In contrast, individuals in cluster 3 had the highest mean age of 67.8 (14.9) years and the highest mean number of MLTC per patient at 8.3 (3.5) LTCs per individual. Almost all individuals in cluster 3 (98.9%) and all in cluster 2 had at least 2 LTCs. Patients who were former or current smokers and were prescribed antipsychotic, antidepressant, or mood stabilisers/anti-epileptic medications were more likely to belong to clusters 2 and 3 than to cluster 1. The BMI was poorly coded for females, with about

Table 1. Descriptive statistics of all adults with learning disabilities and in the three Multiple Long Term Conditions (MLTC) clusters. The columns of 'relatively healthy' clusters for males and females are highlighted in grey.

	MALES			
	All males	**Cluster 1**	**Cluster 2**	**Cluster 3**
Cluster 1: High reflux/ medium mental illness; **Cluster 2**: High cardio vascular and respiratory conditions; **Cluster 3**: Relatively healthy				
Total	6830	1882	702	4246
Mean Age (± std)	55.5 (13.9)	55.8 (13.1)	64.8 (13.1)	53.8 (13.8)
Mean MLTC count	4.16 (2.8)	5.4 (3)	6.8 (3.2)	3.2 (2.1)
Multimorbidity	5757 (84.3%)	1794 (95.5%)	690 (98.3%)	3273 (77.1%)
Medications				
1 Presence	2811	837	281	1693
0 Absence	4019	1045	421	2553
Welsh Index of Multiple Deprivation (WIMD)				
1	1659	499	186	974
2	1345	397	148	800
3	1084	291	116	677
4	1022	268	96	658
5	679	175	69	435
unknown	1041	252	87	702
Alcohol History				
0 Nondrinker	4137	1171	429	2537
1 Ex/Current Drinker	601	237	93	271
Unknown	2092	474	180	1438
Smoking History				
0 Never smoker	3787	950	327	2510
1 Ex/Current smoker	2722	891	346	1485
Unknown	321	41	29	251
Physical Activity				
0 None	2723	809	329	1585
1 Physically active	715	198	58	459
Unknown	3392	875	315	2202
Body Mass Index (BMI)				
underweight	56	18	9	29
normal weight	181	81	15	85
pre-obesity	152	50	18	84
obesity class I	502	154	65	283
obesity class III	70	25	10	35
unknown	5869	1554	585	3730
Age Group				
<40	999	235	30	734
≥40	5831	1647	672	3512
Mortality count	2112	489	429	1194
Mean mortality age (± std)	63.4 (14)	63.8 (13.7)	66.7 (13.2)	62 (14)
Hospitalisation records	2587 (37.9%)	707 (37.6%)	399 (56.8%)	1481 (34.9%)
Mean admission counts (± std)	5.1 (11.2)	6.84 (13.)	8.89 (10.1)	3.721 (10.2)

(*continued*)

Table 1. (*continued*)

	All females	Cluster 1	Cluster 2	Cluster 3
FEMALEsS				

Cluster 1: Relatively healthy; **Cluster 2**: High reflux disorders/ mental illness/pain/respiratory conditions; **Cluster 3**: High cardio-vascular and respiratory conditions

	All females	Cluster 1	Cluster 2	Cluster 3
Total	6239	5025	673	541
Mean Age (± std)	58.1 (14.9)	57 (14.8)	58.6 (12.4)	67.8 (14.9)
Mean MLTC count (± std)	4.9 (3.1)	4.1 (2.5)	8.1 (3)	8.3 (3.5)
Multimorbidity	5474 (87.7%)	4266 (84.9%)	673 (100%)	535 (98.9)
Medications				
0 Absence	3346	2837	239	270
1 Presence	2893	2188	434	271
Welsh Index of Multiple Deprivation (WIMD)				
1	1536	1162	235	139
2	1237	981	135	121
3	1003	834	84	87
4	927	766	82	77
5	667	548	61	58
unknown	869	734	76	59
Alcohol History				
0 Nondrinker	4227	3383	490	354
1 Ex/Current Drinker	264	161	64	39
Unknown	1748	1481	119	148
Smoking History				
0 Never smoker	3894	3292	308	294
1 Ex/Current smoker	2096	1504	358	234
Unknown	249	229	7	13
Physical Activity				
0 None	2650	2048	353	249
1 Physically active	513	412	68	33
Unknown	3076	2565	252	259
Welsh Index of Multiple Deprivation (WIMD)				
underweight	36	32	<10	*
normal weight	168	133	<30	*
pre-obesity	149	116	22	11
obesity class I	656	469	124	63
obesity class III	141	103	24	14
unknown	5089	4172	476	441
Age Group				
<40	683	621	42	20
≥40	5556	4404	631	521
Mortality count	1959	1494	141	324
Mean mortality age (± std)	66.57 (14.9)	65.5 (15.0)	65.3 (13.5)	71.9 (13.6)
Hospitalisation records	1997 (32%)	1534 (30.5%)	196 (29.1%)	267 (49.4%)
Mean admission counts (± std)	5.2 (11.4)	4 (6.4)	9.4 (12)	11.5 (29.4)

81.6% classified as 'unknown'. However, among those with a known status, higher rates were observed in the obesity class compared to other BMI classes.

Regarding hospitalisation, cluster 3 had the highest rate, with 49.4% of its members experiencing at least one hospital admission related to the considered LTCs. In contrast, the rate was lowest in cluster 2, with 29.1% having at least one hospital admission. Cluster 1 had the lowest mean (± std) count of admissions since birth for the considered LTCs at 4 (6.4) admissions per individual, while cluster 3 had the highest at 11.5 (29.4) admissions per individual.

The mean age at mortality was lower in clusters 1 and 2 at 65.5 (15) and 65.3 (13.5) years, respectively. Deceased patients in cluster 3 had a higher mean age of mortality at 71.9 (13.6) years. While females across the 'relatively healthy' cluster and the more unhealthy patients (characterised by higher MLTC and older age) had a higher age at mortality compared to males, both sexes were characterised by lower life expectancy compared to the general population, particularly in some clusters. The higher rate of avoidable deaths in the most disadvantaged clusters may be associated with certain conditions or groups of conditions.

The next subsection explores the most common combinations and trajectories of MLTC in the dominant clusters for males and females.

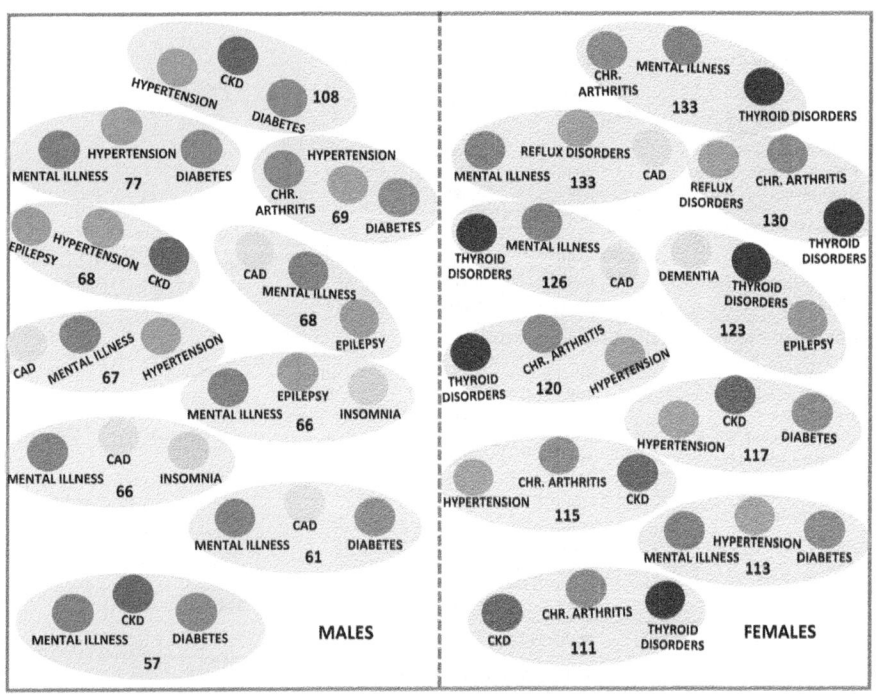

Fig. 4. Common combinations of 3 co-occuring LTCs. **Remark**: figure shows LTC combinations without directions of disease progression. CHR.=chronic; CKD= Chronic Kidney disease; CAD = chronic airway diseases.

3.3   What Were the Most Common Combinations of Multiple LTCs and the Most Frequent Trajectories for the Most Dominant Clusters?

The 'relatively healthy' clusters: cluster 3 for males and cluster 1 for females had the highest number of individuals compared to other clusters. These clusters were characterised by younger patients, fewer mean MLTC counts, and lower mean hospitalization rates. However, the mean age at mortality was the youngest in these clusters compared to the others. This section examines the most common combinations of LTCs and the predominant order of these conditions for individuals in the 'relatively healthy' clusters.

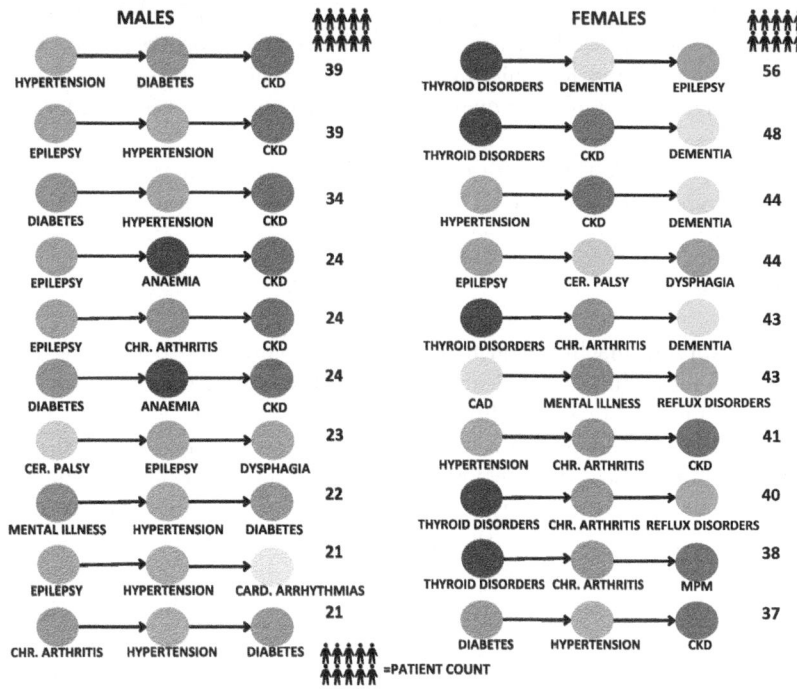

Fig. 5. Trajectories of 3 LTCs for the dominant cluster. CHR.=chronic; CKD= Chronic Kidney disease; CER.PALSY = cerebral palsy, CAD = chronic airway diseases, MPM = menopausal and perimenopausal conditions.

For males in cluster 3, the most prevalent standalone LTC without any co-occurring condition was mental illness with 184 patients, closely followed by epilepsy with 183 patients. Figure 4 depicts the top ten common combinations of three co-occurring conditions for both sexes. The most frequent combination for the males was [CKD, diabetes, hypertension], with 108 patients having these conditions. This was followed by the combination of [diabetes, hypertension, and mental illness], with 77 patients. Other subsequent combinations are illustrated in Fig. 4. Figure 5 illustrates the top ten trajectories for all possible combinations of three LTCs. While all trajectories in Fig. 5 could include other LTC within their sequence, this illustration emphasises the direction of the three selected conditions amidst other co-occurring conditions. The most frequent trajectory was hypertension $\longrightarrow$ diabetes $\longrightarrow$ CKD with 39 patients, followed by the trajectory of epilepsy $\longrightarrow$ hypertension $\longrightarrow$ CKD(39 patients), and diabetes $\longrightarrow$ hypertension $\longrightarrow$ CKD with 34 patients.

For females in cluster 1, thyroid disorders were the most common standalone condition with 122 individuals, followed by epilepsy and mental illness with 110 and 81 patients, respectively. The top combinations of three co-occurring LTC were [chronic arthritis, mental illness, thyroid disorders] and [chronic airway diseases, mental illness, reflux disorders], both with 133 individuals as depicted in Fig. 4. This was followed by [chronic arthritis, reflux disorders, thyroid disorders](130 patients), and [chronic airway diseases, mental illness, thyroid disorders](126) (Fig. 4). The most frequent trajectories over all possible combinations of three LTCs, as depicted in Fig. 5, were thyroid disorders $\longrightarrow$ dementia $\longrightarrow$ epilepsy (56 patients), thyroid disorder $\longrightarrow$ CKD $\longrightarrow$ dementia (48 patients), followed by hypertension $\longrightarrow$ CKD $\longrightarrow$ dementia (48 patients).

4   Conclusion

This study applied machine learning clustering techniques to identify distinct subgroups of individuals with learning disabilities based on their patterns of MLTC. The analyses revealed three main clusters for both males and females. For males, the GMM identified a 'relatively healthy' cluster (Cluster 3) characterised by younger ages, lower MLTC counts, and fewer hospitalizations. However, this cluster also exhibited the lowest mean age at mortality, suggesting high rate of potentially avoidable deaths. The most common MLTC combinations of three conditions involved chronic kidney disease, diabetes, and hypertension, with CKD frequently appearing as the latter of other conditions in the most frequent trajectories.

Among females, the BIRCH algorithm revealed a 'relatively healthy' cluster (Cluster 1) with younger ages and lower MLTC counts. Similar to males, this cluster had the lowest mean age at mortality. The top MLTC combinations included thyroid disorders co-occurring with conditions like CKD, arthritis, dementia, and reflux disorders. Thyroid disorders frequently preceded dementia and epilepsy in common trajectories. While the healthier clusters exhibited better outcomes in terms of ofMLTC counts and hospitalizations, the findings highlighted concerns regarding premature mortality, even among individuals with fewer conditions. The identification of predominant ofMLTC combinations and trajectories provides valuable insights for targeted interventions, optimised care pathways, and resource allocation tailored to the specific needs of individuals with learning disabilities. This study contributes to a better understanding of the complex health profiles and unique challenges faced by this population, paving the way for enhanced healthcare policies, personalised medicine approaches, and improved quality of life for individuals with learning disabilities.

Acknowledgments. Data-driven machinE-learning aided stratification and management of multiple long-term COnditions in adults with intellectual disabilitiEs (DECODE) project (NIHR203981) is funded by the NIHR AI for Multiple Long-term Conditions (AIM) Programme. The views expressed are those of the author(s) and not necessarily those of the NIHR or the Department of Health and Social Care. This work uses data provided by patients and collected by the NHS as part of their care and support. We also want to acknowledge all data providers who make anonymised data available for research.

Disclosure of Interests. The authors have no competing interests to declare that are relevant to the content of this article.

References

1. Abakasanga, E., Kousovista, R., Cosma, G., Jun, G.T., Kiani, R., Gangadharan, S.: Identifying clusters on multiple long-term conditions for adults with learning disabilities. Proceedings of the AIiH: International Conference on AI in Healthcare (2024), accepted for publication
2. Arthur, D., Vassilvitskii, S.: k-means++: the advantages of careful seeding. In: Proceedings of the Eighteenth Annual ACM-SIAM Symposium on Discrete Algorithms, SODA 2007, pp. 1027-1035. Society for Industrial and Applied Mathematics, USA (2007)
3. Chalitsios, C.V., et al.: Multiple long-term conditions in people with psoriasis: a latent class and bidirectional mendelian randomization analysis. Br. J. Dermatol. **190**(3), 364–373 (2024)
4. Cooper, S.A., et al.: Multiple physical and mental health comorbidity in adults with intellectual disabilities: population-based cross-sectional analysis. BMC Fam. Pract. **16**(1), 110 (2015)
5. Emerson, E., Hatton, C.: Health inequalities and people with intellectual disabilities. Cambridge University Press (2014)
6. Ford, D.V., et al.: The SAIL databank: building a national architecture for e-health research and evaluation. BMC Health Serv. Res. **9**, 1–12 (2009)
7. Heslop, P., Hoghton, M.: The learning disabilities mortality review (LeDeR) programme. British J. General Pract. **68**(suppl 1) (2018)
8. Huang, Z.: Extensions to the k-means algorithm for clustering large data sets with categorical values. Data Min. Knowl. Disc. **2**(3), 283–304 (1998)
9. Jolly, K.: Machine learning with scikit-learn quick start guide: classification, regression, and clustering techniques in Python. Packt Publishing Ltd (2018)
10. Kinnear, D., Morrison, J., Allan, L., Henderson, A., Smiley, E., Cooper, S.A.: Prevalence of physical conditions and multimorbidity in a cohort of adults with intellectual disabilities with and without down syndrome: cross-sectional study. BMJ Open **8**(2) (2018)
11. Kirkova, J., Aktas, A., Walsh, D., Davis, M.P.: Cancer symptom clusters: clinical and research methodology. J. Palliat. Med. **14**(10), 1149–1166 (2011)
12. Lyons, R.A., et al.: The SAIL databank: linking multiple health and social care datasets. BMC Med. Inform. Decis. Mak. **9**, 1–8 (2009)

13. Malhat, M.G., Mousa, H.M., El-Sisi, A.B.: Clustering of chemical data sets for drug discovery. In: 2014 9th International Conference on Informatics and Systems, pp. DEKM–11–DEKM–18 (2014)
14. Mann, C., Jun, G.T., Tyrer, F., Kiani, R., Lewin, G., Gangadharan, S.K.: A scoping review of clusters of multiple long-term conditions in people with intellectual disabilities and factors impacting on outcomes for this patient group. J. Intellectual Disabilities **27**(4), 1045–1061 (2023), pMID: 35695384
15. McLachlan, G., Peel, D.: Finite Mixture Models. Wiley Series in Probability and Statistics, Wiley (2004)
16. Miaskowski, C., et al.: Disease and treatment characteristics do not predict symptom occurrence profiles in oncology outpatients receiving chemotherapy. Cancer **120**(15), 2371–2378 (2014)
17. Papachristou, N., et al.: Comparing machine learning clustering with latent class analysis on cancer symptoms' data. In: 2016 IEEE Healthcare Innovation Point-Of-Care Technologies Conference (HI-POCT), pp. 162–166 (2016)
18. Papachristou, N., et al.: Congruence between latent class and K-modes analyses in the identification of oncology patients with distinct symptom experiences. J. Pain Symptom Manage. **55**(2), 318-333.e4 (2018)
19. Rodgers, S.E., Demmler, J.C., Dsilva, R., Lyons, R.A.: Protecting health data privacy while using residence-based environment and demographic data. Health & Place **18**(2), 209–217 (2012)
20. Rousseeuw, P.J.: Silhouettes: a graphical aid to the interpretation and validation of cluster analysis. J. Comput. Appl. Math. **20**, 53–65 (1987)
21. Shakeel, P.M., Baskar, S., Dhulipala, V.R.S., Jaber, M.M.: Cloud based framework for diagnosis of diabetes mellitus using k-means clustering. Health Inform. Sci. Syst. **6**(1), 16 (2018)
22. Sharma, A., et al.: Cluster analysis of cardiovascular phenotypes in patients with type 2 diabetes and established atherosclerotic cardiovascular disease: a potential approach to precision medicine. Diabetes Care **45**(1), 204–212 (10 2021)
23. Zhang, T., Ramakrishnan, R., Livny, M.: BIRCH: an efficient data clustering method for very large databases. In: Proceedings of the 1996 ACM SIGMOD International Conference on Management of Data. SIGMOD 1996, pp. 103-114. Association for Computing Machinery, New York (1996)

A Deep Learning Framework for Assessing the Risk of Transvenous Lead Extraction Procedures

Fazli Wahid[1], YingLiang Ma[1(✉)], Vishal Mehta[2], Sandra Howell[2], Steven Niederer[2,3], and C. Aldo Rinaldi[2]

[1] School of Computing Sciences, University of East Anglia, Norwich, UK
{f.wahid,yingliang.ma}@uea.ac.uk
[2] School of Imaging Sciences and Biomedical Engineering, King's College London, London, UK
[3] National Heart and Lung Institute, Imperial College London, London, UK

Abstract. This paper introduces a deep-learning framework augmented with human guidance for evaluating the risk associated with Transvenous Lead Extraction (TLE). TLE is one type of minimally invasive cardiac procedures, and it is to remove old pacing wires inside the heart. The deep-learning framework automatically extracts geometric features from a single plain chest X-ray image obtained before the procedure. It then utilizes these features in conjunction with clinical data to predict the procedural risk. All geometric features were recommended by a senior clinician and include the positions of coils, the number of leads inside the superior vena cava and the angle of leads. The proposed framework was trained and tested using a database comprising records from 1,053 patients who underwent TLE procedures. Notably, the framework was successfully trained despite the highly imbalanced nature of the data. An accuracy of 0.91 was achieved and the framework can predict 88% of major complication cases. By combining geometric features with clinical data, we were able to deliver a significantly better accuracy and a higher recall rate for detecting high-risks patients, when compared with existing approaches. The methodology described in this paper can be applied to the risk assessment for other cardiac procedures.

Keywords: Deep learning · Risk assessment · Geometric feature extraction

1 Introduction

Transvenous lead extraction (TLE) is a minimally invasive cardiac procedure performed to remove implanted leads (wires) from the veins and heart. In recent decades, there has been widespread adoption of cardiac implantable electronic devices. As a result, an increasing number of patients may need lead extraction procedures due to various factors such as infection, lead malfunction, or the need for device upgrades [1]. While the success rate of the TLE procedure remains high, it can be complex and may result in severe complications, and in some cases, procedure-related death. Clinical studies conducted

© The Author(s), under exclusive license to Springer Nature Switzerland AG 2024
X. Xie et al. (Eds.): AIiH 2024, LNCS 14976, pp. 17–30, 2024.
https://doi.org/10.1007/978-3-031-67285-9_2

in European centers have reported a 1.7% rate of major complications including deaths [2]. Therefore, it is essential to assess the risk for each individual patient before the TLE procedure. Sidhu et al. [3] has proposed an Electra Registry Outcome Score (EROS) to create a risk assessment tool using a limited number of variables and an accuracy of 0.70 was achieved. Recently, Vishal et al. [4] has trained three machine learning (ML) models and tested them on a ELECTRa database [3]. The best performing ML model is the logistic regression (accuracy: 0.74) and followed by the self-normalising neural network (0.73) and support vector machine (0.72). The results are marginally improvement from EROS.

We hypothesized that adding geometric features extracted from a plain chest X-ray image will further improve the accuracy. Therefore, a new deep-learning framework is created to extract geometric features from images and to be trained on two kinds of data inputs. One type of data is related to personal health conditions such as whether the patient has heart failure, chronic respiratory diseases or infected device as well as how long leads has been implanted and more. Those data have been used in previous ML models [4]. The other type of data is geometric features extracted from one plain chest X-ray image acquired before the procedure. The geometric features were first suggested by the senior clinician. Those features are the lead angulations at different locations, the coil position related to the superior vena cava (SVC) and the number of overlapping leads in the SVC. In this paper, robust computer vision algorithms were designed, which are based on deep learning techniques for image segmentation. The computer vision algorithms were able to automatically compute the positions of the leads or coils inside the X-ray image and derive other geometric information such as angulation. After conducting correlation tests between individual geometric features and the outcome of major complications, less significant geometric features were removed. Finally, the ML model was trained using the remaining geometric features along with data regarding personal health conditions.

The main contribution of this paper is the methodology for developing a deep learning framework that combines geometric features with other clinical data to achieve higher accuracy in detecting high-risk patients. The proposed approach is not limited to the TLE procedure using the chest X-ray image and it could apply to assess the risk of other cardiac interventional procedures using X-ray or CT images.

2   Automatic Object Detection

2.1   Selecting Geometric Features

From the existing literature [5] as well as the experiences from a senior clinician, four geometric features from the plain chest X-ray image were selected. As illustrated in Fig. 1, geometric features are the coil (thick wire) position related to the SVC, the number of leads in the SVC, the lead angulation near the entry point of the SVC and the angulation of the pacing lead in the right ventricle (RV). To determine the approximated location of the SVC inside the chest X-ray image, a generic anatomy model is overlaid with the chest X-ray image. From Fig. 2(a), the location of the SVC (green box) is the top left corner of the heart region (red box). The height of the green box is approximately half the height of the heart region. The width of the green box is approximately one third of the heart region. The method was verified by overlaying 3D anatomy models (extracted from pre-procedure CT scan) with the chest X-ray image (Fig. 2b).

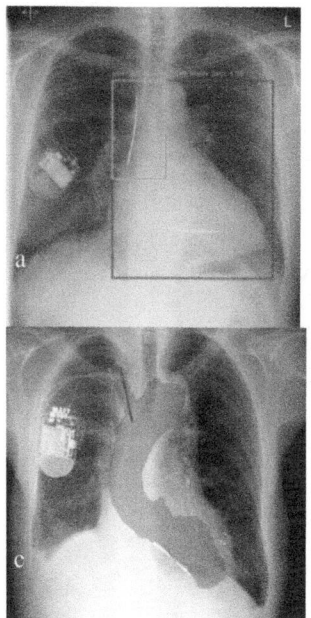
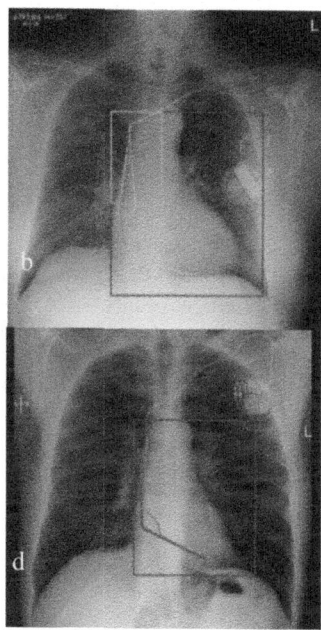

Fig. 1. The red box is the bounding box of the outline of the heart. The green box is the approximated location of the SVC. (a) The yellow lines are the positions of coils. (b) The colorful line segmentations inside the green box indicate how many wires are inside the SVC. (c) The angle formed by two red line is the lead angulation near the entry point of the SVC. The blue shadow represents the overlay of a heart model extracted from the CT images of the same patient. (d) The angle formed by two red line is the angulation of the pacing lead in the right ventricle. (Color figure online)

SVC is a major blood vessel inside the heart and it provides an important pathway for inserting the pacing leads into the right atrium and other heart chambers. The SVC is the most common location requiring surgical repair as the result of a major complication after the TLE procedure [5]. The common reason for the major complication inside SVC is the fibrotic tissue around the lead or the coil [10]. It does more likely happen to the coil which has a large surface area. The fibrotic tissue likely causes mechanical damages such as tear during the procedure.

2.2   The Detection of the Approximate Location of SVC

To automatically located the SVC in the X-ray image, the heart region needs to be detected. A transfer learning approach was used to detect the heart region via bounding box regression, which is based on a modified VGG16 model. As shown in Fig. 3, the last 3 pre-trained fully-connected layers have been removed and replaced with 4 full-connected layers (128x1, 64x1, 64x1 and 4x1). The last layer outputs four float values,

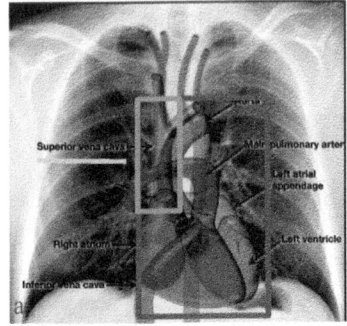 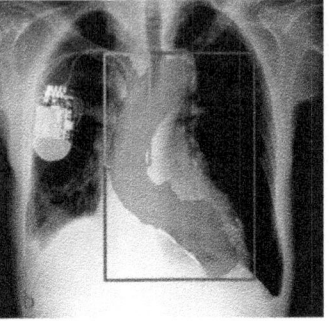

Fig. 2. (a) A medically accurate illustration of the anatomy of the heart. The red box is the region of the heart and the green box is the location of the SVC. (b) Overlaying 3D anatomy models with the X-ray image. (Color figure online)

which are the coordinates of two corners positions of the bounding box. The modified VGG16 model uses the pre-trained weights (ImageNet) [6] and it was re-trained using the manual annotations of the heart region in X-ray images.

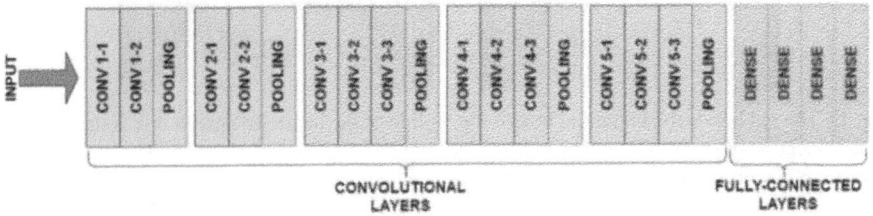

Fig. 3. The architecture of the modified VGG16 model.

Table 1. Results of precisions and recalls.

IoU Threshold	50%	75%
Precision	1.0	0.887
Recall	1.0	1.0

We have a database of 1,053 chest X-ray images from 1,053 patients and images were acquired before the TLE procedures. In addition, a public database of chest X-ray images [7] are also used and there are 5,863 images. The images from the public database were used solely to train and test the heart region detection method. They cannot be used for other detection or geometric feature extraction methods because they do not contain any pacing leads or coils. All images were split into two groups. 70% of images were used for training, 20% of images were used for validation and 10% of images were used for the accuracy testing. The bounding boxes of heart regions were manually annotated by a clinical expert. The loss function for the modified VGG16 model is the mean squared error (MSE) and the optimizer is adaptive moment estimation (Adam). The learning rate was set to 0.001. The accuracy of heart region detection is measured by two metrics: precision and recall. Precision is the ability of a model to identify only the relevant objects. Recall is the ability of a model to find all ground truth bounding boxes. Both precision and recall were calculated at $T(IoU) = 0.5$ and $T(IoU) = 0.75$. IoU is the Intersection Over Union, which measures how well the prediction bounding box aligns with the ground truth box. Table 1 presents the result. Examples of IoU and approximate location of the SVC were presented in Fig. 4.

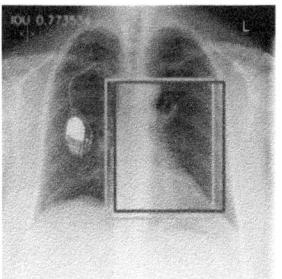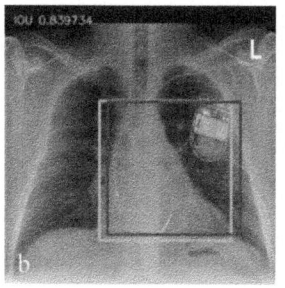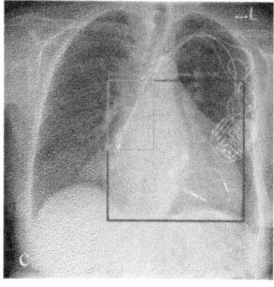

Fig. 4. Detecting the heart region. (a) (b) The results of IOU. The green box is the ground truth and the red box is the detected bounding box. (c) The green box is the bounding box of the SVC and the red box is the bounding box of the heart region. (Color figure online)

2.3   The Detection of Pacing Leads and Coils

The next task to determine the position of pacing leads and coils. For the risk assessment, we categorized leads into two types of leads: the normal pacing lead and the pacing lead with coils. The normal leads are thin metal wires. On the other hand, the pacing lead with coils has one or two segments of coils. Coils have a large surface area of electrodes and they often conduct strong currents to depolarize the heart. They can be recognized on x-ray images as focal areas of wire thickening. The positions of pacing leads and coils in X-ray image need to be automatically localized in order to compute the position of coil, the number of normal pacing leads inside the SVC and the lead angulation. In order to achieve these tasks, a lightweight multiple-output convolutional neural network (MO-Net) based on the UNet-like architecture was proposed. MO-Net has two outputs. One is for the segmentation result and the other one is for localizing the tip position of the pacing lead inside the RV. The number of trainable parameters is 14.3M. Comparing to VGG16 (138M), AlexNet (62M) and ResNet-50 (23M), MO-Net is a lightweight network. As shown in Fig. 5, the main body of MO-Net is a UNet-like architecture, which consists of a downsampling path and an upsampling path. A box-regression branch starts at the bottom of UNet. The branch consists of a further convolution layer and two Max pooling layers to extract features and reduce the spatial dimensionality.

Both segmentation and box regression pathways share the same downsampling path, which consists of a series of convolution layers and Max pooling layers. There are two advantages to this approach. The first one is to reduce the computation load to achieve fast detection speeds. The convolution layers generate filters to extract features from the input image. As the segmentation and box regression targets the same objects, similar features such as wire edges and corners will be extracted by convolution layers on the downsampling path. It is reasonable to allow the segmentation and box regression pathways to share a series of convolution layers so that the computation load is significantly reduced. The second advantage is to enable transfer learning. The MO-Net is trained on one type of target objects and it can be re-trained on another type of objects using transfer learning. The time of re-training could be significantly shortened if pre-trained weights (e.g. ImageNet) are loaded.

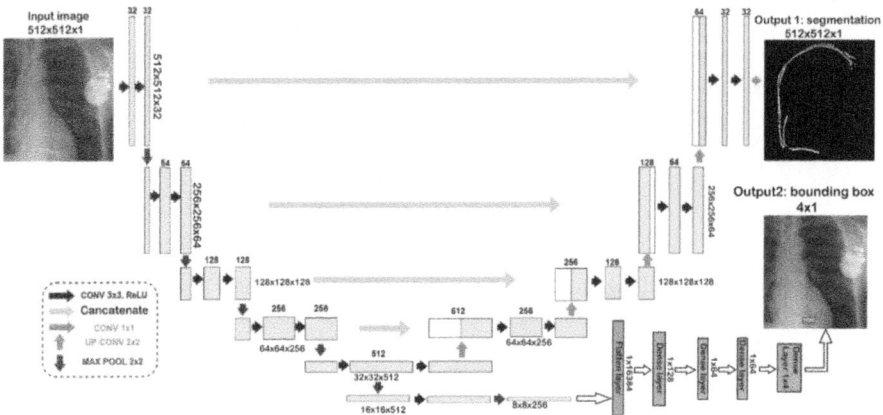

Fig. 5. The architecture of MO-Net.

Manual Labeling. The manual labeling of pacing leads and wires in X-ray images is very time-consuming and tedious. To speed the process up, vessel enhancement filters [8] were used to extract catheters and wires. The resulting image was automatically binarized by an adaptive binarization method [9]. Not all wires were labeled in our training data. As we are only interested in pacing wires inside the heart, the pacemaker and nearby wire segments were also removed as they are not useful for finding geometric features. Therefore, an experienced clinician manually removed the non-target objects. Figure 6 presented the process of manual segmentation.

Training and Results. The ratio for train-validation-test split is 7:2:1 and it is same as the ratio used in the detection of heart region. The loss function for the segmentation output is the dice similarity coefficient (DSC). The optimizer is Adam. The MO-Net was trained using 737 images. Images with the resolution of 512×512 were directly input into the network without any down-sampling as the leads might not be visible in the low resolution images. The data augmentation technique was used to increase the number of training images. The contrast or brightness of the 737 images were reduced by a random factor between 0.6 to 0.9 to create additional 1,474 training images. The reason for reducing contrast or brightness is to improve the performance of coil detection for low-contrast or dark X-ray images. The MO-Net model was implemented using TensorFlow

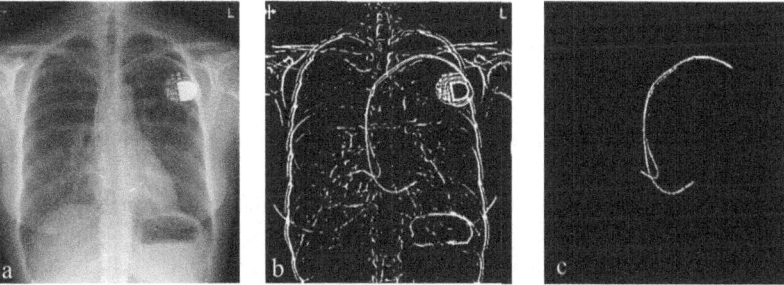

Fig. 6. Manual segmentation of pacing leads. (a) The original image. (b) Image after applying the vessel enhancement filter. (c) The final result of manual segmentation.

API and training was carried out using a GPU cluster (GPU: Nvidia RTX 6000 with 24 GB GPU memory). The training process took about 2.5 h. The trained MO-Net was tested on remaining 316 images. An accuracy of 0.76 ± 0.11 was achieved for the segmentation of leads and coils and it was measured in DSC against the ground truth. Although the MO-Net is not always able to detect the completed length of leads, it is sufficient for our next task: extracting geometric features. More importantly, the recall of coils is 1.0 and it means that all coils within X-ray images have been successfully detected as the coils are high-contrast objects and relatively easy to be detected. Secondly, the accuracy of the tip region detection for the pacing lead is measured by IoU. An accuracy of 0.82 ± 0.07 was achieved. An example of segmentation results and lead tip detection inside the RV are presented in Fig. 7.

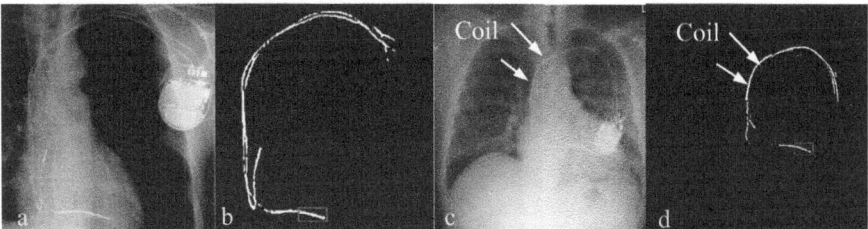

Fig. 7. The results of detecting leads and coils. (a) (c) The original image. (b) (d) The segmentation results output and lead tip detection output by the MO-Net. (c) The coil is clearly within the detected segmentations.

2.4   The Detection of Coils

Although the previous segmentation results already include the pacing leads and coils, the coils have not been detected as separate objects. Determining the coil's placement relative to the SVC is essential for evaluating the risks associated with TLE procedures. [10] reported that the fibrotic tissue surrounding the coil is one of leading factors contributing to the mechanical damages such as tear during the procedure. To detect only the coil, a standard U-Net model is used and the input image is an image mask, which is generated from the previous segmentation results. An image dilation operation with the kernel size of 10×10 were applied on the binary images [11], which were the previous segmentation results for pacing leads and coils. Finally, the dilated binary images were applied on the original images to generate the masked images and they were used as the input images for the U-Net model.

To reduce the distraction from the thin lead wires, the input images were down-sampled to 256×256 before inputting them into the U-Net model. The same data augmentation technique was applied to the training images. The contrast or brightness of the 737 images were reduced by a random factor between 0.6 to 0.9 to create additional 1,474 training images. Therefore, total 2,211 training images were created. The trained U-Net was tested on remaining 316 images. An accuracy of 0.87 ± 0.10 was achieved for the detection of coils and it was measured in DSC against the ground truth. To measure the performance of U-Net with or without data augmentation, key metrics such as accuracy, precision, recall and F1-score were calculated and presented in Table 2. A true positive detection is defined as at least 75% length of the target coil object was detected. A false positive detection is defined as the other wire object was detected as the target coil object. An example of coil segmentation is presented in Fig. 8.

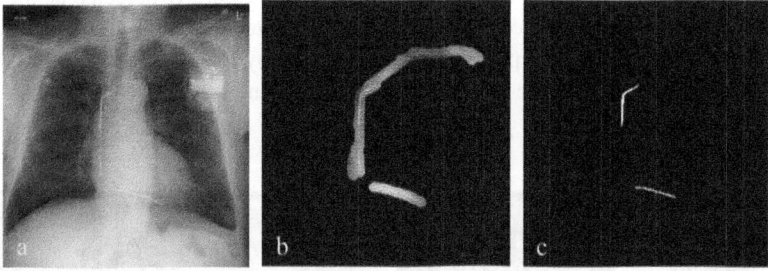

Fig. 8. An example of coil detection. (a) The original image. (b) The masked image. (c) The segmentation of only coils.

Table 2. Results of precisions and recalls.

Data augmentation	Accuracy	Precision	Recall	F1 score
without	0.88	0.89	0.92	0.90
with	0.98	0.98	0.99	0.98

3   The Extraction of Geometric Features

The geometric features are the lead coil position related to the superior vena cava (SVC), the lead angulations at different locations and the number of overlapping leads in the SVC.

3.1 The Determination of the Coil Position Related to the SVC

To quantify the exact location of the detected coil, the centerline extract method described in [9] was used. As illustrated in Fig. 9a, the binarized image of detected coils has been skeletonized so that the centerlines are represented as one-pixel-wide objects. Then a contour finding algorithm [12] was used to extract an array of 2D points of the centerlines. The 2D points were sorted along the long axis of the bounding box of the SVC (the green box in Fig. 9a). By comparing the array of 2D points and the bounding box of the SVC, we can work out the percentage of the coil inside the SVC.

3.2 The Lead Angulations

There are two lead angulations could contribute to the tissue damage during the TLE procedures [13]. As illustrated in Fig. 9b, one is the angulation (highlighted in red) near the entry point of the SVC. The other is the angulation (highlighted in green) within the RV. When any of those two angles become acute, it could increase the risk. The acute angle is the angle of less than 90°.

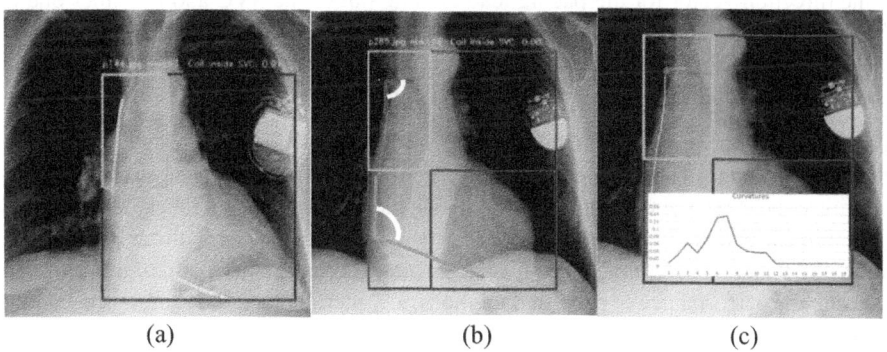

(a)	(b)	(c)

Fig. 9. (a) The workflow of the determination of the coil position related to the SVC. (b) Lead angulations. (c) Find the turning point. (Color figure online)

The Angulation Near the Entry Point of the SVC. In order to compute the angle, the turning point need to be located first. This can be done by computing the local curvature estimation. To compute the local curvature efficiently, an approximation method was developed. In mathematics, the local curvature is defined as $1/R$, where R is the radius of an approximation circle which is fitted with the curve. As shown in Fig. 10, the approximation circle touches the curve on the point where the local curvature calculation is required. Assume that that Pt_1 and Pt_2 are both on the approximation circle and the curve. Therefore, $R = 0.5C/sin\alpha$. As $\alpha + \beta = 90°$, $sin\alpha = cos\beta$. The equation can be rewritten as $R = 0.5C/cos\beta$. To compute $cos\beta$, the dot product of vector V_1 and V_2 should be used. The relationship is $cos2\beta = \vec{V_1} \cdot \vec{V_2}/\|\vec{V_1}\|\|\vec{V_2}\| = 2cos^2\beta - 1$. Finally, local curvature can be computed as $Curv = 1/R = \sqrt{(\vec{V_1} \cdot \vec{V_2}/\|\vec{V_1}\|\|\vec{V_2}\| + 1)/2}/0.5C$. Finally, the turning point is where the local curvature reaches the maximum level. The angulation was calculated by using two vectors (one from each side). Each vector is located where the local curvature reaches a local minimum. Figure 9c show an example of the computation of the local curvatures and the detected turning point.

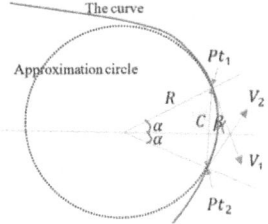

Fig. 10. Illustration for local curvature approximation.

The Definitions of Lead Angulations. The angulation of the pacing lead in the RV is relatively easy to compute, which is defined as the angle between two vectors. One is the direction vector for the pacing lead coming out of the SVC and the other one is the direction vector for lead tip, which can be computed from the second output from MO-Net. In order to increase the robustness, the principal component analysis (PCA) was performed on the wire data to generate the direction vectors [14].

The Results. The proposed methods for detecting acute angles were tested on all 1,053 chest X-ray images. The ground truth was the manual labelling of acute angles in two positions: the entry point of the SVC and inside the RV. The manual labels were created by a clinical expert. In the manual labels, there are 143 images with an acute angle inside the RV and only 7 images with an acute angle near the entry point of the SVC. To measure the performance of proposed methods, key metrics such as accuracy, precision, recall and F1-score were calculated and presented in Table 3.

Table 3. Key metrics for the performance of acute-angle detection methods.

Location	Accuracy	Precision	Recall	F1 score
SVC	0.70	0.83	0.71	0.77
RV	0.91	0.97	0.92	0.95

3.3   Detecting the Number of Leads in the SVC

As the common reason for the major complication inside the SVC is the fibrotic tissue around the lead or the coil, it is also necessary to determine the approximate number of leads inside the SVC. A coil or more than two leads detected inside the SVC is considered as the risk factor for TLE procedures [10]. It is not possible to determine the exact number of leads inside the SVC robustly due to leads quite often overlaps each other and group together. Therefore, one way of determining the risk factor is whether more than two leads inside the SVC or not (the standard pacemaker has only two leads). The other way is whether 50% coil is within the SVC. To count the number of leads inside the SVC, the lead segmentation from the first output of MO-Net was binarized first and the centerlines were localized using the method in [9]. Running a line scanning algorithm within the bounding box of the SVC to count how many leads are inside the SVC. The detection method was tested on 809 chest X-ray images, which do not have a coil inside the SVC. The ground truth was the binary label for each image. There are 61 images (out of 809 images) with the binary label set to true by a clinical expert if there are more than 2 leads inside the SVC. The performance metrics of accuracy, precision, recall and F1-score of the detection method are 0.782, 0.879. 0.836 and 0.857, respectively.

4 Feature Selection and Machine Learning Model

4.1 Feature Selection

There are several geometric features suggested by the senior clinician and the values of those features generated by the detection algorithms are binary values. Therefore, the Jaccard similarity coefficient (JSC) [15] was used to test the correlation between individual geometric feature and the binary outcome of procedure complication, as the JSC is a statistical measure for correlating the similarity between binary data samples. However, JSC cannot be directly applied to our highly imbalanced data. In our data, 97.6% of sampling data are in the majority class, with only 2.4% of the sampling data in the minority class (major complication cases). Therefore, the imbalanced ratio is 40.7:1. Highly imbalanced data could distort the results of the correlation tests towards the majority class [16]. To balance the test data, Adaptive Synthetic (ADASYN) sampling techniques [17] were used. As shown in Table 4, the feature of acute angle near the entry point of the SVC has the lowest JSC score and the detection method for that feature is also not robust (recall is just 0.714). Therefore, it was removed from the feature list.

Table 4. The results of the JSC tests.

Geometric Features	JSC Score
50% of coil or >2 leads inside the SVC	0.351
The acute angle inside the RV	0.029
The acute angle near the entry point of the SVC	0.005

4.2 Machine Learning Model for Risk Assessment

Once the geometric features were selected, they were combined with personal health data to feed into a machine learning model to predict the TLE procedure risk. The personal health data includes gender, age, history of heart failure, respiratory disease status, heart ejection fraction, and other relevant information. The XGBoost classifier [18] was chosen to predict the risk of TLE procedures as because it works well with imbalance datasets and binary classifications [19]. There are total 1053 sets of data from 1,053 TLE clinical cases and the outcome from 25 cases (2.4%) are a major complication or procedure related death. To balance the data, ADASYN were applied to the data and generated additional 1,003 sets of data which was labelled as the cases of a major complication or procedure related death. The balanced data were split into two groups. 70% of data were used for training and 30% of data were used for testing.

In order to compare the performance of model prediction, the XGBoost classifier was trained on the data related to personal health data and geometric features. Geometric features were detected by our computer vision algorithms. Those datasets were used for training and testing the XGBoost classifier. After the training, the model prediction is assessed on the test data only. As shown in Table 5, the balanced accuracy of model prediction using geometric features has improved substantially, when compared with the model prediction without using any of geometric features. Finally, the ranking of feature importance was shown in Fig. 11.

Table 5. The results of the model prediction. AUC is the area under curve.

Geometric features	Accuracy	Recall (major)	Recall (minor)	F1 score	AUC
Without	0.74	0.82	0.62	0.73	0.77
with	0.91	0.91	0.88	0.90	0.96

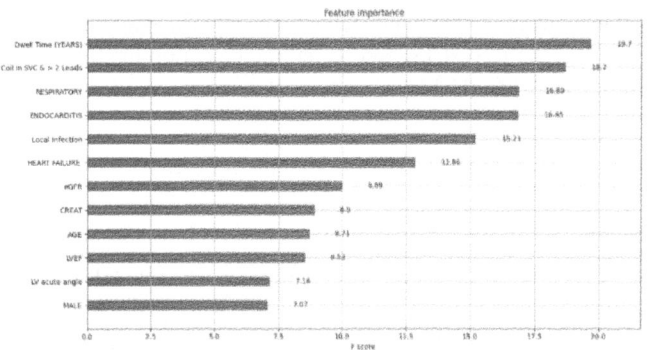

Fig. 11. Feature importance. There are two geometric features in the list: "Coil in SVC & >2 leads" and "RV acute angle".

5   Conclusions

This paper presents a novel deep-learning framework for predicting the risk of the TLE procedures. Robust deep-learning methods were developed to extract geometric features from plain chest X-ray images and the selection of geometric features was carried out by using the statistical analysis. By combining the geometric features with the personal health data, we were able to achieve a higher classification accuracy for detecting high-risk cases in the TLE procedures. The proposed framework not only has substantially improved the chance to identify the high-risk patients but also reduce the chance of falsely identifying low-risk patients as high-risk patients. Our approach only use plain chest X-ray images as the additional data source and the chest X-ray images are routinely acquired before the TLE procedures. Therefore, our approach does not require additional data and will not change current clinical practices for the TLE procedures. The results have demonstrated "lead dwell time" and "coil & more than 2 leads in SVC" were primary features predicting major complication cases in the XGBoost classifier (Fig. 11). This supports current clinical guidance and suggests clinical judgement remains paramount in appropriate patient risk stratification.

Our methodology for feature extraction, feature selection and model building is not limited to the risk prediction of the TLE procedures. The same methodology could be applied to other high-risk cardiac interventional procedures as well as applied to other commonly used medical images such as CT images or X-ray fluoroscopic images.

Acknowledgement. This work is funded by a EPSRC grant (EP/X023826/1). The study was also supported by the Wellcome/EPSRC Centre for Medical Engineering (WT203148/Z/16/Z) and the National Institute for Health Research (NIHR) Biomedical Research Centre based at Guy's and St Thomas' NHS Foundation Trust and King's College London. The views expressed are those of the author(s) and not necessarily those of the NHS, the NIHR or the Department of Health.

References

1. van Erven, L., et al.: Attitude towards redundant leads and the practice of lead extractions: a European survey. Europace **12**(2), 275–276 (2010)
2. Bongiorni, M.G., et al.: The European lead extraction ConTRolled (ELECTRa) study: a European heart rhythm association (EHRA) registry of transvenous lead extraction outcomes. Eur. Heart J. **38**(40), 2995–3005 (2017)
3. Sidhu, B.S., et al.: Risk stratification of patients undergoing transvenous lead extraction with the ELECTRa registry outcome score (EROS): an ESC EHRA EORP European lead extraction ConTRolled ELECTRa registry analysis. Europace **23**(9), 1462–1471 (2021)
4. Mehta, V.S., et al.: Machine learning–derived major adverse event prediction of patients undergoing transvenous lead extraction: using the ESC EHRA EORP European lead extraction ConTRolled ELECTRa registry. Heart Rhythm **19**(6), 885–893 (2022)
5. Tułecki, Ł, et al.: A study of major and minor complications of 1500 transvenous lead extraction procedures performed with optimal safety at two high-volume referral centers. Int. J. Environ. Res. Public Health **18**(19), 10416–10429 (2021)

6. Tariq, M., Palade, V., Ma, Y., Altahhan, A.: Diabetic retinopathy detection using transfer and reinforcement learning with effective image preprocessing and data augmentation techniques. In: Hatzilygeroudis, I.K., Tsihrintzis, G.A., Jain, L.C. (eds.) Fusion of Machine Learning Paradigms. ISRL, vol. 236, pp. 33–61. Springer, Cham (2023). https://doi.org/10.1007/978-3-031-22371-6_3

7. Chest X-Ray Image database. https://www.kaggle.com/datasets/paultimothymooney/chest-xray-pneumonia

8. Ma, Y., et al.: A tensor-based catheter and wire detection and tracking framework and its clinical applications. IEEE Trans. Biomed. Eng. **69**(2), 635–644 (2022)

9. Ma, Y., Alhrishy, M., Narayan, S.A., Mountney, P., Rhode, K.S.: A novel real-time computational framework for detecting catheters and rigid guidewires in cardiac catheterization procedures. Med. Phys. **45**(11), 5066–5079 (2018)

10. Tułecki, Ł, et al.: Analysis of risk factors for major complications of 1500 transvenous lead extraction procedures with especial attention to tricuspid valve damage. Int. J. Environ. Res. Public Health **18**(17), 9100–9113 (2021)

11. Ma, Y., Mehta, V.S., Rinaldi, C.A., Hu, P., Niederer, S., Razavi, R.: Automatic detection of coil position in the chest X-ray images for assessing the risks of lead extraction procedures. In: Bernard, O., Clarysse, P., Duchateau, N., Ohayon, J., Viallon, M. (eds.) FIMH 2023. LNCS, vol. 13958, pp. 310–319. Springer, Cham (2023). https://doi.org/10.1007/978-3-031-35302-4_32

12. Wu, X., Housden, J., Ma, Y., Razavi, B., Rhode, K., Rueckert, D.: Fast catheter segmentation from echocardiographic sequences based on segmentation from corresponding X-ray fluoroscopy for cardiac catheterization interventions. IEEE Trans. Med. Imaging **34**(4), 861–876 (2015)

13. Bashir, J., et al.: Classification and surgical repair of injuries sustained during transvenous lead extraction. Circ. Arrhythm. Electrophysiol. **9**(9) (2016)

14. Panayiotou, M., et al.: A statistical method for retrospective cardiac and respiratory motion gating of interventional cardiac X-ray images. Med. Phys. **41**(071901), 1–13 (2014)

15. Chung, N., et al.: Jaccard/Tanimoto similarity test and estimation methods for biological presence-absence data. BMC Bioinform. **20**(644) (2019)

16. Lai, C., et al.: A robust correlation analysis framework for imbalanced and dichotomous data with uncertainty. Inf. Sci. **470**, 58–77 (2019)

17. He, H., et al.: ADASYN: adaptive synthetic sampling approach for imbalanced learning. In: IEEE International Joint Conference on Neural Networks, pp. 1322–1328 (2008)

18. Chen, T., et al.: XGBoost: a scalable tree boosting system. In: Proceedings of the 22nd ACM SIGKDD International Conference on Knowledge Discovery and Data Mining (KDD 2016), pp. 785–794 (2016)

19. Ogunleye, A., et al.: XGBoost model for chronic kidney disease diagnosis. IEEE/ACM Trans. Comput. Biol. Bioinf. **17**(6), 2131–2140 (2020)

AI-Aided Medical Imaging and Analysis

Assessing the Impact of Deep Learning Backbones for Mass Detection in Breast Imaging

Edouard Chatzopoulos[ID] and Sébastien Jodogne[(✉)][ID]

Institute of Information and Communication Technologies, Electronics and Applied Mathematics (ICTEAM), UCLouvain, 1348 Louvain-la-Neuve, Belgium
`sebastien.jodogne@uclouvain.be`

Abstract. Breast cancer is a significant global health concern, where early detection is crucial for effective treatment and better patient outcomes. Deep learning has emerged as a promising tool for the automated analysis of breast imaging, with the potential to reduce the workload of radiologists and enhance diagnostic sensitivity. The RetinaNet architecture is especially appealing for mass detection in mammograms, merging the advantages of single-shot detectors with the feature extraction capabilities of a feature pyramid network. This paper demonstrates the critical importance of selecting the backbone feature extractor embedded in RetinaNet. It is also shown that fine-tuning pre-trained backbones on the specific domain of interest significantly contributes to enhancing performance. This study addresses a critical gap by offering an evaluation of different feature extraction backbones and training methodologies for RetinaNet models applied to high-resolution breast imaging.

Keywords: Breast imaging · Mass detection · Deep learning · RetinaNet

1 Introduction

Breast cancer remains a significant global health concern, with early detection being a crucial factor for an effective treatment and improved patient recovery, reducing mortality by a substantial factor when implemented [33]. This process, however, is heavily reliant on the expertise of radiologists and their availability [27]. In recent years, the integration of machine learning in breast imaging has shown promising results in the automated detection of breast masses and microcalcifications. It could reduce the workload or stress experienced by radiologists due to the growing number of images they need to handle, as well as improve their sensitivity [28]. In particular, the research in the landscape of deep learning algorithms for breast mass detection has grown exponentially, reflecting the urgent need for accurate, open, and efficient diagnostic tools.

© The Author(s), under exclusive license to Springer Nature Switzerland AG 2024
X. Xie et al. (Eds.): AIiH 2024, LNCS 14976, pp. 33–47, 2024.
https://doi.org/10.1007/978-3-031-67285-9_3

Deep learning applied to breast imaging is characterized by a wide variety of architectures, ranging from simple networks derived from natural image processing [1] to increasingly specific and complex systems [11,28,30]. However, when implementing these networks, it is common to use the default configuration of the architecture [12,25], without considering the effect of its different components on the performance of the system.

In this paper, we evaluate the effectiveness of different variants of the RetinaNet architecture [17] for the detection of breast masses on mammograms. Indeed, the distinguishing feature of the RetinaNet architecture lies in its capability to incorporate various backbone models utilized for the binary classification of patches within images. It remains an open question as to which of these backbones yields optimal performance in breast imaging applications. Furthermore, we demonstrate the importance of adopting a learning methodology that first fine-tunes pre-trained backbones on the application domain, before training the entire RetinaNet model. These contributions offer guidelines to train simple, adaptable deep learning models whose performance reaches the state-of-the-art for mass detection in breast imaging.

2   Related Work

In this section, the main deep learning architectures that are commonly applied to mass detection in mammograms are presented. These algorithms are categorized according to the underlying architectures. Moreover, the challenges and limitations associated with the existing methods are highlighted, which will call for the novel approach that is introduced in the subsequent sections.

A first approach to computer-aided decision (CAD) based on deep learning in mammograms consists in considering mass detection as an image classification task. This restricts detection to a binary decision based on presence or absence of masses in either the entire mammogram or a predefined region of interest (ROI). This approach is simple in terms of training requirements, as it only necessitates binary annotations. However, it is far from ideal to reduce the amount of work of radiologists. Indeed, if radiologists wish to delve deeper into the decision made by the system, they have no indication about which part of the image is identified as suspicious, which necessitates further scrutiny in analysis. This lack of interpretability can be mitigated by introducing explainability components to the neural networks with techniques such as Grad-CAM [26] or weakly supervised feature localization with attention maps [7]. However, such approaches attempt to trace back the inner working of the models exclusively from the value of their existing weights and can be improved by further guiding the model with more complete annotations, including information about the localization of masses.

Another common approach consists of using segmentation-based methods, such as the well-known U-Net architecture [24]. Such methods output binary segmentation masks that closely outline the contours of the anomalies, which provides information about the localization. These methods are widely used in the context of deep learning applied to medical imaging, as they allow a precise targeting of affected tissues. In the context of breast imaging, this approach is often chosen for the detection of microcalcifications because of their wide variety in terms of shapes and dimensions, as well as because of the importance of the shape for diagnostic purposes [4]. Unfortunately, the training of segmentation-based neural networks requires a substantially greater amount of effort compared to binary classification. Indeed, significant expertise and time are required to accurately delineate the contours of each anomaly present in the images.

An intermediate option between binary classification and segmentation-based methods is object detection. The task of object detection consists in locating bounding boxes around the elements of interest. The training of a neural network for lesion detection only requires approximate annotations provided as bounding boxes, which drastically reduces the time commitment from radiologist while maintaining a satisfactory level of explainability and localization. Work in tumor detection using bounding boxes is extensive and includes a variety of detection networks such as YOLO [21], Faster R-CNN [22], and PAA [13]. Among these methods, single-shot detection networks such as YOLO and RetinaNet are often used because of their fast inference speed. For instance, a modified version of YOLOv3 was used to obtain a model less biased towards low recall caused by the vast number of easy negative cases in mammogram databases [31]. However, YOLO networks often lack performance when it comes to the detection of small objects. Faster R-CNN, a two-shot detection network, has been proved to overcome such issues on the OMI-DB database [1]. An even deeper three-stage network based on PAA has also been shown to improve detection capabilities [11].

In this context, the RetinaNet detection network is an appealing alternative, as it combines the detection performance of Faster R-CNN with an efficient single-shot detector [17]. The RetinaNet architecture consists in incorporating a classifier network as the backbone of a feature pyramid network (FPN), which enables feature extraction at various scales. These features are fed to subsequent layers to predict the localization and class of detected targets in a single stage. RetinaNet has been used with a satisfactory level of success in literature. However, it is often restricted to images with small resolution to reduce the hardware requirements [23]. Consequently, the large resolution of mammograms (around 3000×4000 pixels) has remained a big challenge for a long time, often restraining the use of convolutional neural networks to very reduced resolutions.

To overcome this limitation, Jung et al. combined a mammogram of reduced size with 25 overlapped sections of the mammogram at full resolution [12]. The final prediction was taken as the combination of the predictions using a standard RetinaNet network with a ResNet50 backbone over the different views of the same breast. The rapid advancement of GPU capabilities, as well as the emergence of more efficient classification networks like ConvNeXt, are quickly overcoming the limitations related to the size of mammograms and can further improve the detection capabilities of RetinaNet. Unfortunately, there is currently a lack of systematic evaluation of feature extraction backbones and of training methodologies for RetinaNet models applied to breast mass detection at high resolutions. This paper aims to contribute to filling this gap. Since the release of

RetinaNet, newer networks such as FreeAnchor [32] and TOOD [6] have demonstrated promising detection capabilities. However, the objective of this study is not to identify the best-performing detection network, but to explore simple architectural and training modifications that improve detection performance.

3   Materials and Methods

Designing a deep learning model for the detection of breast masses involves a multitude of decisions about the data pre-processing, about the design of the network architecture, as well as about the training methodology. This section provides a comprehensive description of the steps that were followed to train a RetinaNet model for breast imaging that integrates different backbones.

3.1   Dataset

One of the largest and most widely used mammogram datasets is the "Digital Database for Screening Mammography" (DDSM) [10]. The dataset that was used to train our RetinaNet models is the "Curated Breast Imaging Subset" (CBIS-DDSM) dataset [15], a revised and standardized subset of DDSM. This dataset is composed of 6775 digitized film mammograms from 1566 patients. The original DDSM dataset contains either imaging studies with no signs of tumor, or imaging studies with masses or microcalcifications. This contrasts with the revised version that excludes the normal exams, and only contains images of breasts with either masses or microcalcifications. Furthermore, images in the revised dataset are encoded using the DICOM interoperable format and underwent some additional corrections. In this work, only the images of the CBIS-DDSM dataset containing masses are taken into consideration. Several preprocessing steps are then applied to the source dataset, as described below:

Corrections to the Dataset: Despite its high-quality data curation process, the CBIS-DDSM dataset contains some inconsistencies. Indeed, a portion of the segmentation masks delineating tumors do not match the dimensions of the mammograms. As a result, superimposing the coordinates of some masks can result in an erroneous position of the tumor on the source mammogram. In such cases, a simple resizing of the mask to the dimensions of the associated mammogram was proved to solve the issue. Consequently, in this work, wherever the source mask does not match the resolution of the mammogram, a resized version of the mask is used.

Dataset Split: To prevent any contamination between the training, the validation, and the test sets, the source dataset is split at the patient level instead of the image level. This patient-wise separation of the original dataset ensures that the model is not evaluated on an image containing a mass already seen from another angle or on breast tissue from the same patient. To this end, the whole CBIS-DDSM dataset is merged, then uniformly split at the patient level according to a 80%/10%/10% train/validation/test distribution.

Patch Generation for Normal Tissues: In the early phases of the training, a part of the model is trained on a patch classification task. It is therefore needed to generate 256×256 image patches that include either breast masses or normal breast tissues. Since the CBIS-DDSM dataset lacks images of normal breast tissues, such patches are extracted from all mammograms from the dataset. To avoid selecting tissue containing lesions, a segmentation mask encompassing all anomalies in the mammogram is generated. This mask is subsequently dilated using a 256×256 pixel kernel to incorporate a safety margin around the tumors. To also avoid sampling too much background instead of healthy tissue, this dilated mask is then merged via a binary "OR" operation with a background mask, obtained through binary Otsu's thresholding of the breast image. The resulting mask is inverted to produce a segmentation mask of the normal breast tissue, with safety margins. The patch center is then uniformly drawn in this mask, to create a patch that contains normal breast tissue, while ensuring the absence of known lesions.

Patch Generation for Breast Masses: In order to generate patches containing masses, all the masses available in the training set are randomly sampled. Two different strategies are then applied depending on the size of the sampled masses. The first strategy is used for masses with an area that is greater than 40% of the area of the patch. In this case, the center of the patch is drawn uniformly among the points of the patch situated inside the tumor. The second strategy is used for smaller masses, for which centering the patch inside the mass would result in highly similar patches when sampling the same tumor. A random perturbation is generated uniformly in the range from -25% to $+25\%$ of the patch side, in both the x and y directions. The center of the patch is then defined as the sum of the barycenter of the tumor mask and this random offset. The percentage of the area of the tumor visible on this patch is then computed and patching is repeated from the start if the ratio is smaller than 80% until this criterion is met. The combination of those two strategies ensures to combine coverage of the entirety of large masses, while benefiting from greater peripheral coverage next to smaller masses.

Data Augmentation: To augment the number of training images and reduce overfitting, a combination of different data augmentation techniques is used. The images are randomly flipped with a probability of 50% in both the horizontal and vertical direction. The patches are resized with a scale uniformly distributed between 80% and 120%. Patches are rotated by an angle that is randomly selected between $0°$, $90°$, $180°$, and $270°$. Affine transformations are then applied to the patches to add an additional rotation in the $-5°$ to $+5°$ range, a relative translation in the 0% to 5% range in both directions, and a shearing in the $-5°$ to $+5°$ range in both directions. If the modified image is greater than the original dimensions, a center crop is applied with the original image dimension to reduce memory footprint of large images.

Contrast Enhancement: To enhance the local contrast in dense breast tissues, each image is processed with an adaptive histogram equalization algorithm for both training and inference. The algorithm used for this purpose is Contrast Limited Adaptive Histogram Equalization (CLAHE) [20]. CLAHE is applied

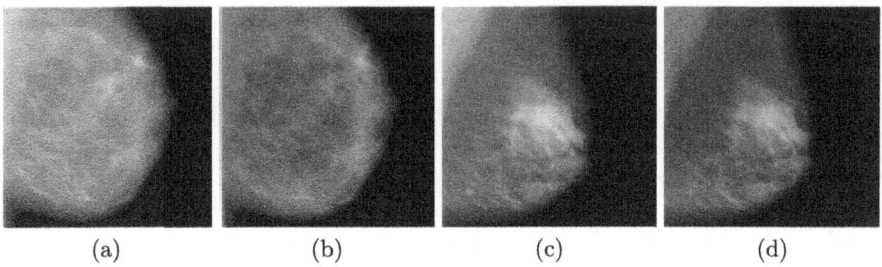

(a)   (b)   (c)   (d)

Fig. 1. Examples of portions of mammograms from CBIS-DDSM before (a and c), and after (b and d) applying CLAHE.

with a grid size of 8×8 and a clip limit of 1. To apply the algorithm, the image must first be converted to integer, and converted back in the 0 to 1 range in floating point after the contrast enhancement before being fed to the network. The effect of contrast enhancement is illustrated in Fig. 1.

3.2   Deep Learning Models

The model used in this work is an adapted version of RetinaNet [17] using different feature extraction backbones. RetinaNet is a single-stage detector network based on a feature extraction backbone extended with two different heads for classification and regression. The features of the classification network are extracted at three different scales by the feature pyramid network (FPN) [16] and fed to the two heads of the network. This multi-scale feature extraction allows combining the higher-resolution features of the first layers, which is required for the precise detection of small tumors and precise contours, while using the more abstract features of the deeper layers to obtain better classification of the lesions. The classification head of the network is responsible for detecting candidate lesions, and eventually predicting their class, while the regression head is tasked with predicting the dimensions and position of the bounding boxes.

As RetinaNet relies on its backbone to produce features relevant for lesion detection, the backbone model can have an important influence on the quality of the detection, as well as on the memory footprint of the model and on the execution time that is needed for inference. In this work, backbone with different sizes and characteristics are integrated to the network and compared on the task of detection of breast masses. The following backbones have been investigated:

ResNet: ResNet is a well-known type of classification network that is widely used on image classification tasks [9]. Its architecture is simple, using four blocks of convolutional layers and a classification head. The RetinaNet architecture is traditionally built on the top of a ResNet50 backbone.

ResNeXt: ResNeXt networks are improved versions of ResNet that exploit a new dimension, the so-called *cardinality* [29]. Compared to ResNet blocks, the

Table 1. The set of hyperparameters used for the different training phases. Phases 1A and 1B consist in training the patch classifier alone. Phases 2A and 2B correspond to the training of the RetinaNet network.

Training phase	1A	1B	2A	2B
Task	Patch binary classification	Patch binary classification	Mass detection	Mass detection
Loss function	Binary cross entropy loss	Binary cross entropy loss	Focal loss	Focal loss
Trained layers	Final fully-connected layer	Complete backbone	Heads of RetinaNet	Complete RetinaNet
Batch size	32	32	1	1
Learning rate	1e-4	1e-4	1e-4	1e-5
Weight decay	5e-4	5e-4	1e-4	1e-4
Optimizer	RAdam	RAdam	SGD	SGD
Learning rate scheduler	Cosine annealing	Cosine annealing	Cosine annealing	Cosine annealing
Epochs	100	100	100	100
Batch normalization state	Unfrozen	Unfrozen	Frozen	Frozen

blocks are reduced in the channel dimension, but each block is duplicated C times (C being the value of the cardinality) and the output of every sub-block is aggregated. Even under the condition of maintaining complexity, increasing the cardinality can improve classification accuracy of the network.

ConvNeXt: ConvNeXt networks represent another evolution of ResNet that aims to reach the same high classification performance as vision transformers [5], while maintaining the simplicity of traditional convolutional networks [18]. Their biggest addition is a special type of convolution named "depth-wise convolution" which increases the receptive field of the network without increasing computational complexity. Because of an alternating between two distinct types of blocks inside the ConvNeXt network, connecting the FPN of RetinaNet to a ConvNeXt network is not as straightforward as with ResNet or ResNeXt networks. Indeed, instead of feeding the output of the last three blocks of the network to the FPN, we need to feed one out of every two blocks. This is because only blocks 0, 2, 4, and 6 down-sample the dimension of the feature maps, and therefore extracting two consecutive layers does not result in extracting different resolution feature maps for the different levels of the FPN. For this reason, in this work, the layers extracted by the FPN are the outputs of layers 3, 5, and 7.

3.3 Training

The training of the RetinaNet model is divided into four parts, two for training the backbone on a patch classification task, and two for training the complete RetinaNet network. The training starts with a backbone that is pre-trained on the ImageNet dataset [3]. In the first training phase (1A), all the layers of the backbone network are frozen, except for its classification head that is fine-tuned to distinguish patches containing normal tissues from patches corresponding to tumor masses. In the second phase (1B), all other layers of the backbone are unfrozen, and the model is fine-tuned on the patch classification task with a lower learning rate. Once the backbone is trained, it is extended with a FPN

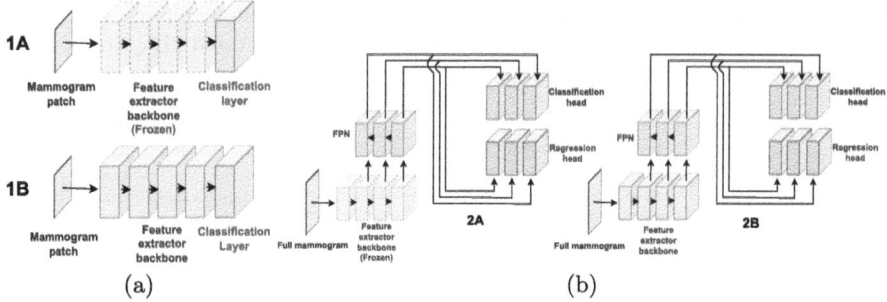

Fig. 2. Configuration of the network (a) in phases 1A and 1B, and (b) in phases 2A and 2B. The frozen layers are displayed with dotted contours and a reduced opacity.

and integrated as the feature extractor of the RetinaNet model. In the third learning phase (2A), the resulting RetinaNet model is trained on the task of mass detection, while keeping the weights of the backbone frozen. In the final phase (2B), the weights of the backbone are unfrozen, and the learning rate is lowered again to fine-tune the entire RetinaNet network. For the last two phases, the batch normalization layers are kept in a frozen state to prevent instabilities that could result from training batch normalization with a unit batch size. Table 1 reports the hyperparameters that were used throughout the distinct phases. The four training phases are illustrated in Fig. 2.

3.4   Metrics

This study employs commonly used metrics to assess the accuracy and reliability of the networks. In the context of breast mass detection, a True Positive (TP) happens when the model correctly predicts the presence of a mass. An Intersection over Union (IoU) threshold at 0.2 between the true bounding box of a mass and the predicted one is used to consider them matching, which is consistent with standard conventions for mass detection in mammograms [11]. A False Positive (FP) happens when the model incorrectly predicts the presence of a mass. The False Positive per Image rate (FPI) is the average number of FP for a prediction on any given image. The True Positive Rate (TPR) represents the ratio of the total number of TP, against the sum of all TPs and FPs. This ratio is also known as sensitivity. Finally, the Free response Receiver Operating Curve (FROC), is the plot of sensitivity versus the average number of false positives per image. This metric is analogous to the Receiver Operating Curve (ROC) in image-level evaluation, but for lesion-level evaluation.

4   Results

In the following section, we present the results of our study on the impact of numerous factors on the performance of the breast mass detection network.

We examine the effect of backbone pre-training, the influence of backbone fine-tuning within the detection network, and compare different backbone architectures for the RetinaNet model. Additionally, we analyze the performance relative to network size and compare our results with other works on the same dataset. This systematic evaluation provides insights into the optimal configurations and strategies for enhancing the accuracy of breast mass detection.

4.1 Effect of Backbone Pre-training

This section explores the benefits of pre-training the model used in the backbone of the detection network on the task of patch classification, instead of using a network that is pre-trained on ImageNet as such. Indeed, most earlier works simply fine-tune the complete RetinaNet network, without training the underlying feature extractor on the domain of interest first. Figure 3 (a) depicts the FROC curve for the RetinaNet model trained in two ways: firstly, using the four-stage approach suggested in this paper, and secondly, using only stages 2A and AB with the pre-trained backbone. A significant jump in performance can be observed at every point of the FROC curve if pre-training the backbone on the patch classification task. These results indicate that first training the backbone sub-network on the specific task of mammography mass classification can help the network converge to a better optimum in the lesion detection task. Note that both networks were trained until convergence, therefore the improvement in performance is not due to a longer training time.

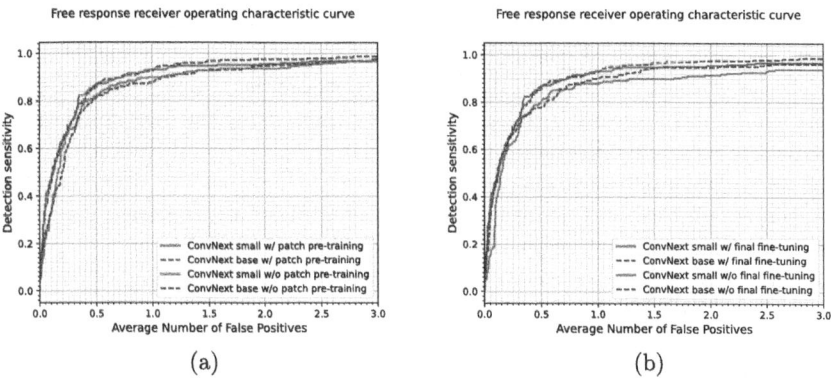

(a)   (b)

Fig. 3. (a) Effect of pre-training the backbone on a patch classification task before its integration in RetinaNet. The baseline shown in red is the result of using a backbone pre-trained on ImageNet only. (b) Effect of the addition of the final fine-tuning stage of the whole network (phase 2B) on ConvNeXt base and on ConvNeXt small. The baseline shown in red is the result of bypassing the final fine-tuning. (Color figure online)

4.2 Effect of Backbone Fine-Tuning Inside the Detection Network

The previous section indicates the interest of fine-tuning the patch classifier. One might intuitively believe that since this backbone is already fine-tuned, unfreezing its weights during the final stage of RetinaNet training would yield no additional benefits. Figure 3 (b) displays the comparison of the FROC curve of two models, before and after stage 2B. This experiment shows that even after pre-training the backbone classifier in stages 1A and 1B, the addition of stage 2B allows to further ameliorate the TPR of the network at any FPI.

This result indicates that unfreezing the weights of the backbone in the final training phase of the model is beneficial, even in the case of a feature extractor trained to convergence on the same dataset. This may be due to the additional layers corresponding to the FPN and to the two RetinaNet heads, which add several layers of abstraction to the deeper feature of the network, hereby requiring a finer adjustment of the shallower features of the network. These findings, combined with those of Sect. 4.1, indicate that the optimal convergence of the model cannot rely solely on a feature extraction backbone trained on the target dataset, nor can it rely solely on the RetinaNet model to fine-tune this backbone on its own. For optimal detection performance, a combination of these two factors seems to be required.

4.3 Backbone Comparison

The detection performance of the RetinaNet model depends upon the choice of the backbone. In this section, to assess the significance of this decision, various feature extraction backbones are compared for the task of detecting breast masses. Figure 4 compares the performance of RetinaNet models embedding six different backbones (ResNet50, ResNet101, RestNeXt50, ConvNeXt base, ConvNeXt small, and ConNeXt tiny) after training them using the four-stage method described in Sect. 3.3. This figure indicates that the traditional RetinaNet model based on a ResNet50 backbone is competitive with respect to other combinations, but its performance is overtaken by a handful of alternatives.

Among these alternatives, the models based on ConvNeXt seem to perform best, with performance consistently above the ResNet50 baseline, with a sensitivity up to 18% greater for the same FP rate. For the same FPI of 0.5, the ConvNeXt base network reaches a TPR of 0.87, while the ResNet50-based network peaks at 0.74 TPR, with an increase of 17.6% in sensitivity. ResNet101, a larger variant of the model, provides only a slightly higher overall sensitivity. However, some models that are more recent than ResNet, such as ResNeXt50, appear to be behind in terms of performance on this specific task, as can be seen by the overall lower FROC score compared to the networks configured with the other backbones. Despite the apparent advantage of the ResNeXt model in some image classification tasks [29], this superiority does not seem to transfer to mass detection in the CBIS-DDSM dataset within a RetinaNet detection model.

These findings are further validated by the mean Average Precision (mAP) of the various models at an IoU threshold of 0.2. The ResNet50-based model achieves a mAP of 0.6806, while the ResNet101-based model attains a mAP of 0.6897, indicating a marginal performance difference between the two models. In contrast, the ConvNeXt-based models exhibit significantly higher mAP values, with the tiny, small, and base variants respectively achieving mAPs of 0.7264, 0.7649, and 0.7736, which highlights their superior detection performance.

4.4 Performance Relative to the Size of the Network

In Fig. 5, a modest correlation between model size and detection capabilities can be observed, although it is not entirely consistent. Indeed, bigger models in general achieve higher scores, with the largest model demonstrating the best performance and the smallest model showing the poorest. However, the networks based on ConvNeXt small and ConvNeXt tiny exceed the performance of the larger ResNet101 network at every measured threshold. This could be a result of their larger receptive field and their novel convolution method, allowing them to make better use of the large resolution of the mammogram. Moreover, the performance of RetinaNet-based on ConvNeXt small and ConvNeXt tiny is comparable to that of the ConvNeXt base model, despite the latter being larger by a factor of 77% and 192% respectively. The lack of a larger improvement in performance relatively to the size of the model indicates that with the right architecture, a small model is sufficient for mass detection on small mammogram datasets such as CBIS-DDSM. Further research would be necessary to determine whether this fact holds true for larger datasets or more complex tasks.

As expected, the inference time of the models is strongly correlated with the size of the network, with the ConvNeXt-based model respectively averaging 88ms, 143ms and 211ms per iteration for the base, small, and tiny variations on a NVIDIA RTX A4500 GPU. The ResNet-based models average 75ms and 102ms per iteration for the 50 and 101 variations on the same hardware. These inference times are all of the same order, but could be of importance in the case of inference on slower hardware.

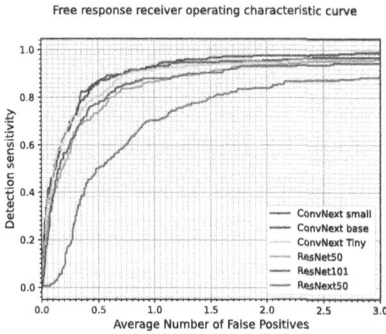

Fig. 4. Comparison of the FROC of the RetinaNet model with five different backbones. All networks are trained using the four-stage training.

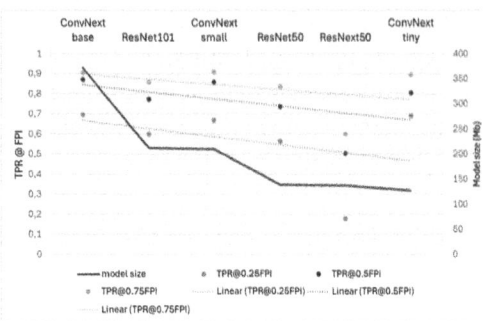

Fig. 5. Comparison of TPR for different rates of FPI in relation to total model size.

Table 2. Comparison of the proposed method vs. CAD systems trained and evaluated on CBIS-DDSM, expressed as true positive rate at given false positive per image rate.

Method	Model type	Size of test set	TPR @ FPI
Yu et al. [30]	GFNet	348	0.89 @ 2.21 0.90 @ 2.91
Lbachir et al. [14]	HRAK + BTC + SVM	152	0.91 @ 0.65
Peng et al. [19]	Faster R-CNN + ResNeXt	Unknown	0.94 @ 2.2805
Cao et al. [2]	Faster R-CNN+FPN+FL+NL trained w/ CBIS-DDSM+INbreast+BCD	~320	~0.8 @ 0.4
Ours	RetinaNet + FPN + ConvNeXt base	249	0.8 @ 0.38 0.89 @ 0.57 0.95 @ 1.07

4.5   Comparison with Other Works on CBIS-DDSM

Table 2 shows a comparison of the proposed method against other similar CAD systems trained on CBIS-DDSM. Our method is on par with the state of the art, offering either higher TPR at comparable FPI, or similar TPR at a lower FPI. These results show that despite its size, CBIS-DDSM remains a challenging dataset. This difficulty can partly be attributed to the dataset being composed of digitized scans. These scans, originating from analog sources, exhibit lower contrast and more artifacts compared to fully digital mammograms. Access to high-quality datasets continues to be one of the major obstacles to perfecting CAD for breast cancer screening [8].

5   Conclusion

This paper introduces an efficient, comprehensive methodology to train a RetinaNet network on the task of mass detection in breast imaging. The achieved performance aligns with the state-of-the-art results on the CBIS-DDSM dataset. The importance of selecting a proper backbone network for use as a feature extractor has been highlighted. It has also been shown that fine-tuning pre-trained backbones on the specific domain of interest is a crucial element for enhancing the performance of RetinaNet models. We argue that transparently disclosing such training methodology is crucial for ensuring the reproducibility of deep learning algorithms in medical imaging.

The scope of this work is currently limited to the detection of breast masses and ignores microcalcifications or other types of lesions. Future work will train RetinaNet models that are at the same time applicable to the detection of breast masses and microcalcifications, and that predicts the malignancy of the lesions. The potential of alternative multi-scale feature extractors such as Bidirectional FPN will also be explored, as well as multi-view feature extraction to enhance the detection of challenging lesions such as architectural distortions and focal asymmetries. Finally, it is planned to publicly release pre-trained RetinaNet models as free and open-source software. This initiative aims to contribute to the advancement and implementation of computer-aided detection in breast imaging, offering benefits in education and research contexts.

References

1. Agarwal, R., Díaz, O., Yap, M.H., Lladó, X., Martí, R.: Deep learning for mass detection in full field digital mammograms. Comput. Biol. Med. **121**, 103774 (2020)
2. Cao, Z., et al.: Deep learning based mass detection in mammograms. In: 2019 IEEE Global Conference on Signal and Information Processing (GlobalSIP), pp. 1–5 (2019)
3. Deng, J., Dong, W., Socher, R., Li, L.J., Li, K., Fei-Fei, L.: ImageNet: a large-scale hierarchical image database. In: IEEE CVPR 2009, pp. 248–255. IEEE (2009)
4. Dengler, J., Behrens, S., Desaga, J.: Segmentation of microcalcifications in mammograms. IEEE Trans. Med. Imaging **12**(4), 634–642 (1993)
5. Dosovitskiy, A., et al.: An image is worth 16×16 words: transformers for image recognition at scale. In: International Conference on Learning Representations (2021)
6. Feng, C., Zhong, Y., Gao, Y., Scott, M.R., Huang, W.: TOOD: task-aligned one-stage object detection. In: ICCV 2021, pp. 3490–3499 (2021)
7. Gupta, S., Lakhotia, S., Rawat, A., Tallamraju, R.: ViTOL: vision transformer for weakly supervised object localization. In: Proceedings of the IEEE/CVF CVPR Workshops, pp. 4101–4110 (2022)
8. Hassan, N., Hamad, S., Mahar, K.: Mammogram breast cancer CAD systems for mass detection and classification: a review. Multimedia Tools Appl. **81**(14), 20043–20075 (2022)
9. He, K., Zhang, X., Ren, S., Sun, J.: Deep residual learning for image recognition. In: IEEE CVPR 2016, pp. 770–778. IEEE (2016)
10. Heath, M., Bowyer, K., Kopans, D., Moore, R., Kegelmeyer, W.P.: The digital database for screening mammography. In: Proceedings of the 5th International Workshop on Digital Mammography, pp. 212–218 (2001). http://www.eng.usf.edu/cvprg/Mammography/Database.html
11. Jiang, J., Peng, J., Hu, C., Jian, W., Wang, X., Liu, W.: Breast cancer detection and classification in mammogram using a three-stage deep learning framework based on PAA algorithm. Artif. Intell. Med. **134**, 102419 (2022)

12. Jung, H., et al.: Detection of masses in mammograms using a one-stage object detector based on a deep convolutional neural network. PLoS ONE **13**(9), 1–16 (2018)
13. Kim, K., Lee, H.S.: Probabilistic anchor assignment with IoU prediction for object detection. In: Vedaldi, A., Bischof, H., Brox, T., Frahm, J.M. (eds.) ECCV 2020, pp. 355–371. Springer International Publishing, Cham (2020). https://doi.org/10.1007/978-3-030-58595-2_22
14. Lbachir, I.A., Daoudi, I., Tallal, S.: Automatic computer-aided diagnosis system for mass detection and classification in mammography. Multimedia Tools Appl. **80**(6), 9493–9525 (2021)
15. Lee, R., Gimenez, F., Hoogi, A., Miyake, K., Gorovoy, M., Rubin, D.: A curated mammography data set for use in computer-aided detection and diagnosis research. Sci. Data **4**(1) (2017)
16. Lin, T.Y., Dollar, P., Girshick, R., He, K., Hariharan, B., Belongie, S.: Feature pyramid networks for object detection. In: IEEE CVPR 2017, pp. 936–944. IEEE (2017)
17. Lin, T.Y., Goyal, P., Girshick, R., He, K., Dollár, P.: Focal loss for dense object detection. IEEE Trans. Pattern Anal. Mach. Intell. **42**(2), 318–327 (2020)
18. Liu, Z., Mao, H., Wu, C.Y., Feichtenhofer, C., Darrell, T., Xie, S.: A ConvNet for the 2020s. In: IEEE/CVF CVPR 2022, pp. 11966–11976 (2022)
19. Peng, J., Bao, C., Hu, C., Wang, X., Jian, W., Liu, W.: Automated mammographic mass detection using deformable convolution and multiscale features. Medical Biol. Eng. Comput. **58**(7) (2020)
20. Pizer, S.M., et al.: Adaptive histogram equalization and its variations. Comput. Vis. Graph. Image Process. **39**(3), 355–368 (1987)
21. Redmon, J., Divvala, S., Girshick, R., Farhadi, A.: You only look once: unified, real-time object detection. In: 2016 IEEE CVPR, pp. 779–788 (2016)
22. Ren, S., He, K., Girshick, R., Sun, J.: Faster R-CNN: towards real-time object detection with region proposal networks. In: Cortes, C., Lawrence, N., Lee, D., Sugiyama, M., Garnett, R. (eds.) Advances in Neural Information Processing Systems, vol. 28. Curran Associates, Inc. (2015)
23. Ribeiro, R.F., Torres, H.R., Oliveira, B., Morais, P., Vilaça, J.L.: Comparative analysis of deep learning methods for lesion detection on full screening mammography. In: 2023 45th Annual International Conference of the IEEE Engineering in Medicine & Biology Society (EMBC), pp. 1–4 (2023)
24. Ronneberger, O., Fischer, P., Brox, T.: U-net: Convolutional networks for biomedical image segmentation. In: Navab, N., Hornegger, J., Wells, W.M., Frangi, A.F. (eds.) MICCAI 2015, pp. 234–241. Springer International Publishing, Cham (2015). https://doi.org/10.1007/978-3-319-24574-4_28
25. Ryspayeva, M., Molinara, M., Bria, A., Marrocco, C., Tortorella, F.: Transfer learning in breast mass detection on the OMI-DB dataset: a preliminary study. In: Rousseau, J.J., Kapralos, B. (eds.) Pattern Recognition, Computer Vision, and Image Processing. ICPR 2022 International Workshops and Challenges, pp. 529–538. Springer Nature Switzerland, Cham (2023). https://doi.org/10.1007/978-3-031-37660-3_37
26. Selvaraju, R.R., Cogswell, M., Das, A., Vedantam, R., Parikh, D., Batra, D.: Grad-CAM: visual explanations from deep networks via gradient-based localization. In: IEEE ICCV 2017, pp. 618–626 (2017)
27. Sickles, E.A., Wolverton, D.E., Dee, K.E.: Performance parameters for screening and diagnostic mammography: specialist and general radiologists. Radiology **224**(3), 861–869 (2002). PMID: 12202726

28. Wu, N., Phang, J., Park, J., Shen, Y., Huang, Z.: Deep neural networks improve radiologists' performance in breast cancer screening. IEEE Trans. Med. Imaging **39**(4), 1184–1194 (2020)
29. Xie, S., Girshick, R., Dollar, P., Tu, Z., He, K.: Aggregated residual transformations for deep neural networks. In: IEEE CVPR 2017, pp. 5987–5995. IEEE Computer Society, Los Alamitos, CA, USA (2017)
30. Yu, X., Zhu, Z., Alon, Y., Guttery, D.S., Zhang, Y.: GFNet: a deep learning framework for breast mass detection. Electronics **12**(7) (2023)
31. Zhang, L., Li, Y., Chen, H., Wu, W., Chen, K., Wang, S.: Anchor-free YOLOv3 for mass detection in mammogram. Expert Syst. Appl. **191**, 116273 (2022)
32. Zhang, X., Wan, F., Liu, C., Ji, R., Ye, Q.: FreeAnchor: learning to match anchors for visual object detection. In: Wallach, H., Larochelle, H., Beygelzimer, A., d'Alché-Buc, F., Fox, E., Garnett, R. (eds.) NeurIPS 2019, vol. 32. Curran Associates, Inc. (2019)
33. Zielonke, N., Gini, A., Jansen, E.E., Anttila, A., Segnan, N., et al.: Evidence for reducing cancer-specific mortality due to screening for breast cancer in Europe: a systematic review. Eur. J. Cancer **127**, 191–206 (2020)

Transferable Variational Feedback Network for Vendor Generalization in Accelerated MRI

Riti Paul[1], Sahil Vora[1], Kevin Pak Lun Ding[1], Ameet Patel[2], Leland Hu[2], Baoxin Li[1], and Yuxiang Zhou[2(✉)]

[1] School of Computing and Augmented Intelligence, Arizona State University, Tempe, AZ 85281, USA
{rpaul12,svora7,kevinding,baoxin.li}@asu.edu
[2] Department of Radiology, Mayo Clinic, 57 77 E. Mayo Boulevard, Phoenix, AZ 85054, USA
{Patel.Ameet,Hu.Leland,Zhou.Yuxiang}@mayo.edu

Abstract. Magnetic Resonance Imaging (MRI) is a widely used diagnostic tool in medicine. The long acquisition time of MRI remains to be a practical concern, leading to suboptimal patient experiences. Existing deep learning models for fast MRI acquisition struggle to handle the problem of data heterogeneity due to scanners from different vendors. This study explores the transfer learning capabilities of variational deep learning architectures to address this problem. Using standard ACR protocols, we acquired 135 ACR phantom samples from GE and Siemens 3.0T MR scanners and conducted comprehensive experiments to compare the reconstruction quality of the images produced by different models. Our experiments identified vendor differences as a major challenge in the generalization of accelerated MRI. We propose a feature refinement-based transfer learning method that outperforms the baseline networks by ∼2.0 dB (PSNR), 1.8% (SSIM) for GE, and ∼3.0 dB (PSNR), 0.8% (SSIM) for SIEMENS. Furthermore, we used experience replay to address the problem of catastrophic forgetting. We established it as a robust baseline through experiments with strong results (PSNR and SSIM performance drop reduced by 25.55% and 9.5%, respectively).

Keywords: Accelerated MRI Reconstruction · Generalization · Transfer Learning

1 Introduction

Magnetic resonance imaging (MRI) is an important non-invasive clinical procedure that can produce high-resolution and reproducible images for different parts of the anatomy. The availability of such images plays an important role in medical diagnosis. However, compared to other imaging techniques like CT or X-rays, the scan time of MRI is significantly longer (can sometimes take up to 2 h), which leads to exhaustion and discomfort of patients, inducing artifacts due to voluntary movements of the patients and involuntary physiological movements. To minimize the acquisition time, methods involving sub-sampling k-space [5,9,23,31,32] and deep-learning-based reconstruction [3,10,15,16,24,25,30,35] have been popularized recently. In recent years, variational learning with unrolled gradient descent scheme has seen an increased interest [4,10,16,30,33]. The authors of [10] applied a variational network on the CS-MRI [17] algorithm, outperforming standard or traditional reconstruction algorithms.

The nonlinear capacity of deep neural networks facilitates learning intricate down-sampled/fully sampled mappings, enhancing their effectiveness in accelerated MRI reconstruction. Despite their capacity, these networks require abundant training data to effectively learn parameters and generalize to new data. However, public availability of well-annotated medical imaging datasets are limited due to patient privacy concerns and the labor-intensive nature of manual annotation.

The 2020 fast MRI challenge highlighted vendor variation as a significant obstacle to generalization across MRI data. In [19], a new competition track, "Transfer", evaluated participants' models on data from different vendors (GE, Philips), unseen during training. Results from the "Transfer" track showed that many finalist submissions faced challenges in adapting to GE test data. These variations, whether inter or intra-dataset, lead to differing distributions between training and test datasets, causing a domain shift that negatively affects model generalization.

Diversifying the training data by creating compound datasets is a possible solution [6], but recent medical imaging studies [1,22] have shown that it does not guarantee improved generalization. Deep networks have limited generalization abilities, making them struggle to adapt to data acquired from different vendors. Consequently, such architectures create artifacts and noise in accelerated reconstructions, making them inadmissible for diagnostic and clinical use. Transfer learning allows any pre-trained model to transfer knowledge across domains and adapt to novel domains with relatively limited datasets. Consequently, it imbibes the model with the ability to handle data heterogeneity and variability. Research from the past few years has examined whether transfer learning is always successful [8,11–14,20,38]. The contribution of feature reuse in meta-learning (MAML [7]) was examined and found to be a dominant factor in [26]. [27] investigates transfer learning from a trained ImageNet model to the medical domain. However, most existing works on transfer learning in MRI reconstruction focus on protocol or domain transfer. This work focuses on vendor transfer in the MRI reconstruction domain, which to the best of our knowledge is the first work in this area. In this work, our key contributions are:

- We propose an attentive feature refinement-based transfer learning approach for vendor transfer in medical image accelerated MRI reconstruction, and the results demonstrate that our proposed approach improves reconstruction quality significantly with limited data.
- We assess the influence of pretrained networks and vendor differences on the generalization of reconstruction.

– We address catastrophic forgetting in accelerated MRI reconstruction. Through experiments, we establish experience replay as a strong baseline, reducing performance drop by 25.55% (**P**eak **S**ignal **N**oise-to-**R**atio) and 9.5% (**S**tructural **SIM**ilarity).

2   Materials and Methods

2.1   Background and Problem Formulation

MR scanners perform the acquisition in k-space, also known as the frequency domain, to obtain MR images. The relation between a given k-space data k and the corresponding image x can be represented by the following equation, $k = \mathcal{F}(x)$, where F is an operator denoting Fourier transform. We can obtain only part of the k-space data to accelerate the acquisition of MRI. Consider a binary mask matrix M, the under-sampled k-space data $\tilde{k}_i$ for the ith coil can be described as $\tilde{k}_i = M \odot k_i$ where $\odot$ is the Hadamard product.

To obtain the fully sampled images, the root-sum-of-squares [29] reconstruction approach can be applied to the data in the spatial domain:

$$X = \left(\sum_{i=0}^{n_c} |x_i|^2 \right)^{1/2} \tag{1}$$

where X and n_c represent the reconstruction images from the fully sampled k-space data and the number of coils, respectively. We follow the same procedure for undersampled reconstruction.

In this work, we focus on mitigating the distribution gap between vendors through transfer learning where the objective is to enhance the model's performance on the target dataset by using existing knowledge from a source dataset for similar tasks. Pertaining to the definition, we assessed the impact of transfer learning techniques in the task of *accelerated reconstruction across different vendors*. We used multicoil T1-weighted phantom MRI data from SIEMENS and GE scanners as our two domains and analyzed the transfer in both directions. The architecture that we adopted for the task is represented as $VFN(k_{LR}; \theta)$, where k_{LR} denotes the undersampled kspace input to the network, and θ refers to the parameters of the network. We will refer to the source and target datasets as D_S and D_T. Following the same standard, we define θ_S and θ_T as VFN parameters trained on D_S and D_T, respectively. In the following sections, we briefly describe the base architecture for our task and the proposed feature transfer.

2.2   Base Architecture: Variational Feedback Network

We adopted VFN [4] (Fig. 1(c)) as the base architecture to conduct and evaluate the effectiveness of our proposed transfer learning strategy. VFN builds upon the End-to-End Variational Network (E2EVarNet) [2], which consists of multiple cascades modeled after a single gradient step. However, there are two fundamental differences between E2EVarNet and VFN architecture. The authors of VFN

[4] proposed modifying the U-Net architecture to consider two inputs instead of one to enable feedback connection in each cascade. Therefore, the gradient update step of each cascade becomes

$$x_{t+1} = x_t - \eta^t A^*(A(x_t) - \tilde{k}) + CNN(x_t, f_t) \tag{2}$$

where x_t and f_t denote the reconstruction and a high-level feature map extracted from the previous cascade (t, in this case). Only for the first cascade, f_t is *None*. $\tilde{k}$ is the subsampled kspace data, used to enforce data consistency in the frequency domain. The η^t values and parameters of the CNNs are learned from the data. A is the forward linear operator that multiplies the data (x_t) by the sensitivity maps (learnable), applies 2D Fourier transform, and then under-samples the data. A^* is the hermitian of the forward operator A. VFN also reuses the cascades multiple times, annotating it as "folds", and returning multiple reconstructions instead of one (as is in the case of [2]). The loss is averaged over the set of reconstructions predicted by the folds.

2.3 Proposed Feature Transfer Learning Architecture

We extend the transfer learning capability of VFN beyond existing transfer learning methods (i.e., weights finetuning) by selecting and adapting pretrained features that benefit reconstruction quality. Low-resolution k-space data is acquired by masking high-resolution k-space data. The subsampled data contains only $\frac{1}{K}$ of the frequency lines in raw data, affecting reconstruction quality for higher accelerations. To combat this problem, we propose refining the low-resolution data with high-level feature transfer from source domains for the same task of accelerated MRI reconstruction. Generally, any pretrained models' reconstruction (Fig. 3(b)) is capable of recovering high-frequency details partially when compared with zero-filled undersampled reconstruction (Fig. 3(i)). We reap the benefits of a source-pretrained model reconstruction and attention-based networks to select high-frequency details missing in the low-resolution data and refine it.

Let's assume we have a pre-trained network $VFN(.;\theta_S)$ trained on a source dataset D_S. We are also provided a target dataset D_T. We exploit the high-level features and reconstructions from $VFN(.;\theta_S)$ network to refine target tasks. To refine the undersampled data, we propose a feature extraction and refinement (FER) module described below in detail, followed by the details of the attention module $Att(.)$.

Feature Extraction and Refinement Module (FER). The proposed feature extraction module consists of a conventional U-Net (upper channel, Fig. 1) and a multilevel attentive U-Net network (bottom channel, Fig. 1). A traditional U-Net network was used to recognize transferable features from the pretrained reconstructions, denoted by FE_{PR}. For low-resolution (LR) feature refinement, we used a multilevel attentive U-Net structure that adapts the pretrained reconstructions' features and refines each instance's low-resolution features. This network is denoted by FR_{LR}.

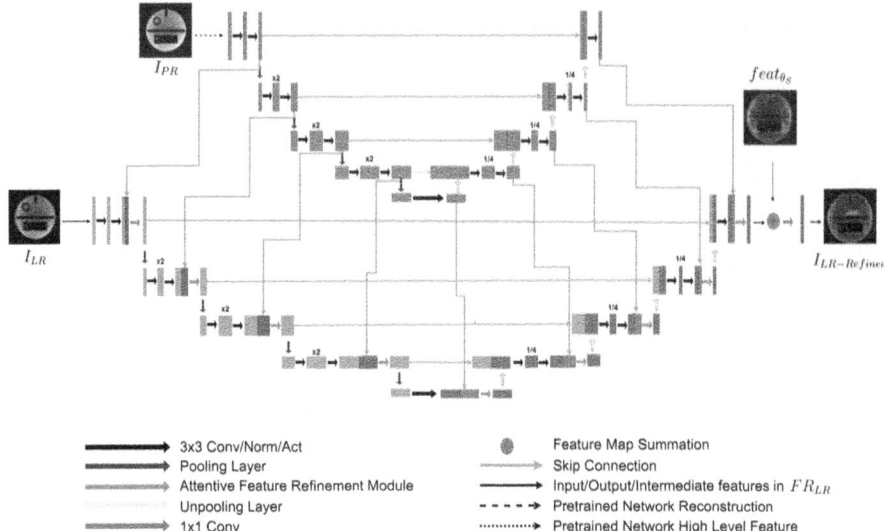

Fig. 1. Architecture illustration of the proposed $FER(.)$ module for refining low-resolution image data. The top U-Net channel is FE_{PR} for pretrained feature extraction, and the bottom attentive U-Net is FR_{LR} for undersampled feature refinement. Legends are provided in the figure. Best viewed in color.

This section provides an overview of the low-level feature refinement process in the proposed FER module at any depth L. FE_{PR} consists of an encoder and decoder architecture. The encoder is a series of *Conv-Conv-Pool* combinations where an instance normalization and leaky ReLU layer follow each convolution layer. The number of such combinations depends on the depth selected for each U-Net structure. In our method, we have chosen depth $D = 4$. The decoder is a series of *Unpool-Conv-Conv* modules with a skip connection from the encoder at the corresponding depth. The feature extracted from pretrained model reconstruction at depth L of FE_{PR} is defined as:

$$f_{PR}^{L} = Pooling(ConvBlock^{L}(f_{PR}^{L-1})) \tag{3}$$

Moving onto the encoding block architecture for FR_{LR} at depth L, the *Conv-Conv* block is identical to that of FE_{PR}, followed by a skip connection, the proposed attention module and finally, the pooling layer. This *Conv-Conv-Skip-Att* block can be formulated as:

$$f_{LR}^{L} = ConvBlock^{L}(f_{LR-Refined}^{L-1}) \tag{4}$$

$$f_{LR-Refined}^{L} = Pooling(Att(Skip(f_{LR}^{L}, f_{PR}^{L}))) \tag{5}$$

This process of extracting features and refining them using attention is repeated for every encoder and decoder depth. The combination of undersampled and pretrained reconstructions' features at multiple depths makes the attention modules pay different attention per channel and across all channel features. Inherently, it optimizes the contribution of transferable features from pretrained reconstructions.

The $FR_{LR}(.)$ output is concatenated with the high-level features extracted from the pre-trained model $VFN(.; \theta_S)$ and passed through the 1×1 convolution to provide a refined LR input feature. $feat_{\theta_S}$ is the high-level feature extracted from $VFN(.; \theta_S)$. We use the degraded image I_{LR} which can be derived from the undersampled k-space data k_{LR} from D_T, pretrained network reconstruction I_{HR}, and $feat_{\theta_S}$ create a refined feature vector $I_{LR-Refined}$. As opposed to existing VFN architecture, which takes in only I_{LR} as the input to the first cascade, we provide an additional input $I_{LR-Refined}$. Therefore, instead of $VFN(k_{LR})$ for cascade 1, we adapt it to $VFN(k_{LR}, I_{LR-Refined})$ for transferring features. The adapted VFN architecture is shown in Fig. 2. Please note

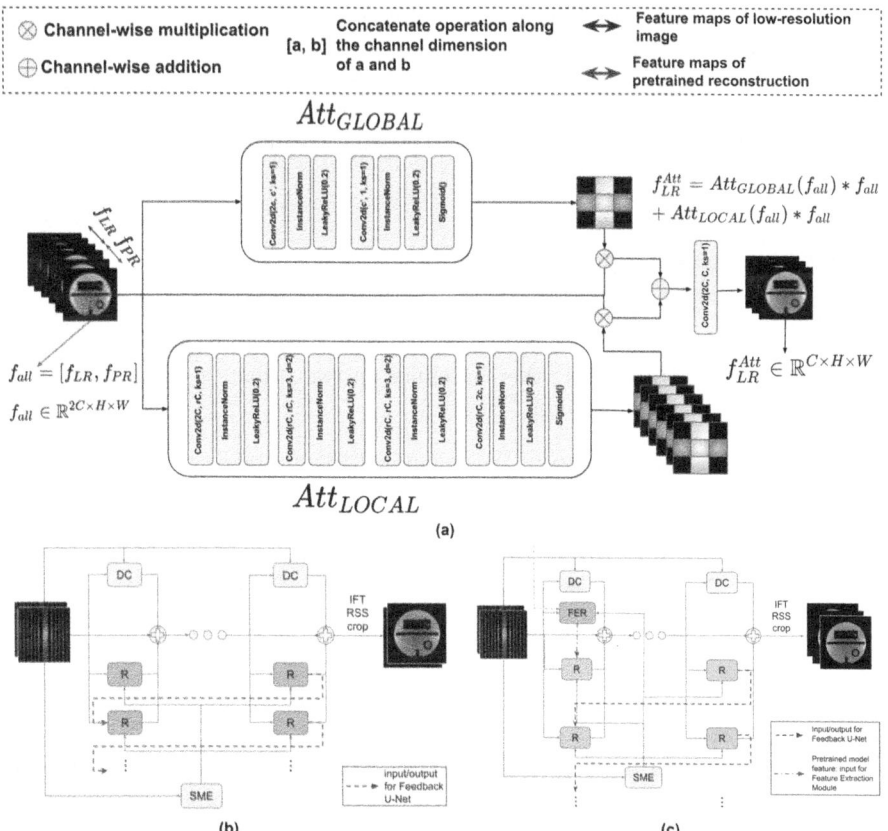

Fig. 2. Architecture illustration of **(a)** Proposed $Att(.)$ module for local and global attention in $FER(.)$. **(b)** $VFN(.)$ network of [4] and **(c)** $VFN - FT$ - integration of FER with $VFN(.)$. Legends are provided for each diagram separately. Best viewed in color.

that $I_{LR-Refined} = FER(I_{LR}, I_{HR}, feat_{\theta_S})$. Figure 1 represents the proposed FER module. The learning objective of the feature extraction and refinement module here is to filter relevant, high-level features from existing pre-trained network reconstructions to enhance the quality of the low-resolution data. The refined low-resolution data is an additional feature that helps converge faster and significantly enhances reconstruction quality in fewer training iterations. Integration of $VFN(.)$ with $FER(.)$ is refereed to as $VFN - FT(.)$.

Attention Module ($Att(.)$)

We now provide details about the attention module $Att(.)$ in Eq. 5. The proposed attention module is a convolutional network consisting of local and global attention branches. It accepts the concatenated (along channel dimension) feature maps of both the pretrained reconstruction and the low-resolution image as input to the local and global modules. The local attention network produces a heatmap for each channel of the input feature maps. It helps localize and highlight features per channel. We use a combination of conventional and dilated convolution layers, which helps capture neighboring and distant pixel characteristics and their relationships. In contrast, the global attention module produces a unified heatmap for all channels, which is applied over all the feature maps. Figure 1(b) depicts the proposed attention module architecture for feature refinement.

3   Experiments and Results

3.1   Datasets

We evaluate our method and other baselines on two private phantom datasets, which are listed as the following:

- **SIEMENS ACR Phantom**: We assembled 135 multicoil T1-weighted (slice thickness=5mm, TR=700 ms, TE=10 ms, FOV=250 × 250 mm^2) phantom samples (11 slices per sample, matrix resolution: 256 × 256) from the SIEMENS scanner.
- **GE ACR Phantom**: We assembled 135 multicoil T1-weighted phantom samples (slice thickness=5mm, 11 slices per sample, matrix resolution: 256 × 256, TR=700 ms, TE=10 ms, FOV=250 × 250 mm^2) from the GE scanner.

We divided the acquired data into training (100 volumes), validation (20 volumes), and evaluation (15 volumes) sets. To augment the available SIEMENS and GE datasets, we applied simple transformations (rotations), resulting in augmented datasets comprising 400 and 80 samples for training and validation, respectively. For both source and target datasets, we obtained 4x under-sampled data by applying equispaced masks to the original fully-sampled data, which was retrospectively down-sampled by four times.

Table 1. Comparison of parameters and training/inference time of proposed $VFN - FT(.)$ against $VFN(.)$.

Metrics	$VFN(\theta_T)$	$VFN - FT(\theta_T)$
Parameters	2.0 Million	3.3 Million
Average Time/Epoch	24 minutes	26 minutes
Training epochs (to converge)	50	40
Inference Time	1.2 secs/slice	1.2 secs/slice

The equispaced masks (Fig. 3(j)) included 8% of the k-space lines as fully sampled central region, known as the Auto Calibration Signal (ACS). We prefer to experiment on actual human data, but keeping the same acquisition standards across various vendors, let alone for a single patient or volunteer, is challenging. Collecting phantom data to eliminate variations in real patient data is sensible. Also, to control the interference of other factors in the data acquisition and generalization, we acquire all data with the same acquisition parameters in both SIEMENS and GE.

3.2 Training Protocol

We extend the Variational Feedback Network [4] with the proposed FER module. We use SSIM (Structural Similarity Index) [36] as the loss function. As there are T outputs for this network (with T folds), we define our loss function as $L(\{x^t\}_{t=1}^T, x^*) = 1 - \frac{1}{T}\sum_{t=1}^T SSIM(x^t, x^*)$, where $x^1, ..., x^T$ and x^* represent the reconstructions of the model and the ground truth, respectively. We use x^T as our final output. We use instance normalization [34] and leaky ReLU [18] for the normalization and activation layers. For the FER block, max pooling and bilinear interpolation are used for pooling and unpooling, and the number of channels of the features after the first convolution is set to 18. The depth of the block is 4 (i.e., there are 4 pooling layers and 4 unpooling layers).

The variational network uses two cascades and two folds (T=2). All networks are trained with batch size = 1 and initial learning rate as $3e^{-4}$, updated by $1e^{-1}$ every 40 epochs. Usually, in transfer learning, it is recommended to use a lower learning rate while finetuning. However, via our trials, we discovered that $3e^{-4}$ is a good choice for generalized performance during transfer learning. All networks are implemented using Pytorch 1.7 [21] with Python 3.8 on Ubuntu 20.04. A computer system with nVidia Tesla K40C and Intel(R) Xeon(R) E5-2630 CPU is used for the experiments. Due to hardware resource limitations, we had to restrict the batch size to 1. In Table 1, we compare the parameters, training, and inference time for $VFN(.)$ and $VFN - FT(.)$.

3.3 Vendor Transfer

In this section, we evaluate the generalization performance across different vendors' acquisitions. We conduct experiments on implicit transfer between SIEMENS and GE-acquired data by evaluating the test set on $VFN(\theta_{S_{aug}})$ and $VFN(\theta_T)$, where S_{aug} and T represent 400 and 100 volumes of SIEMENS and GE training data, respectively. Both networks are trained from scratch for 50 epochs. Results in Table 2 (Columns: $VFN(\theta_{S_{aug}})$, $VFN(\theta_T)$) indicate a challenge in generalization across SIEMENS and GE vendors. This difficulty is attributed to the distribution shift in the data acquired from the two vendors. Vendor differences are a major cause of the statistical shift, as different MRI scanners produce images of different characteristics related to manufacturer-specific MRI physics [19,37]. Deep learning models rely on data-driven statistical modeling, where differences in data distributions across vendors hinder generalization, leading to implicit transfer failure (Table 2) even with *structurally identical* data. Thus, training the network on data from the same vendor domain as the test is crucial for improving reconstruction quality, although acquiring a large dataset may not always be feasible.

We propose a feature transfer-learning approach for accelerated MRI to address the data scarcity problem and experiment with a 100-volume configuration of the target dataset, $D_T = \{100\}$. First, we consider the transfer from SIEMENS to GE vendor data. For evaluation purposes, we compare the following DNNs (deep neural networks):

- $VFN(\theta_T)$ **[Baseline]**: $VFN(.)$ trained on 100 volumes of GE ACR Phantom volumes (D_T).
- $VFN - PT(\theta_T)$ **[Baseline]**: $VFN(\theta_{S_{aug}})$ parameters fine-tuned with target samples D_T.
- $VFN - WS(\theta_T)$ [27] **[Baseline]**: Parameters of $FER(.,.,.)$ were initialized randomly. $VFN(.,.)$ parameters were initialized with *iid* weights from $N(\mu, \sigma^2)$, where μ and σ^2 are the mean and variance of the weights of $VFN(\theta_{S_{aug}})$ (per layer).
- $VFN - Transfusion(\theta_T)$ [27] **[Baseline]**: Only the lowest layers of the network are initialized with the weights of the pretrained network $VFN(\theta_{S_{aug}})$. In our case (cascades=2), pretrained weights were only initialized for the first cascade.
- $VFN - FT(\theta_T)$ **[Proposed]**: $VFN(\theta_{S_{aug}})$ is used as a pretrained feature extractor to refine undersampled data (using proposed attentive FER module) for target samples. Parameters of $FER(.,.,.)$ and $VFN(.,.)$ are initialized randomly.

All experiments are conducted for an acceleration factor of 4. Our experiments (Table 2) demonstrate that the proposed method successfully transfers information from source to target and significantly enhances the quality of the reconstructions. Figure 3 demonstrates the visual quality of test reconstruction across all networks. We successfully transferred from GE to the SIEMENS vendor to ensure that our results were not biased by selecting a specific MR vendor as the test set. We additionally note that, in the context of vendor transfer, the practice of scaling the pretrained weights ($VFN-WS$) or transferring a modified pretrained feature ($VFN-FT$) yields greater success compared to directly transferring the unaltered pretrained weights ($VFN - PT$ or $VFN - Transfusion$). This observation is reasonable, given that the performance of implicit transfer is subpar, suggesting a lack of compatibility between the datasets from the two vendors.

Table 2. Quantitative evaluation of transfer methods and base networks for transfer in both directions (SIEMENS to GE and vice-versa).

Test Dataset	Metrics	Base Networks			Transfer Learning			
		$VFN(\theta_{S_{aug}})$	$VFN(\theta_T)$	$VFN(\theta_{S_{aug}+T})$	$VFN-PT(\theta_T)$	$VFN-WS(\theta_T)$	$VFN-Transfusion(\theta_T)$	$VFN-FT(\theta_T)$
		Transfer from SIEMENS to GE: $D_{S_{aug}}$ = 400 SIEMENS, D_T = 100 GE						
GE	PSNR	35.7 +/- 13.05	43.73 +/- 15.6	44.16 +/- 13.06	42.61 +/- 13.76	42.88 +/- 14.98	40.43 +/- 16.16	**44.72 +/- 16.38**
	SSIM	0.9024 +/- 0.12	0.9718 +/- 0.06	0.9806 +/- 0.03	0.9631 +/- 0.08	0.9462 +/- 0.1118	0.9236 +/- 0.1495	**0.9893 +/- 0.09**
SIEMENS	PSNR	**42.2 +/- 15.67**	32.89 +/- 7.88	41.06 +/- 12.48	28.75 +/- 4.901	28.37 +/- 4.518	30.31 +/- 10.54	34.98 +/- 8.22
	SSIM	0.9588 +/- 0.07	0.863 +/- 0.15	**0.969 +/- 0.06**	0.8384 +/- 0.15	0.7971 +/- 0.1677	0.7995 +/- 0.2541	0.8801 +/- 0.16
		Transfer from GE to SIEMENS: $D_{S_{aug}}$ = 400 GE, D_T = 100 SIEMENS						
GE	PSNR	43.9 +/- 15.33	33.32 +/- 13.76	**44.15 +/- 14.81**	37.68 +/- 13.83	38.01 +/- 13.98	33.92 +/- 15.47	37.49 +/- 13.91
	SSIM	0.9718 +/- 0.06	0.8617 +/- 0.19	**0.9774 +/- 0.04**	0.9177 +/- 0.13	0.9208 +/- 0.1416	0.7915 +/- 0.279	0.884 +/- 0.19
SIEMENS	PSNR	32.63 +/- 6.95	38.69 +/- 9.96	40.22 +/- 12.14	41.22 +/- 15.31	41.76 +/- 16.5	40.12 +/- 15.29	**42.52 +/- 17.22**
	SSIM	0.8694 +/- 0.15	0.9525 +/- 0.08	0.9542 +/- 0.07	0.9549 +/- 0.10	0.9566 +/- 0.1079	0.9388 +/- 0.1346	**0.9573 +/- 0.08**

a Base GE $(VFN(\theta_T))$ 50.72/0.9955
b Base SIEMENS$(VFN(\theta_{S_{aug}}))$ 40.08/0.9594
c Base GE+SIEMENS $(VFN(\theta_{S_{aug}+T}))$ 49.91/0.9937
d VFN-PT$(VFN-PT(\theta_T))$ 49.02/0.9953
e Scaled-PT$(VFN-WS(\theta_T))$ 50.59/0.9926
f Transfusion$(VFN-Transfusion(\theta_T))$ 47.56/0.9803
g VFN-FT $(VFN-FT(\theta_T))$ 52.57/0.9962
h Fully sampled kspace
i Undersampled kspace
j Undersampling mask

Fig. 3. Vendor transfer from SIEMENS to GE. The sample-specific reconstruction quality is mentioned in the format of PSNR/SSIM. VFN-FT performs significantly better with high PSNR and SSIM. The proposed method can also predict the high-resolution details that seem blurred/smudged (indicated with magnified ROI) in other networks.

Impact of Pretrained Networks: To analyze the impact of a pretrained model during transfer learning, we train two source models, with $D_{S_{aug}}$ = 400 and D_S = 100, for SIEMENS and GE. During transfer learning to a different target dataset with D_T = 100, we observe that transferring from the augmented dataset ($D_{S_{aug}}$) trained pretrained models perform better (significantly for GE, marginally for SIEMENS). Since augmentation doesn't alter the distribution of the data, the results match the expectation. However, it does lead to the conclusion that a diverse pretraining dataset will lead to better transferability and, therefore, generalization.

Impact of Matrix Resolution: Our training datasets comprise samples with a resolution 256×256 and a field of view (FOV) of 250. To assess the performance of VFN across varying matrix sizes in the test dataset, we acquired test samples of different sizes (Table 3) with the same FOV. We evaluate the performance of a VFN trained on SIEMENS(/GE) data from scratch across all matrix sizes in the test dataset to mitigate the influence of other factors. Results reveal a significant performance deviation in the 128×128 test set compared to the 256×256 test set. Diversity in the matrix size of acquired data with static FOV impacts pixel size. Additionally, 4x undersampling on smaller matrix sizes reduces the ACS lines, further impacting generalization. Regardless of vendor, Table 3 indicates performance degradation across different matrix sizes.

3.4   Learning Without Forgetting in Accelerated MRI

The reconstruction quality of transfer learning networks dropped significantly while reconstructing the source test dataset (Table 2) due to catastrophic forgetting. To create a generalizable model, we need access to ample multi-vendor data which is challenging due to patient privacy and annotation costs. Therefore, in this section, we explore the possibility of developing a single network that can generalize across test samples from different vendors. Experience replay [28] is one of the most prominent and successful techniques to solve the problems associated with transfer learning. In this work, we adopt the strategy of vanilla experience replay by randomly sampling N source(SIEMENS) training samples to be used along with M target(GE) training samples($N << M$). **Please note that we only use the reconstructed output (from pre-trained networks) as our ground truth for the source samples in the replay buffer during training.**

Table 3. $VFN(\theta_S)$ is trained on 100 T1 siemens/ge ACR samples, all of matrix size 256×256. The test sets have been separated according to the matrix size. Each column header denotes the matrix size of the corresponding test set.

Test Dataset	Metrics	Transfer from SIEMENS to GE: $D_{S_{aug}} = 400$ SIEMENS, $D_T = 100$ GE	
		Pretrain: $VFN(\theta_{S_{aug}})$ $VFN - FT(\theta_T)$	Pretrain: $VFN(\theta_S)$ $VFN - FT(\theta_T)$
GE	PSNR	44.72 +/- 16.38	43.89 +/- 16.63
	SSIM	0.9893 +/- 0.09	0.9789 +/- 0.08
		Transfer from GE to SIEMENS: $D_{S_{aug}} = 400$ GE, $D_T = 100$ SIEMENS	
		Pretrain: $VFN(\theta_{S_{aug}})$ $VFN - FT(\theta_T)$	Pretrain: $VFN(\theta_S)$ $VFN - FT(\theta_T)$
SIEMENS	PSNR	42.52 +/- 17.22	42.49 +/- 17.08
	SSIM	0.9573 +/- 0.08	0.9562 +/- 0.08

Let each dataset have a universal label, Y_i, assigned to it that recognizes the task/dataset. It further implies that $\forall x \in D_i$, label=Y_i. Let us denote λ_S and λ_T as the weight for losses encountered due to replay buffer (source) and target samples, respectively.

$$L_{Total} = \lambda_S * L(\{x_i^t\}_{t=1}^T, x_i').\mathbb{I}_{y_i \in Y_S} + \lambda_T * L(\{x_i^t\}_{t=1}^T, x_i^*).\mathbb{I}_{y_i \in Y_T} \qquad (6)$$

Table 4. Impact of pretrained networks on feature transfer learning. $VFN(\theta_S)$ is trained on a source dataset $D_S = 100$ samples of siemens/ge.

Network	Metrics	128×128	256×256	512×512
SIEMENS - $VFN(\theta_S)$	PSNR	31.92 +/- 0.23	42.48 +/- 0.51	41.646 +/- 0.69
	SSIM	0.8994 +/- 0.01	0.9912 +/- 0.00	0.9667 +/- 0.00
GE - $VFN(\theta_S)$	PSNR	34.13 +/- 0.23	47.61 +/- 3.21	-
	SSIM	0.9335 +/- 0.01	0.9914 +/- 0.00	-

where x_i', x_i^* and x_i^t represent the pretrained reconstruction for replay buffer samples, the ground truth reconstruction for the target samples and predicted reconstruction, respectively.

For evaluation, we compare the following network configurations: 1) $VFN(\theta_{T100})$: VFN trained on 100 GE T1 Phantom samples from scratch, 2)$VFN(\theta_{S10+T100})$: VFN trained on 10 SIEMENS T1 (with ground truth) and 100 GE T1 Phantom samples from scratch, 3) $VFN(\theta_{S400+T100})$: VFN trained on 400 SIEMENS T1 (with ground truth) and 100 GE T1 Phantom samples from scratch, 4)$VFN - FT(\theta_{T100})$: $VFN(\theta_{S400})$ fine-tuned with 100 GE T1 Phantom samples using proposed algorithm and 5) $VFN - FT(\theta_{S10+T100})$: $VFN(\theta_{S400})$ fine-tuned with $10(N)$ SIEMENS T1 (with pretrained network $VFN(\theta_{S400})$ reconstructions as the ground truth) and $100(M)$ GE T1 Phantom samples using the proposed algorithm. $VFN - FT(\theta_{S10+T100})$ is trained with Eq. 6 as the training objective. Table 5 summarizes the evaluation metrics for the networks listed above. A comparison of the different settings reveals certain behaviors, summarized as follows:

- **Networks trained on compound datasets may yield sub-optimal performance**: To evaluate the performance of transfer learning with memory replay, we compare its performance against $VFN(\theta_{S10+T100})$ and $VFN(\theta_{S400+T100})$. Results indicate that the reconstruction quality of $VFN - FT(\theta_{S10+T100})$ is significantly better than both baselines due to the presence of pretrained knowledge and our proposed feature extraction and refinement module. It provides the flexibility to adapt the pretrained features in order to optimize performance.
- **Vanilla Experience Replay is a strong baseline for accelerated MRI reconstruction**: To evaluate the quantity of degradation, we propose the performance drop as a metric for this work, which is given by: $\frac{Metric(x_i)-Metric(x_j)}{Metric(x_i)} * 100\%$, where $Metric$ is PSNR/SSIM and x_i, x_j represent the reconstructions of network snapshots after task i, j. For $VFN - FT(\theta_{S10+T100})$, the SSIM and PSNR performance drop (SIEMENS) are 0.2% and 4.35%, respectively. For $VFN - FT(\theta_{T100})$ (no experience replay), the PSNR and SSIM performance drop are 29.9% and 9.75%. Both are compared against $VFN(\theta_{S400+T100})$. Clearly, $VFN - FT(\theta_{S10+T100})$ mitigates the for-

getting significantly with a strictly limited capacity ($N = 10$) for pretrained source reconstructions as samples. Due to space constraints, we are unable to include further visualizations.

- **Significance of λ_S**: Usage of a lower λ_S allows the network to learn the target dataset more effectively and control the interference caused by the source samples. $\lambda_S = 1.0$ is optimal for the combined test dataset. It outperforms both $VFN(\theta_{T100})$ and $VFN(\theta_{S10+T100})$ in that case. The results are shared in Table 5.

Table 5. Quantitative analysis of transfer learning with limited source samples (experience replay). Usage of a lower λ_S reduces the effect of the source samples on the learned weights and allows the network to learn the target dataset more efficiently. $\lambda_T = 1.0$ for all the transfer learning networks.

Test Dataset	Metrics	Baselines			TL w/o Source	TL w Source		
						$VFN-FT(\theta_{S10+T100})$		
		$VFN(\theta_{T100})$	$VFN(\theta_{S10+T100})$	$VFN(\theta_{S400+T100})$	$VFN-FT(\theta_{T100})$	$\lambda_S = 1.0$	$\lambda_S = 0.1$	$\lambda_S = 0.01$
GE	PSNR	47.61 +/- 3.24	47.32 +/- 3.69	46.76 +/- 3.06	49.61 +/- 3.58	49.88 +/- 3.16	**49.99 +/- 3.56**	49.93 +/- 3.49
	SSIM	0.9914 +/- 0.00	0.9915 +/- 0.00	0.9911 +/- 0.03	0.9942 +/- 0.03	0.9946 +/- 0.003	0.9952 +/- 0.009	**0.9961 +/- 0.01**
SIEMENS	PSNR	33.07 +/- 0.47	43.16 +/- 0.55	**48.32 +/- 0.51**	35.67 +/- 0.44	48.08 +/- 0.53	45.14 +/- 0.45	41.85 +/- 0.36
	SSIM	0.8746 +/- 0.00	0.9899 +/- 0.00	**0.9960 +/- 0.00**	0.9006 +/- 0.00	0.9957 +/- 0.00	0.9941 +/- 0.00	0.9882 +/- 0.0
GE+SIEMENS	PSNR	40.34 +/- 7.96	45.18 +/- 3.56	47.04 +/- 2.04	42.63 +/- 7.73	**49.23 +/- 2.24**	47.35 +/- 3.34	45.49 +/- 4.48
	SSIM	0.9440 +/- 0.06	0.9907 +/- 0.00	0.9936 +/- 0.00	0.9474 +/- 0.05	**0.9957 +/- 0.00**	0.9924 +/- 0.01	0.9932 +/- 0.01

3.5   Further Discussion

Our experiments revealed that, while vendor difference is a challenge in MRI reconstruction tasks, the problem may be mitigated by the proposed feature transfer method, which surpasses standard fine-tuning mechanisms' performance visually and quantitatively. We also found that the diversity and quantity of the pretraining dataset are important factors affecting knowledge transfer and, eventually, reconstruction quality. Furthermore, transfer learning with limited source (experience replay) is a better alternative to training with compound datasets. The training protocol we have established for experience replay does not violate the privacy concerns of sensitive data (since we use predictions as pseudo-ground truth during training) and maintains decent performance on combined test data of both vendors.

4   Conclusion

In this work, we present insight into the generalization ability of a learned variational feedback network for MR image reconstruction concerning deviations in the vendors. We demonstrated successful vendor transfer with our proposed algorithm. We also tackle the continual accelerated MRI reconstruction problem using experience replay. Our experiments show that experience-replay-based learning significantly improves the performance of older test datasets over the baselines. Incorporating diffusion-based networks and leveraging their generalization capacity is a future direction for this work. The sequential transformation process in diffusion models may provide the opportunity to handle even multiple undersampling in a single network.

References

1. AlBadawy, E.A., Saha, A., Mazurowski, M.A.: Deep learning for segmentation of brain tumors: impact of cross-institutional training and testing. Med. Phys. **45**(3), 1150–1158 (2018)
2. Chen, E.Z., Chen, T., Sun, S.: MRI image reconstruction via learning optimization using neural odes. arXiv preprint arXiv:2006.13825 (2020)
3. Ding, P.L.K., Li, B., Chang, K.: Convex dictionary learning for single image super-resolution. In: 2017 IEEE International Conference on Image Processing (ICIP), pp. 4058–4062 (2017). https://doi.org/10.1109/ICIP.2017.8297045
4. Ding, P.L.K., Paul, R., Patel, A., Zhou, Y., Li, B.: Variational feedback network for accelerated MRI reconstruction. ISMRM & SMRT Annual Meeting & Exhibition (2021). https://doi.org/10.13140/RG.2.2.26769.10087
5. Donoho, D.L.: Compressed sensing. IEEE Trans. Inf. Theory **52**(4), 1289–1306 (2006)
6. Ellis, R.: Leveraging Large Scale Data Sets: a Transfer Learning Approach for 7T Super Resolution. University of California, San Francisco (2021)
7. Finn, C., Abbeel, P., Levine, S.: Model-agnostic meta-learning for fast adaptation of deep networks. In: International Conference on Machine Learning, pp. 1126–1135. PMLR (2017)
8. Geirhos, R., Rubisch, P., Michaelis, C., Bethge, M., Wichmann, F.A., Brendel, W.: Imagenet-trained CNNs are biased towards texture; increasing shape bias improves accuracy and robustness. arXiv preprint arXiv:1811.12231 (2018)
9. Griswold, M.A., et al.: Generalized autocalibrating partially parallel acquisitions (grappa). Mag. Reson. Med. Official J. Int. Soc. Magn. Reson. Med. **47**(6), 1202–1210 (2002)
10. Hammernik, K., Klatzer, T., Kobler, E., Recht, M.P., Sodickson, D.K., Pock, T., Knoll, F.: Learning a variational network for reconstruction of accelerated MRI data. Magn. Reson. Med. **79**(6), 3055–3071 (2018)
11. He, K., Girshick, R., Dollár, P.: Rethinking ImageNet pre-training. In: Proceedings of the IEEE/CVF International Conference on Computer Vision, pp. 4918–4927 (2019)
12. Huh, M., Agrawal, P., Efros, A.A.: What makes ImageNet good for transfer learning? arXiv preprint arXiv:1608.08614 (2016)
13. Kolesnikov, A., et al.: Large scale learning of general visual representations for transfer. **2**(8) (2019). arXiv preprint arXiv:1912.11370
14. Kornblith, S., Shlens, J., Le, Q.V.: Do better ImageNet models transfer better? In: Proceedings of the IEEE/CVF Conference on Computer Vision and Pattern Recognition, pp. 2661–2671 (2019)
15. Kwon, K., Kim, D., Park, H.: A parallel MR imaging method using multilayer perceptron. Med. Phys. **44**(12), 6209–6224 (2017)
16. Liang, D., Cheng, J., Ke, Z., Ying, L.: Deep MRI reconstruction: unrolled optimization algorithms meet neural networks. arXiv preprint arXiv:1907.11711 (2019)

17. Lustig, M., Donoho, D.L., Santos, J.M., Pauly, J.M.: Compressed sensing MRI. IEEE Signal Process. Mag. **25**(2), 72–82 (2008)
18. Maas, A.L., Hannun, A.Y., Ng, A.Y.: Rectifier nonlinearities improve neural network acoustic models. In: Proceedings of ICML, vol. 30, p. 3 (2013)
19. Muckley, M.J., et al.: Results of the 2020 fastMRI challenge for machine learning MR image reconstruction. IEEE Trans. Med. Imaging **40**(9), 2306–2317 (2021)
20. Ngiam, J., Peng, D., Vasudevan, V., Kornblith, S., Le, Q.V., Pang, R.: Domain adaptive transfer learning with specialist models. arXiv preprint arXiv:1811.07056 (2018)
21. Paszke, A., et al.: Automatic differentiation in PyTorch (2017)
22. Pooch, E.H., Ballester, P.L., Barros, R.C.: Can we trust deep learning models diagnosis? The impact of domain shift in chest radiograph classification. arXiv preprint arXiv:1909.01940 (2019)
23. Pruessmann, K.P., Weiger, M., Scheidegger, M.B., Boesiger, P.: Sense: sensitivity encoding for fast MRI. Mag. Reson. Med. Official J. Int. Soc. Magn. Reson. Med. **42**(5), 952–962 (1999)
24. Putzky, P., et al.: i-rim applied to the fastMRI challenge. arXiv preprint arXiv:1910.08952 (2019)
25. Putzky, P., Welling, M.: Invert to learn to invert. In: Advances in Neural Information Processing Systems, vol. 32 (2019)
26. Raghu, A., Raghu, M., Bengio, S., Vinyals, O.: Rapid learning or feature reuse? Towards understanding the effectiveness of MAML. arXiv preprint arXiv:1909.09157 (2019)
27. Raghu, M., Zhang, C., Kleinberg, J., Bengio, S.: TransFusion: understanding transfer learning for medical imaging. In: Advances in Neural Information Processing Systems, vol. 32 (2019)
28. Robins, A.: Catastrophic forgetting, rehearsal and pseudorehearsal. Connect. Sci. **7**(2), 123–146 (1995)
29. Roemer, P.B., Edelstein, W.A., Hayes, C.E., Souza, S.P., Mueller, O.M.: The NMR phased array. Magn. Reson. Med. **16**(2), 192–225 (1990)
30. Schlemper, J., Caballero, J., Hajnal, J.V., Price, A., Rueckert, D.: A deep cascade of convolutional neural networks for MR image reconstruction. In: Niethammer, M., et al. (eds.) IPMI 2017. LNCS, vol. 10265, pp. 647–658. Springer, Cham (2017). https://doi.org/10.1007/978-3-319-59050-9_51
31. Shin, P.J., et al.: Calibrationless parallel imaging reconstruction based on structured low-rank matrix completion. Magn. Reson. Med. **72**(4), 959–970 (2014)
32. Sodickson, D.K., Manning, W.J.: Simultaneous acquisition of spatial harmonics (SMASH): fast imaging with radiofrequency coil arrays. Magn. Reson. Med. **38**(4), 591–603 (1997)
33. Sriram, A., et al.: End-to-end variational networks for accelerated MRI reconstruction. In: Martel, A.L., et al. (eds.) MICCAI 2020. LNCS, vol. 12262, pp. 64–73. Springer, Cham (2020). https://doi.org/10.1007/978-3-030-59713-9_7
34. Ulyanov, D., Vedaldi, A., Lempitsky, V.: Instance normalization: the missing ingredient for fast stylization. arXiv preprint arXiv:1607.08022 (2016)
35. Wang, S., et al.: Accelerating magnetic resonance imaging via deep learning. In: Biomedical Imaging (ISBI), 2016 IEEE 13th International Symposium on, pp. 514–517. IEEE (2016)
36. Wang, Z., Simoncelli, E.P., Bovik, A.C.: Multiscale structural similarity for image quality assessment. In: The Thrity-Seventh Asilomar Conference on Signals, Systems & Computers, 2003, vol. 2, pp. 1398–1402. IEEE (2003)

37. Yan, W., et al.: The domain shift problem of medical image segmentation and vendor-adaptation by Unet-GAN. In: Shen, D., et al. (eds.) MICCAI 2019. LNCS, vol. 11765, pp. 623–631. Springer, Cham (2019). https://doi.org/10.1007/978-3-030-32245-8_69

38. Yosinski, J., Clune, J., Bengio, Y., Lipson, H.: How transferable are features in deep neural networks? In: Advances in Neural Information Processing Systems, vol. 27 (2014)

CVD_Net: Head and Neck Tumor Segmentation and Generalization in PET/CT Scans Across Data from Multiple Medical Centers

Nchongmaje Ndipenoch[1]([✉]), Alina Miron[1], Kezhi Wang[1], Zhan Shu[2], and Yongmin Li[1]

[1] Department of Computer Science, Brunel University London, Uxbridge, UK
Mcndipenoch@hotmail.com
[2] Department of Electrical and Computer Engineering, University of Alberta Edmonton, Edmonton, Canada

Abstract. Accurate diagnosis, analysis, and monitoring of the progress of head and neck squamous cell carcinoma (HNSCC) or tumors using Positron Emission Tomography (PET) and Computed Tomography (CT) is paramount for radiation therapy treatment plans. Deep learning methods have shown promising performances in segmenting HNSCC, but most of the methods are trained and tested on homogeneous datasets (data from the same source), leading to a degradation of performance when tested on independent datasets from different sources, as in real-world scenarios. One of the main causes of the poor generalizability is the variability in the quality of scans from diverse sources. In this work, we propose a novel algorithm, CVD_Net, which is a combination of Convolutional Neural Networks for feature extraction, Vision Transformers to capture long-range dependencies, and domain-specific adapters to mitigate the problem of negative knowledge transfer. The CVD_Net was evaluated on the HECKTOR 2022 dataset collected from nine medical centers around the world, obtaining a mean Dice Score of 0.77492 (comparable to performances from specifically designed state-of-the-art algorithms) when tested on a hidden dataset from three medical centers, two of which are new (not seen during training). Furthermore, the algorithm also demonstrated high generalizability performance when tested on independent data from a new medical center.

Keywords: Segmentation · Transfer learning · Deep Learning · Convolutional neural network · Vision transformers · Domain specific adapters · Head and Neck tumor

1 Introduction

Head and Neck (H&N) cancer is one of the most common worldwide and the fifth leading cause of death globally [15], accounting for 4% of all cancer deaths in the USA [35]. The head and neck squamous cell carcinoma (HNSCC) are the most common form of H&N cancers, typically originating in the squamous cells lining the mucosal surfaces of the mouth, throat, and voice box. Although head and neck cancers can also develop in the salivary glands, sinuses, or muscles and nerves in the head and

© The Author(s), under exclusive license to Springer Nature Switzerland AG 2024
X. Xie et al. (Eds.): AIiH 2024, LNCS 14976, pp. 64–76, 2024.
https://doi.org/10.1007/978-3-031-67285-9_5

neck, these types of cancer are much less prevalent than squamous cell carcinomas [12,36].

Effective treatment plans for H&N cancers exist in the form of surgery, radiation therapy, chemotherapy, targeted therapy, immunotherapy, or a combination of these treatments. However, the effectiveness of these treatments depends on frequent monitoring and early detection of the disease. Additionally, the treatments are expensive and involve regular administration of injections over a prolonged period of time, thereby imposing a socioeconomic burden on patients and the healthcare system.

Detecting, monitoring, and analyzing H&N cancerous cells can be achieved through PET and CT imaging, which provide a cross-sectional, noninvasive, and high-resolution 3D image of the head and neck. Developing an automated tool to assist doctors in analyzing, monitoring, and detecting this disease using PET/CT images is paramount. Deep Learning (DL) methods have shown success in segmenting H&N cancer tumors, but demonstrate poor generalizability performance when tested on data from different medical centers. The scans are multimodal, taken from different medical centers by radiologists with varying expertise using different devices. Consequently, the acquired image quality and scan density can vary widely between different medical centers. Moreover, the quality of annotated images varies depending on the expertise of the annotator.

The two most popular approaches used in DL are based on Convolutional Neural Network (CNN) and Vision Transformer (ViT) [16]. The latter will outperform the former when trained on a very large dataset because ViTs are more data-hungry than CNNs due to their ability to model long-range dependencies, as explained in [16]. In this work, we aim to address the problem of generalizability of H&N tumor segmentation in PET/CT images across variations in data sources by combining CNN, ViT, and Domain-Specific Adapters (DSA) [7].

In this work, we combine CNN, ViT, and DSA to propose a novel algorithm called CVD_Net (Convolutional Neural Network and Vision Transformer with Domain-Specific Batch Normalization) to address the problem of head and neck tumor segmentation from PET/CT images.[1] The rest of the paper is organized as follows. Section 2 provides a brief review of previous studies. Section 3 presents the method and its main components. The experimental results, generalizability, comparisons with SOTA algorithms and visualisation are presented in Sect. 4. Finally, Sect. 5 outlines the conclusion, with our contributions, limitations and future work.

2 Background

The segmentation of medical images has been prevalent for many years. Some of the recent deep learning methods are reviewed in the following. The nnUNet_RASPP [31], a variant of nnUNet [21,25,26], is introduced for retinal Optical Coherence Tomography (OCT) fluid detection, segmentation, and generalisation across variations of data sources. This algorithm extends nnUNet by incorporating residual connections and Atrous Spatial Pyramid Pooling (ASPP) blocks into the network's backbone for the segmentation of three retinal fluids. The Deep_ResUNet++ model is

---

[1] Our code is available at: https://github.com/ndipenoch/CVD-Net.

introduced in [32] for the simultaneous segmentation of layers and fluids in reti-nal OCT images. The algorithm incorporates an atrous spatial pyramid pooling block, squeeze-and-excite block, residual connections, and dense layer into the U-Net architecture. This model simultaneously segments four retinal layers and three fluids from the Annotated Retinal OCT Images (AROI) database [27], achieving a mean Dice score above 0.90 for each segment. The CoNet (Coherent Network) is introduced in [30] for retinal image segmentation of small datasets. This algorithm integrates atrous spatial pyramid pooling into the U-Net architecture to simultane-ously segment seven retinal layers and one fluid class. The model is evaluated on the Duke DME dataset [11], which comprises of 110 B-scans from 10 patients suf-fering from Diabetic Macular Edema (DME), achieving a mean Dice score of 0.88. The CoTr (CNN-Transformer) model is introduced in [39] for the segmentation of 3D medical images. The authors combined CNN and Transformer architectures to segment eleven abdominal organs from CT scans. The method is evaluated on the Synapse dataset [1]. Experimental results demonstrate that the algorithm achieves performance comparable to SOTA algorithms.

The Segment Anything Model (SAM), a foundational model developed by researchers at Meta, is introduced in [22]. Inspired by the concept of strong zero-shot and few-shot generalisation [5] from the natural language processing (NLP) com-munity, the authors trained the model on 1 billion masks and 11 million images of diverse objects using vision Transformers [6,10], aiming to generalize to new tasks and data distributions beyond those seen during training. MA-SAM, a variant of SAM tailored for 3D medical image segmentation, is presented in [9]. While SAM is built for the segmentation of 2D images, MA-SAM integrates the crucial third dimen-sion into the network's architecture for the segmentation of 3D medical images. The algorithm is validated on four medical image segmentation tasks across 10 public datasets, including CT, MRI, and surgical video data.

The automatic segmentation of head and neck tumors and nodal metastases in PET-CT scans is presented in [4]. The authors combined NiftyNet [17] and 3D V-Net [28], using U-Net [34] as the backbone. The method consists of four downsampling blocks for compression, four upsampling blocks for decompression, and one final prediction residual convolutional block. In both the upsampling and downsampling paths, the convolutional filters were set to $2 \times 2 \times 2$ with a stride of 2, ReLU activations, and final softmax activation. The algorithm was evaluated on the Head-Neck-PET-CT dataset [37] from the Cancer Imaging Archive (TCIA) [13].

The segmentation of gross tumor volume for head and neck cancer radiother-apy using a deep dense multimodality network is introduced in [18]. The method employs DenseNet [19] as the backbone, consisting of forty-nine convolution layers. The algorithm was evaluated on the Head-Neck-PET-CT dataset [37], which was split into training (140 patients), validation (35 patients), and testing (75 patients) sets. It achieved a mean Dice score of 0.73.

The second edition of the HEad and neCK TumOR (HECKTOR) challenge is pre-sented in [3]. The first task of the challenge involves the automatic segmentation of Head and Neck primary Gross Tumor Volume (GTVt) in PET/CT images. The offline version of the challenge attracted 103 teams, resulting in 448 submissions. Here, we review some of the methods used by the top teams in the first task of this challenge.

Team Pengy secured the first position, achieving a mean Dice score of 0.778. They utilized nnUNet [21], a self-configuring pipeline for medical image segmentation. SJTU [2] ranked second with a mean Dice score of 0.7733. Their method employed ResUNet [14] as a backbone, comprising three parts: the first part for extracting the region of interest (ROI), the second part for training a model based on the ROI, and the third part for refining the trained model. HiLab [24] presented an ensemble of five deep learning methods and an attention mechanism, achieving a mean Dice score of 0.773. BCIOqurit [40] extended nnUNet [21] by incorporating squeeze and excitation normalization [20] into the algorithm backbone, achieving a mean Dice score of 0.7709. Another nnUNet based method was presented by team Aarhus Oslo [33], achieving a mean Dice score of 0.779. Team Aarhus Oslo obtained the best DS but also had a high rate of missing predictions on one or multiple patients, hence it was ranked fifth by the organizers. The Fuller MDA [33] introduced an ensemble of 3D residual U-Nets trained on a 10-fold cross-validation and majority voting, obtaining a mean dice score of 0.7702.

3 Method

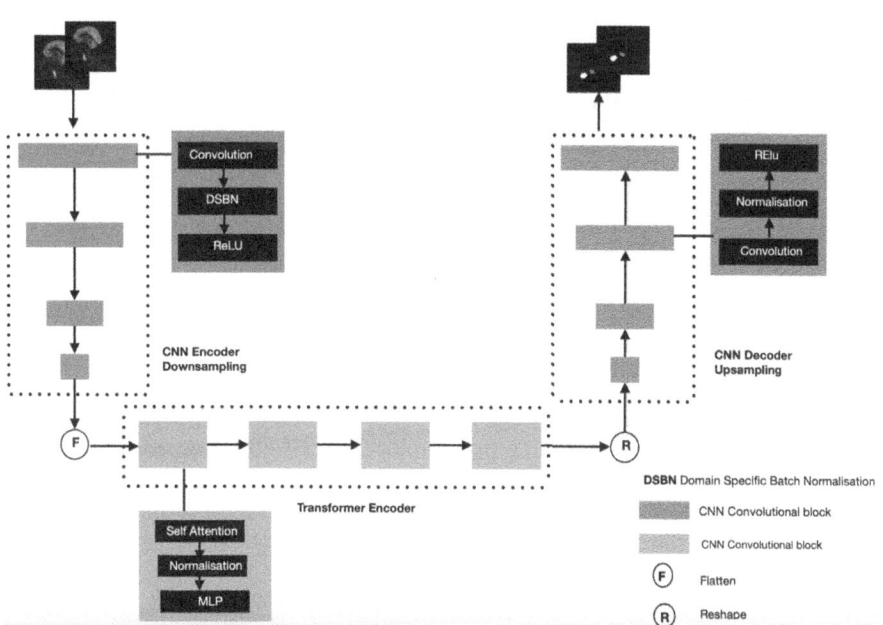

Fig. 1. A high-level illustration of the CVD_Net architecture. The convolutional blocks at the CNN encoder for feature map extraction are shown in gray, those at the CNN decoder for upsampling in green, and the Transformer blocks to capture long-range dependencies at the encoder in yellow. F stands for flattening the maps before feeding into the Transformer encoder, and R stands for reshaping the maps before feeding into the CNN decoder. (Color figure online)

CVD_Net is composed of four main components: a CNN encoder, a domain-specific batch normalization, a Transformer encoder, and a CNN decoder as demonstrated in Fig. 1. Details of these components are as follows.

3.1 CNN Encoder

The CNN Encoder is used to extract features from the input images and it is composed of three convolutional blocks in series with residual connections. Each of the block is followed by a batch normalization and and Rectified Linear Unit (ReLU) activation. Given a raw image $X \in \mathbb{R}^{H \times W \times D}$ whose spatial resolution is H × W and the depth (number of slices) D. The feature maps produced by the CNN Encoder (F_CNN) can be formally expressed as :

$$\{f\}L_{l=1} = F^l_{CNN}(x; \Theta) \in \mathbb{R}^{C \times D \times \frac{2}{l} \times H \times \frac{2}{l+1} \times W \times \frac{2}{l+1}} \tag{1}$$

where $\{f\}L_{l=1}$ is the feature map produced by the CNN Encoder, x is the input image, L indicates the number of feature levels, Θ denotes the parameters of the CNN encoder, and C denotes the number of channels.

3.2 Domain-Specific Batch Normalization (DSBN)

The DSBN [8] is the batch normalization technique used at every convolutional block within the CNN encoder to capture domain-specific information. The DSBN consists of several batch normalization layers, each reserved for a specific domain.

3.3 Transfomer Encoder

The Transformer encoder is used to capture long-range dependencies from the extracted features. It is composed of an input-to-sequence layer and stacked deformable Transformer layers. The extracted features from the CNN encoder are flattened into a 1D vector before being fed into the Transformer encoder. Due to this, they lose some spatial information. To mitigate this problem, we employ sine and cosine functions with different frequencies [38] to compute the positional coordinates of each dimension. The Transformer encoder consists of transformer blocks stacked in series. Each transformer block employs the self-attention mechanism [41] to capture long-range dependencies by computing the weighted sum of the input data based on the similarity between the input features. The self-attention mechanism generates a trainable associative memory with a query (Q) and a pair of key (K)-value (V) pairs to produce an output by linearly transforming the input. This is represented as follows:

$$\text{Attention}(Q, K, V) = \text{Softmax}\left(\frac{QK^T}{\sqrt{d}}\right) V \tag{2}$$

where $\sqrt{d}$ is a scaling factor based on the depth of the network. The output is normalized and fed through a feed-forward multi-layer perceptron (MLP). Skip connections are employed to avoid the vanishing gradient problem.

3.4   CNN Decoder

The output of the transformer encoder is fed to a CNN decoder. The CNN decoder progressively upsamples the feature map through a series of convolutional blocks consisting of a convolutional layer, normalization layer, and a ReLU activation using residual connections. At the end of the decoder path is a classification layer for pixel classification. Assuming there are k classes, including the background, the classification layer predicts k semantic masks. $\hat{S}_l \in \mathbb{R}^{h \times w \times k}$ simultaneously, corresponding to each semantic label as demonstrated on Eqn (3)

$$\hat{S} = argmax(Softmax(\hat{S}_l, d = -1), d = -1) \tag{3}$$

where $d = -1$ indicates the Softmax and argmax operations performed across the last dimension (the channel dimension). The loss functions is the sum of the cross entropy and Dice loss which is express as follows :

$$L = \lambda_1 CE(\hat{S}, D(S)) + \lambda_2 Dice(\hat{S}, D(S)) \tag{4}$$

where CE and Dice represents cross entropy loss and Dice loss, respectively. D denotes as the downsample operation. λ_1 and λ_2 represent the loss weights.

4   Experiments

4.1   Dataset

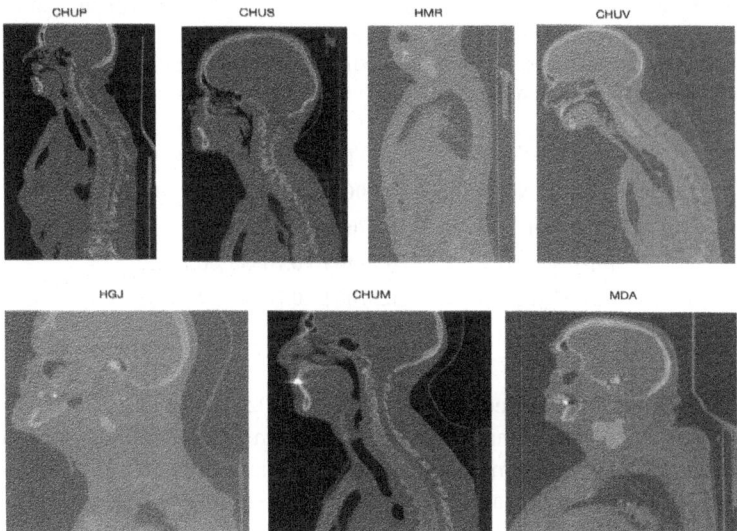

Fig. 2. An example of a sagittal plane taken from each of the eight medical centers in the training dataset highlighting the high variability in the image quality of the dataset. The GTVp is marked in red, and the GTVn is marked in green (Color figure online)

Table 1. The HECKTOR 2022 dataset [3] consists of 883 cases (524 for training and 359 for testing) collected from 9 medical centers using 12 different scanners across 4 different countries. The test dataset was collected from 3 different vendor machines, of which 2 were not used in the training set.

Center	Acronym	Scanners	Training Cases	Testing Cases (Hidden)
Hôpital général juif, Montréal, Canada	HGJ	Discovery ST GE Healthcare	55	None
Centre hospitalier universitaire de Sherbooke, Sherbrooke, Canada	CHUS	GeminiGXL 16 Philips	72	None
Hôpital Maisonneuve-Rosemont, Montréal, Canada	HMR	Discovery STE GE Healthcare	18	None
Centre hospitalier de l'Université de Montréal, Montréal, Canada	CHUM	Discovery STE, GE Healthcare	56	None
Centre Hospitalier Universitaire Vaudois, Switzerland	CHUV	Discovery D690 TOF GE Healthcare	53	None
UniversitätsSpital Zürich, Switzerland	USZ	Discovery HR, RX, LS, TE, 690	None	101
Centre Henri Becquerel, Rouen, France	CHB	GE710 GE Healthcare	None	38
Centre Hospitalier Universitaire de Poitiers, France	CHUP	Biograph mCT 40 ToF GE Healthcare	72	None
MD Anderson Cancer Center, Houston, Texas, USA	MDA	Discovery HR, RX, ST, STE	198	200
Total			524	359

Table 2. Segmentation table of the Dice Scores (DS) by segment classes: primary tumors (GTVp) and Gross Tumor Volumes (GTVn) in columns, and algorithms/teams in rows. The evaluation performance by training on the entire training set from six medical centers and testing on the holding testing set from three medical centers, including two new independent medical centers not included in the training set.

Methods/Teams	GTVp	GTVn	Mean
NVIDIA(Nvauto) [29]	**0.80066**	**0.77539**	**0.78802**
CVD_Net	0.77603	0.77382	0.77492
nnUNet [21]	0.77485	0.76938	0.77212
MA-SAM [9]	0.67052	0.74453	0.70753

The CVD_Net was evaluated on the HECKTOR 2022 dataset [3]. The dataset consists of 883 cases of PET/CT images collected from 9 medical centers from 4 different countries using 12 different medical devices. The dataset is split into 524 training cases from 7 different centers and 359 hidden test cases from 3 different centers, 2 of which are new centers not included in the training sets. The datasets were annotated by human experts for three classes: 0 for background, 1 for primary tumors (GTVp), and 2 for Gross Tumor Volumes (GTVn). A summary of the dataset is shown in

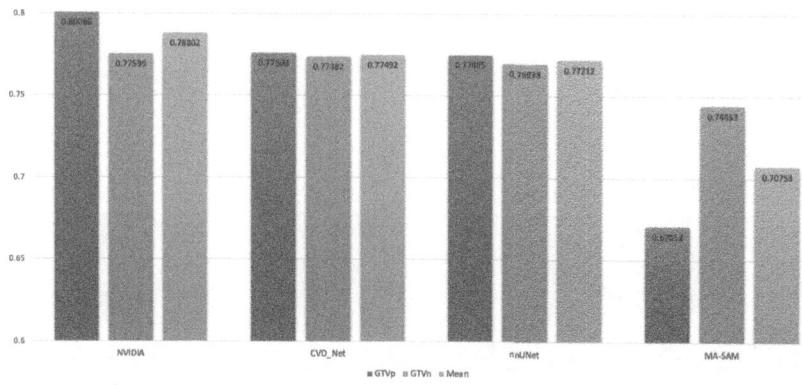

Fig. 3. Avisualisation comparison measured in Dice Scores (DS) by segment classes: primary tumors (GTVp) and Gross Tumor Volumes (GTVn), grouped by algorithms/teams. The evaluation performance by training on the entire training set from six medical centers and testing on the holding testing set from three medical centers, including two new independent medical centers not included in the training set.

Table 3. A table comparing the generalizability performance of segmentation in Dice Scores (DS) by segment classes (columns) and algorithms (rows) for training on the training subset from five medical centres and testing on the holding testing set from an independent centre not seen during training.

Methods	Training Centres	Testing Centre	GTVp	GTVn	Mean
CVD_Net	CHUM, CHUP, CHUS, CHUV, MDA, HGJ	HMR	**0.7628**	**0.7781**	**0.7705**
nnUNet [21]	CHUM, CHUP, CHUS, CHUV, MDA, HGJ	HMR	0.7598	0.7758	0.7678
MA-SAM [9]	CHUM, CHUP, CHUS, CHUV, MDA, HGJ	HMR	0.5718	0.5879	0.5799
CVD_Net	CHUM, CHUP, CHUS, CHUV, MDA, HMR	HGJ	**0.7891**	**0.7634**	**0.7763**
nnUNet [21]	CHUM, CHUP, CHUS, CHUV, MDA, HMR	HGJ	0.7807	0.7597	0.7702
MA-SAM [9]	CHUM, CHUP, CHUS, CHUV, MDA, HMR	HGJ	0.6710	0.5781	0.6255
CVD_Net	CHUM, CHUP, CHUS, CHUV, MDA, HGJ	CHUV	**0.7781**	**0.7672**	**0.7727**
nnUNet [21]	CHUM, CHUP, CHUS, CHUV, MDA, HGJ	CHUV	0.7719	0.7596	0.7658
MA-SAM [9]	CHUM, CHUP, CHUS, HGJ, MDA, HMR	CHUV	0.6212	0.5949	0.6081

Table 1. An illustration depicting the high variability in image quality among images sourced from the seven medical centers in the training set is shown in Fig. 2.

4.2   Training and Testing

The CVD_Net was trained for maximum of 1000 epochs with early stopping [23] to avoid over-fitting. ADAM was the optimizer, and the learning rate was set to 0.01, decreasing according to the following: $(1 - \frac{\text{epoch num}}{1000})^{0.9}$. The sum of the cross-entropy and Dice loss was taken as the loss function. For a fair comparison of the performance of the CVD_Net with other SOTA algorithms, our model was evaluated on a

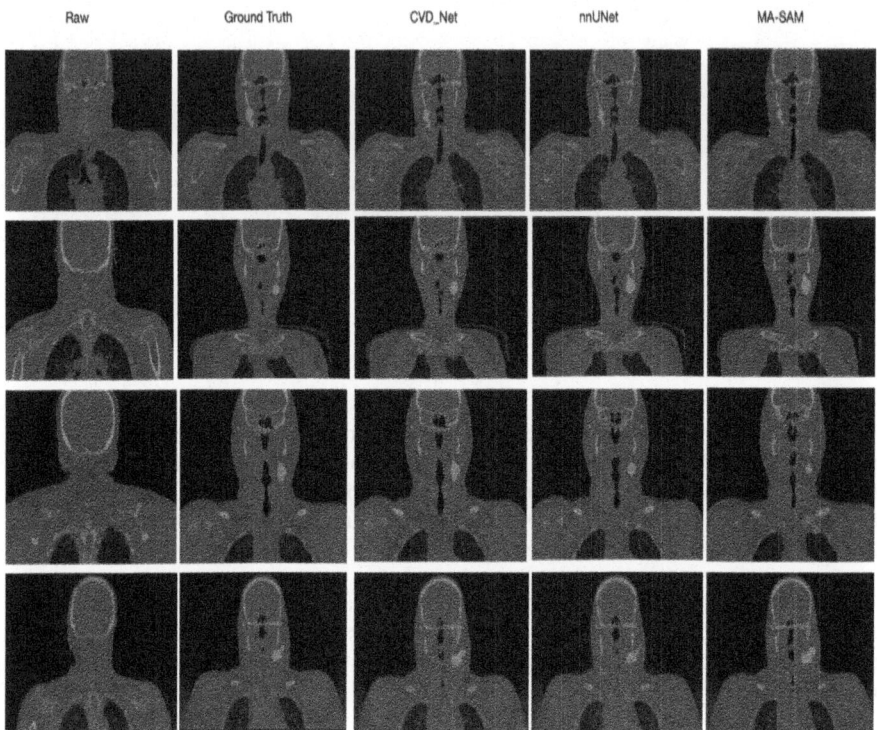

Fig. 4. Coronal planes visualization comparing predictions from different architectures to the ground truth/human annotations and raw images. The GTVp is marked in red, and the GTVn is marked in green. (Color figure online)

blind test set on the organizer's website. The ground truth for this test set is held by the organizers and is not available to the public. The hidden test set includes data from three medical centers, two of which are new centers not used during training. To further evaluate the generalization performance of the CVD_Net, the training dataset was split into two subsets: a training subset and a testing subset. The testing subset consists of data from medical centers not used in the training subset. The evaluation metric used was the Dice Score (DS), which is twice the intersection divided by the union. It measures the overlapping of the pixels, ranging from 0 to 1, with 1 being the perfect score and 0 being the worst. DS was the evaluating metric used by the challenge organizers, so for fair comparison, we have used DS. The models were implemented in Python using the PyTorch library, and were trained on a GPU server with NVIDIA RTX A6000 48GB.

4.3   Results

Experimental results show that when the CVD_Net is trained on the available HECK-TOR 2022 [3] training dataset from six medical centers and tested on the hidden test dataset from three medical centers, of which two medical centers are new and not in the training set, we obtained a mean dice score of 0.77492 (0.77603 for GTVp and 0.77382 for GTVn) as demonstrated in Table 2 with the corresponding bar chart in Fig. 3. To further illustrate the generalization ability of our algorithm, we trained the CVD_Net on a subset of the training dataset and evaluated the performance on a holding subset from independent medical center not seen during training. Additionally, we provide comparisons of our proposed CVD_Net to other SOTA specialized and foundational models in this domain. This is illustrated in Table 3. B-Scans of the coronal view showing the raw data, annotated/ground truth, and corresponding predictions from different models are illustrated in Fig. 4, demonstrating the slight performance advantage of CVD_Net.

5   Conclusions

In this work, we investigated the problem of the generalizability of segmentation of head and neck squamous cell carcinoma (HNSCC) using PET/CT images from nine centers across the world, employing SOTA specialized and foundational models. The main contribution of the work is that we have proposed a novel segmentation algorithm, CVD_Net, which is comprised of a CNN encoder, a domain-specific batch normalization, a transformer encoder and a CNN decoder.

The CVD_Net was evaluated on the HECKTOR 2022 dataset [3] from nine medical centers, achieving a mean Dice score of 0.77492 when tested on the hidden test set from three medical centers, two of which were not included in the training data. Also, we have demonstrated the high generalizability of the CVD_Net by training on a subset from the training set, comprising data from six centers, and testing it on data from a new center (a holding subset of the training dataset). We achieved state-of-the-art (SOTA) performance, surpassing that of large foundation models while using fewer resources. Furthermore we have compared our results to other SOTA algorithms and demonstrated that while large foundation models, show promising generalization performances for this specific problem, specifically designed deep networks such as nnUNet [21] and CVD_Net still offer a slight advantage for addressing this particular problem. We believe that CVD_Net's slight outperformance in this particular problem is achieved by integrating a CNN encoder, domain-specific batch normalization, a Transformer encoder, and a CNN decoder into the model's architecture.

A limitation of CVD_Net is that some of its main components are built on ViT, which is more data hungry than CNN as explained in [16]. In the future, we look forward to evaluating our models on other datasets once they become publicly available.

References

1. Multi-atlas labeling beyond the cranial vault - workshop and challenge. https://www. creatis.insa-lyon.fr/Challenge/acdc/databases.html
2. An, C., Chen, H., Wang, L.: A coarse-to-fine framework for head and neck tumor segmentation in CT and PET images. In: Andrearczyk, V., Oreiller, V., Hatt, M., Depeursinge, A. (eds.) Head and Neck Tumor Segmentation and Outcome Prediction: Second Challenge, HECKTOR 2021, Held in Conjunction with MICCAI 2021, Strasbourg, France, September 27, 2021, Proceedings, pp. 50–57. Springer International Publishing, Cham (2022). https://doi.org/10.1007/978-3-030-98253-9_3
3. Andrearczyk, V., et al.: Overview of the HECKTOR challenge at MICCAI 2021: automatic head and neck tumor segmentation and outcome prediction in PET/CT images. In: Andrearczyk, V., Oreiller, V., Hatt, M., Depeursinge, A. (eds.) Head and Neck Tumor Segmentation and Outcome Prediction: Second Challenge, HECKTOR 2021, Held in Conjunction with MICCAI 2021, Strasbourg, France, September 27, 2021, Proceedings, pp. 1–37. Springer International Publishing, Cham (2022). https://doi.org/10.1007/978-3-030-98253-9_1
4. Andrearczyk, V., et al.: Automatic segmentation of head and neck tumors and nodal metastases in PET-CT scans. In: Medical Imaging with Deep Learning, pp. 33–43. PMLR (2020)
5. Brown, T., et al.: Language models are few-shot learners. Adv. Neural. Inf. Process. Syst. **33**, 1877–1901 (2020)
6. Carion, N., Massa, F., Synnaeve, G., Usunier, N., Kirillov, A., Zagoruyko, S.: End-to-end object detection with transformers. In: Vedaldi, A., Bischof, H., Brox, T., Frahm, J.-M. (eds.) Computer Vision – ECCV 2020: 16th European Conference, Glasgow, UK, August 23–28, 2020, Proceedings, Part I, pp. 213–229. Springer International Publishing, Cham (2020). https://doi.org/10.1007/978-3-030-58452-8_13
7. Chang, W.-G., You, T., Seo, S., Kwak, S., Han, B.: Domain-specific batch normalization for unsupervised domain adaptation. In: Proceedings of the IEEE/CVF Conference on Computer Vision and Pattern Recognition, pp. 7354–7362 (2019)
8. Chang, W.-G., You, T., Seo, S., Kwak, S., Han, B.: Domain-specific batch normalization for unsupervised domain adaptation. In: Proceedings of the IEEE/CVF Conference on Computer Vision and Pattern Recognition, pp. 7354–7362 (2019)
9. Chen, C., et al.: MA-SAM: modality-agnostic SAM adaptation for 3D medical image segmentation. arXiv preprint arXiv:2309.08842 (2023)
10. Cheng, B., Schwing, A., Kirillov, A.: Per-pixel classification is not all you need for semantic segmentation. Adv. Neural. Inf. Process. Syst. **34**, 17864–17875 (2021)
11. Chiu, S.J., Allingham, M.J., Mettu, P.S., Cousins, S.W., Izatt, J.A., Farsiu, S.: Kernel regression based segmentation of optical coherence tomography images with diabetic macular edema. Biomed. Opt. Express **6**(4), 1172–1194 (2015)
12. Chow, L.Q.M.: Head and neck cancer. N. Engl. J. Med. **382**(1), 60–72 (2020)
13. Clark, K., et al.: The cancer imaging archive (TCIA): maintaining and operating a public information repository. J. Digit. Imaging **26**, 1045–1057 (2013)
14. Diakogiannis, F.I., Waldner, F., Caccetta, P., Wu, C.: ResUNet-a: a deep learning framework for semantic segmentation of remotely sensed data. ISPRS J. Photogram. Remote Sens. **162**, 94–114 (2020)
15. Dm, P.: Global cancer statistics, 2002. CA Cancer J. Clin. **55**, 74–108 (2005)
16. Dosovitskiy, A., et al.: An image is worth 16 × 16 words: transformers for image recognition at scale. arXiv preprint arXiv:2010.11929 (2020)

17. Gibson, E., et al.: NiftyNet: a deep-learning platform for medical imaging. Comput. Methods Programs Biomed. **158**, 113–122 (2018)
18. Guo, Z., Guo, N., Gong, K., Li, Q., et al.: Gross tumor volume segmentation for head and neck cancer radiotherapy using deep dense multi-modality network. Phys. Med. Biol. **64**(20), 205015 (2019)
19. Huang, G., Liu, Z., Van Der Maaten, L., Weinberger, K.Q.: Densely connected convolutional networks. In: Proceedings of the IEEE Conference on Computer Vision and Pattern Recognition, pp. 4700–4708 (2017)
20. Iantsen, A., Visvikis, D., Hatt, M.: Squeeze-and-excitation normalization for automated delineation of head and neck primary tumors in combined PET and CT Images. In: Andrearczyk, V., Oreiller, V., Depeursinge, A. (eds.) Head and Neck Tumor Segmentation: First Challenge, HECKTOR 2020, Held in Conjunction with MICCAI 2020, Lima, Peru, October 4, 2020, Proceedings, pp. 37–43. Springer International Publishing, Cham (2021). https://doi.org/10.1007/978-3-030-67194-5_4
21. Isensee, F., Jaeger, P.F., Kohl, S.A.A., Petersen, J., Maier-Hein, K.H.: nnU-Net: a self-configuring method for deep learning-based biomedical image segmentation. Nat. Methods **18**(2), 203–211 (2021)
22. Kirillov, A., et al.: Segment anything. arXiv preprint arXiv:2304.02643 (2023)
23. Li, M., Soltanolkotabi, M., Oymak, S.: Gradient descent with early stopping is provably robust to label noise for overparameterized neural networks. In: International Conference on Artificial Intelligence and Statistics, pp. 4313–4324. PMLR (2020)
24. Lu, J., Lei, W., Gu, R., Wang, G.: Priori and posteriori attention for generalizing head and neck tumors segmentation. In: Andrearczyk, V., Oreiller, V., Hatt, M., Depeursinge, A. (eds.) Head and Neck Tumor Segmentation and Outcome Prediction: Second Challenge, HECKTOR 2021, Held in Conjunction with MICCAI 2021, Strasbourg, France, September 27, 2021, Proceedings, pp. 134–140. Springer International Publishing, Cham (2022). https://doi.org/10.1007/978-3-030-98253-9_12
25. McConnell, N., Miron, A., Wang, Z., Li, Y.: Integrating residual, dense, and inception blocks into the nnUNet. In: IEEE 35th International Symposium on Computer Based Medical Systems (2022)
26. McConnell, N., Nchongmaje Ndipenoch, Yu., Cao, A.M., Li, Y.: Exploring advanced architectural variations of nnUNet. Neurocomputing **560**, 126837 (2023)
27. Melinščak, M., Radmilović, M., Vatavuk, Z., Lončarić, S.: AROI: annotated retinal oct images database. In: 2021 44th International Convention on Information, Communication and Electronic Technology (MIPRO), pp. 371–376. IEEE (2021)
28. Milletari, F., Navab, N., Ahmadi, S.-A.: V-Net: fully convolutional neural networks for volumetric medical image segmentation. In: 2016 Fourth International Conference on 3D Vision (3DV), pp. 565–571. IEEE (2016)
29. Myronenko, A., Siddiquee, M.M.R., Yang, D., He, Y., Xu, D.: Automated head and neck tumor segmentation from 3D PET/CT HECKTOR 2022 challenge report. In: Andrearczyk, V., Oreiller, V., Hatt, M., Depeursinge, A. (eds.) Head and Neck Tumor Segmentation and Outcome Prediction: Third Challenge, HECKTOR 2022, Held in Conjunction with MICCAI 2022, Singapore, September 22, 2022, Proceedings, pp. 31–37. Springer Nature Switzerland, Cham (2023). https://doi.org/10.1007/978-3-031-27420-6_2
30. Ndipenoch, N., Miron, A., Wang, Z., Li, Y.: Retinal image segmentation with small datasets. In: 10th International Conference on Bioimaging (2023)
31. Ndipenoch, N., Miron, A., Li, Y.: Performance evaluation of retinal oct fluid segmentation, detection, and generalization over variations of data sources. IEEE Access **12**, 31719–31735 (2024)

32. Ndipenoch, N., Miron, A., Wang, Z., Li, Y.: Simultaneous segmentation of layers and fluids in retinal oct images. In: 2022 15th International Congress on Image and Signal Processing, BioMedical Engineering and Informatics (CISP-BMEI), pp. 1–6. IEEE (2022)

33. Ren, J., Huynh, B.-N., Groendahl, A.R., Tomic, O., Futsaether, C.M., Korreman, S.S.: PET normalizations to improve deep learning auto-segmentation of head and neck tumors in 3D PET/CT. In: Andrearczyk, V., Oreiller, V., Hatt, M., Depeursinge, A. (eds.) Head and Neck Tumor Segmentation and Outcome Prediction: Second Challenge, HECKTOR 2021, Held in Conjunction with MICCAI 2021, Strasbourg, France, September 27, 2021, Proceedings, pp. 83–91. Springer International Publishing, Cham (2022). https://doi.org/10.1007/978-3-030-98253-9_7

34. Ronneberger, O., Fischer, P., Brox, T.: U-Net: convolutional networks for biomedical image segmentation. In: Medical Image Computing and Computer-Assisted Intervention–MICCAI 2015: 18th International Conference, Munich, Germany, October 5-9, 2015, Proceedings, Part III 18, pp. 234–241. Springer (2015). https://doi.org/10.1007/978-3-319-24574-4_28

35. Siegel, R.L., Miller, K.D., Fuchs, H.E., Jemal, A., et al.: Cancer statistics, 2021. CA Cancer J. Clin. **71**(1), 7–33 (2021)

36. Son, E., Panwar, A., Mosher, C.H., Lydiatt, D.: Cancers of the major salivary gland. J. Oncol. Pract. **14**(2), 99–108 (2018)

37. Vallieres, M., et al.: Radiomics strategies for risk assessment of tumour failure in head-and-neck cancer. Sci. Rep. **7**(1), 10117 (2017)

38. Vaswani, A., et al.: Attention is all you need. In: Advances in Neural Information Processing Systems, vol. 30 (2017)

39. Xie, Y., Zhang, J., Shen, C., Xia, Y.: CoTr: efficiently bridging CNN and transformer for 3D medical image segmentation. In: de Bruijne, M., et al. (eds.) MICCAI 2021. LNCS, vol. 12903, pp. 171–180. Springer, Cham (2021). https://doi.org/10.1007/978-3-030-87199-4_16

40. Yousefirizi, F., et al.: Segmentation and risk score prediction of head and neck cancers in PET/CT volumes with 3D U-Net and Cox proportional hazard neural networks. In: Andrearczyk, V., Oreiller, V., Hatt, M., Depeursinge, A. (eds.) Head and Neck Tumor Segmentation and Outcome Prediction: Second Challenge, HECKTOR 2021, Held in Conjunction with MICCAI 2021, Strasbourg, France, September 27, 2021, Proceedings, pp. 236–247. Springer International Publishing, Cham (2022). https://doi.org/10.1007/978-3-030-98253-9_22

41. Zhou, D., et al.: DeepViT: towards deeper vision transformer. arXiv preprint arXiv:2103.11886 (2021)

Applying Deep Learning Based Super-Resolution to Knee Imaging

Alvaro Rey-Blanes[1] and Enrique Dominguez[1,2(✉)] (iD)

[1] Department of Computer Science, University of Málaga, Málaga, Spain
{alvarorey,enriqued}@uma.es
[2] Biomedical Research Institute of Málaga (IBIMA), Málaga, Spain

Abstract. In the realm of modern health and healthcare, imaging tests play a pivotal role in furnishing essential information for patient diagnosis and treatment. Among these techniques, magnetic resonance imaging (MRI) stands out due to its capacity to visualize the inner workings of the human body using magnetic fields. Advancements in computing have led to enhanced efficiency and image quality in MRI scans conducted within medical facilities. Researchers have focused on MRI processing, specifically leveraging convolutional neural network (CNN) models to enhance the resolution of knee images. In this paper, two novel models have been proposed, along with different experiments and their comparative results, which have been evaluated using standard metrics. These innovative approaches aim to optimize MRI utilization, thereby enhancing diagnostic precision and patient care while mitigating the risks associated with diagnostic test resolution.

Keywords: Super-Resolution · Magnetic Resonance Image · Convolutional Neural Networks

1 Introduction

MRI is an imaging technique used mainly in the biomedical field and is based on the physical phenomenon known as magnetic resonance (MR), which allows us to see those particles that have spin and charge when subjected to a magnetic field. It differs from other techniques such as X-ray (Rx) or computed tomography (CT) in that it does not use ionising radiation but radiofrequency (RF) signals, which means that MRI is a harmless method without any loss of information quality. All in all, with computer processing and improvement, and because it can be used to image almost any anatomical part of the body (apart from the knee), it is a useful technique that is expanding worldwide.

Depending on our medical intentions, the magnetic resonance equipment can be configured to show different anatomical parts. Weights are used by working on the relaxation properties [9] and we can distinguish:

- **T1-Weighted MRI (T1).** This weight uses a time constant given by the return to equilibrium of longitudinal magnetisation. It has a great soft tissue contrast and can be useful on detecting vascularity of injuries. In addition, shorter T1 will be brighter.

X. Xie et al. (Eds.): AIiH 2024, LNCS 14976, pp. 77–88, 2024.
https://doi.org/10.1007/978-3-031-67285-9_6

- **T2-Weighted MRI (T2)**. T2-weighting relies on the relaxation time constant, specifically on the transverse magnetization affected by neighboring spins interactions. Commonly used to evaluate anatomical structures such as meniscus, ligaments, or tendons in knee imaging, T2-weighted MRI highlights brighter signals with longer T2 relaxation times, compared to T1-weighted imaging.
- **Proton Density Weighted MRI (PD)**: As its name indicates, it shows the hydrogen protons concentration on the tissue. The contrast will be given by variations on proton density. It can also differentiate ligaments or meniscus, meaning it is pretty common to use PD-weights on a knee MRI.
- **Short Tau Inversion Recovery MRI (STIR)**. This technique is useful to suppress fat signal, which is usually not necessary in a knee study.

The main use of MRI in the knee is to detect and assess possible tissue damage. While almost all ligament/cartilage/meniscus-related injuries require complementary MRI to observe the status of a malfunctioning tissue, bones and muscles can also be accurately assessed with other imaging techniques, requiring MRI in some specific trauma cases [10,11].

Super-resolution (SR), as a group of techniques for increasing the resolution of an image, has been in use for almost half a century. However, its use has increased in recent years due to improvements in computing power and accessibility combined with the latest technologies in both hardware and software. Its main purpose is to construct high-resolution images (HR) from low-resolution images (LR) [5] in order to obtain finer details or better anatomical detail in the specific medical field. Depending on the approach to enhance the image resolution we can discriminate into five classes of algorithms, interpolation methods (bilinear or bicubic interpolation) [4], reconstruction (iterative back-projection, maximum a posteriori) [3], patch-based methods (anchored neighborhood regression), frequency domain (wavelet-based) and learning based methods as convolutional neural networks (CNN) or generative adversarial networks (GAN) [12], where our solution stands. Current state-of-the-art for CNNs usage regarding MRI SR stands after the first CNN was applied in order to improve image quality on natural images by Dong et al. [1]. This model consisted on a simple three-layer CNN divided on extraction, non-linear mapping and reconstruction layers. Due to the SR convolutional neural network (SRCNN) model results it was followed by its usage in different SR tasks concerning medical images in different anatomical parts as chest [2], brain [6] or knee [7].

2   SR Models

In this section, we propose three different CNNs to increase the resolution of knee images. With the knowledge and observing the available data, we proceed to design the models that will learn the features from our data. First there was made the decision to use 2D-Convolution approach, which focuses on enhancing the resolution of individual MRI segment, treating each as a separate image although MRI is processed as voxels (3D). This is because a 3D convolution has higher computational cost than a 2D convolution, and an anatomical damage can be observed on a single MRI slice. Note that the first or last slices of knee MRI may not have specific anatomical data to improve our training and solution. This would be different in other anatomical evaluations such as brain where specific diagnosis of brain cancer or Alzheimer requires of a volumetric evaluations and size calculation.

2.1   SRCNN

The first proposed model consists on a full convolution layers on three sequential blocks for a total of 57,281 trainable parameters. Figure 1 shows the sequential blocks, which are described as follows:

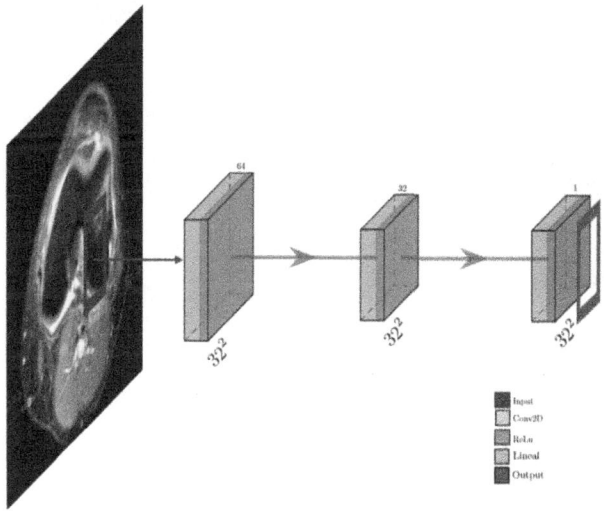

Fig. 1. SRCNN model schema.

- Feature extraction layer, which is the first convolutional layer, consisting on a 1 channel entry (grayscale characteristics of medical image) and 64 outputs channels (filters), 9×9 kernel, 1×1 stride (one pixel movement at a time across the image) and 4×4 as padding to ensure output size.
- Non-linear Mapping Layer with 64 input channels from the previous layer and 32 output channels as filters, a 5×5 kernel size and same stride/padding. The objective of this layer is to consolidate the extracted features.
- Reconstruction Layer receives 32 inputs to create a final 1 output channel. Kernel size is 5×5 to combine detailed acquired features into a final image.

2.2 ExSRCNN

The second model proposed (Fig. 2) for super-resolute medical images consists of a deep feature enhancer that tries to emphasise deep feature extraction through multiple layers and its potential application in enhancing or transforming images based on learnt features. It has a total of 557,953 trainable parameters, and it is divided in the following three blocks:

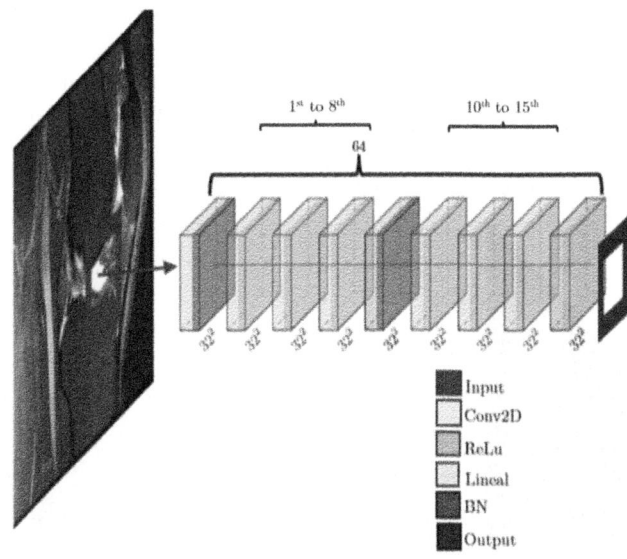

Fig. 2. ExSRCNN model schema simplified reducing redundant intermediate layers.

- Initial Conv2D Layer, consisting of 64, 7 × 7 filters followed by batch normalization, which is added with the aim of improving training stability and boost efficiency.
- Intermediate Convolutional Layers, which is the core of the network's feature extraction capability. It consists of 15 successive stacked 64-channel convolutional layers, with 3 × 3 kernel size filters to learn in fine detail. The main purpose of these consecutive layers is to progressively refine image features while trying to maintain computer efficiency. These blocks also add batch normalization to the 9th layer to help further stabilise, numerical stability, and reduce overfitting risk.
- Output final layer, with 64 channels and 3 × 3 kernel, to synthesize the previously processed features into a 1 channel image.

2.3 RBSRCNN

The last proposed model (Fig. 3) uses a varied structure, integrating the usage of residual blocks to facilitate learning and improve performance, with a total of 353,729 trainable parameters divided now into four differentiable blocks:

- Initial Conv2D Layer, similar to SRCNN feature extraction layer. Usage of 64 filters with a 9×9 kernel to try to capture as many features as possible (simple to complex).
- Residual Blocks consist of four iterations of the same residual block composed by two blocks of 2D convolutional layer (3×3) and batch normalization layer. The whole block will work on 64 input/output channels, and it is intended to refine details, allowing gradient flow during back-propagation to learn identity mappings.
- Non-linear mapping Layer with a 2D convolutional layer (5×5) to map the enhanced features from 64 to 32 channels, and to prepare the data for the final reconstruction.
- Reconstruction Layer is the final step, focused on reconstructing the image using the learnt features. It consists on a 2D convolutional layer (5×5) with a single channel output.

3 Dataset and Experimental Setup

All MRI data used in this work belongs to the Stanford Machine Learning Group, and it is available as the MRNet dataset for research and competition purposes exclusively. This dataset comprises 1,370 test (5.7GB) consisting of normal and abnormal examinations as various injuries including ACL tears (23.3%) and meniscus tears (37.1%). Among these, 1,088 patients underwent examination using GE scanners operating at 1.5T/3.0T magnetic field strengths, utilizing the MRI sequences detailed below:

- Sagittal PD.
- Sagittal T2 + fat saturation.
- Axial PD + fat saturation.
- Coronal T1.
- Coronal T2 + fat saturation.

As previously mentioned, the anatomical plane is entirely represented in MRNet, so an approximate equal number of images from each anatomical plane are going to be used. The proposed models utilize 32×32 patches, with a 50% overlap, meaning each patch shares 16×16 overlapping pixels with its neighboring patches, meaning that a 256×256 would generate 255 patches. The data distribution is as follows:

- Training: 223 images for a total of 56,330 patches that will be used in LR for training.

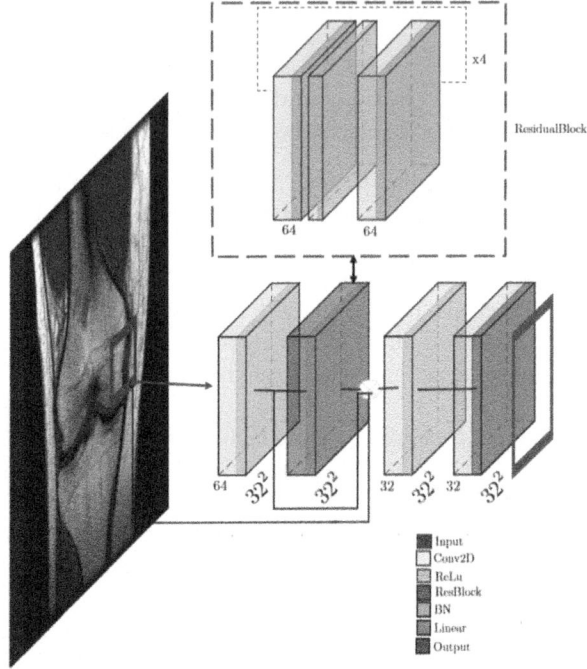

Fig. 3. RBSRCNN model schema.

- Validation: 40 images for a total of 10,240 patches pairs LR-HR, to evaluate the learning status.
- Testing: 42 images for a total of 10,752 patterns pairs LR-HR, to test and assess the best training result for each model and experiment.

Regarding to both the learning rate and the weight decay, they were established to $1 * 10^{-4}$ initially, and adjusted for quicker or slower convergences of the model. Model momentum was set to 0.9 using a batch size of 16. This initial batch size allows to reduce computational risk (memory issues) in older GPUs. For the weights initialisation, all proposed models contain a Kaiming Initialisation due to the large number of *ReLu* activation functions. Basically, it focuses on initializing the weights for the convolutional layers with values drawn from a Gaussian distribution with a mean of 0 and a standard deviation of $\sqrt{\frac{n}{2}}$, where n is the number of incoming nodes of the neurons. Two loss functions were used, Mean Squared Error (MSE) and Mean Absolute Error (MAE), to mathematically evaluate how the model is performing. Adaptive Moment Estimation (Adam), which tries to combine ideas from the Stochastic Gradient Descent (SGD) optimizer and Root Mean Square Propagation (RMSprop), was chosen due to regularly converges faster than SGD and it has an adaptive learning rate that reduces manual adjustment (Table 1).

Table 1. Hardware specifications

Component	Specification
CPU	Intel Core I5-7400 quad core 3GHz base clock
RAM	8 GB DDR4 SODIMM
Storage	100 GB SSD
Graphics	NVIDIA GPU, 6 GB available RAM
Operating System	Ubuntu 18.04.6

In order to evaluate the model, the peak signal noise ratio metrics (PSNR)(1) and the structural similarity index measure (SSIM)(2) were used to obtain an objective evaluation [8].

$$\text{PSNR} = 10 \cdot \log_{10} \left(\frac{\text{MAX}_I^2}{\text{MSE}} \right) \quad (1)$$

where MSE is the mean squared error and MAX_I is the maximum possible pixel value in the image.

$$\text{SSIM}(x, y) = \frac{(2\mu_x\mu_y + c_1)(2\sigma_{xy} + c_2)}{(\mu_x^2 + \mu_y^2 + c_1)(\sigma_x^2 + \sigma_y^2 + c_2)} \quad (2)$$

where the mean values of x and y are represented as μ_x and μ_y respectively. The variances of x and y are denoted as σ_x^2 and σ_y^2 respectively. The covariance between x and y is denoted as σ_{xy}. The constants c_1 and c_2 are used to stabilise the division with weak denominators. Usually defined as $c_1 = (k_1 L)^2$ and $c_2 = (k_2 L)^2$, where L is the dynamic range of pixel values, and $k_1 = 0.01$ and $k_2 = 0.03$ by default.

4   Experimental Results

Validation results provides an initial insight into the progress of the training of the proposed models. Figures 4 and 5 show a tendency for the values to plateau towards the end of 300 epochs, suggesting that this number of epochs is sufficient to obtain better results from the proposed models. In both figures, MAE loss function shows better performance than MSE for each model, where residual blocks based models come out to the top performers. In contrast to the observed performance of models like the ExSRCNN (experiments 2.A, B)), which demonstrate rapid initial improvements followed by a plateau in later epochs, SRCNN models display more moderate metrics. Despite their recognized potential in superresolution tasks, SRCNN models maintain relatively simple architectures.

Testing is conducted by using completely unseen data to ensure the reliability and credibility of the obtained results. Table 2 shows that residual blocks models outperform the other proposed models, and the MAE loss function provides better results than MSE, which is widely used in many other works in the literature (Figs. 6 and 7).

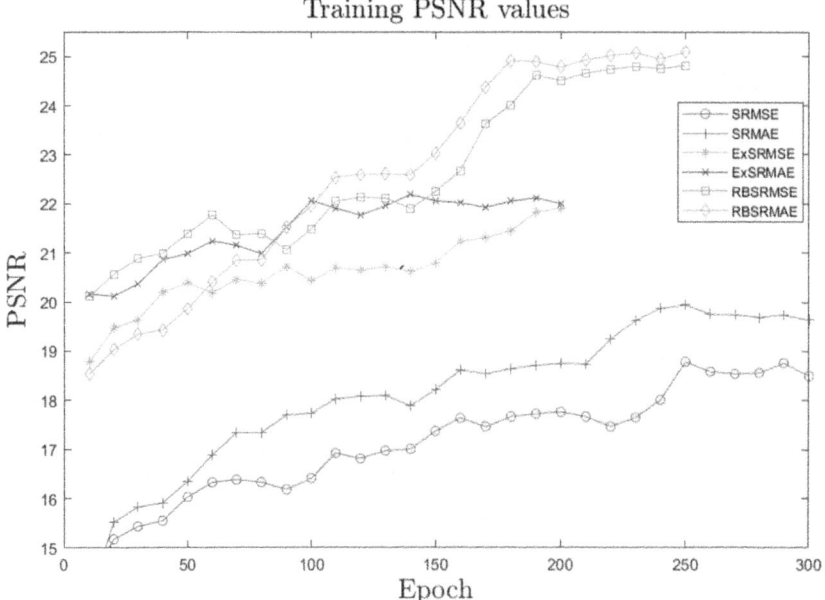

Fig. 4. Validation PSNR Values along epochs

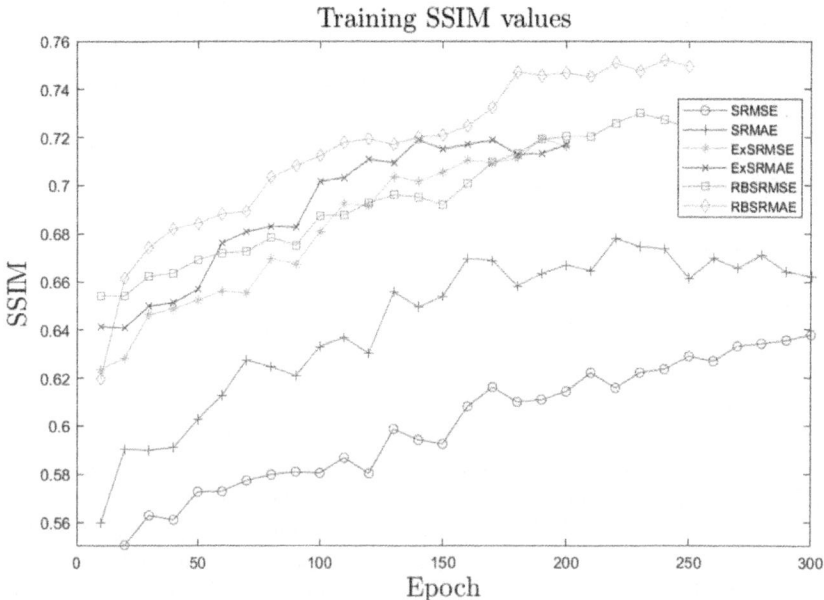

Fig. 5. Validation SSIM Values along epochs

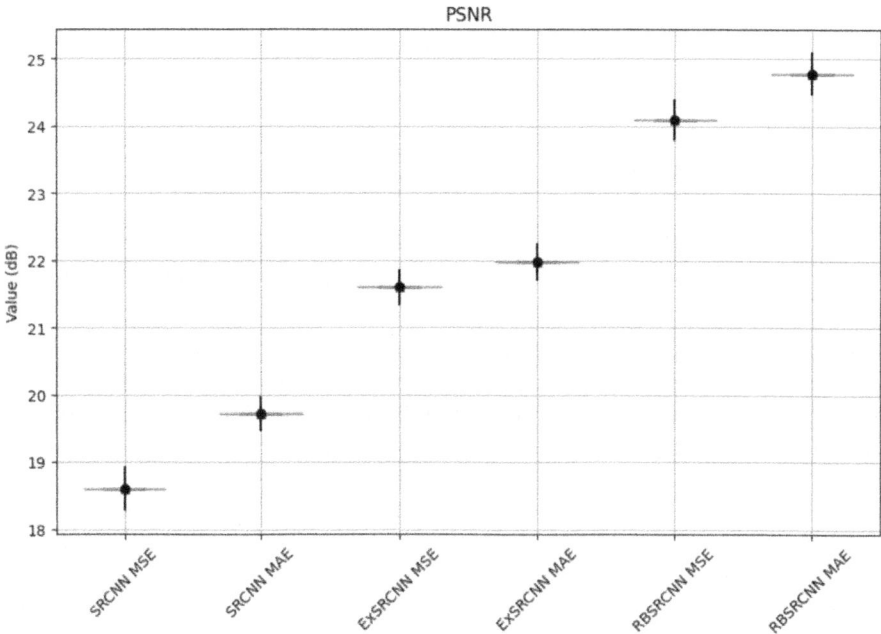

Fig. 6. Graphical view of PSNR for each model with their standard deviation

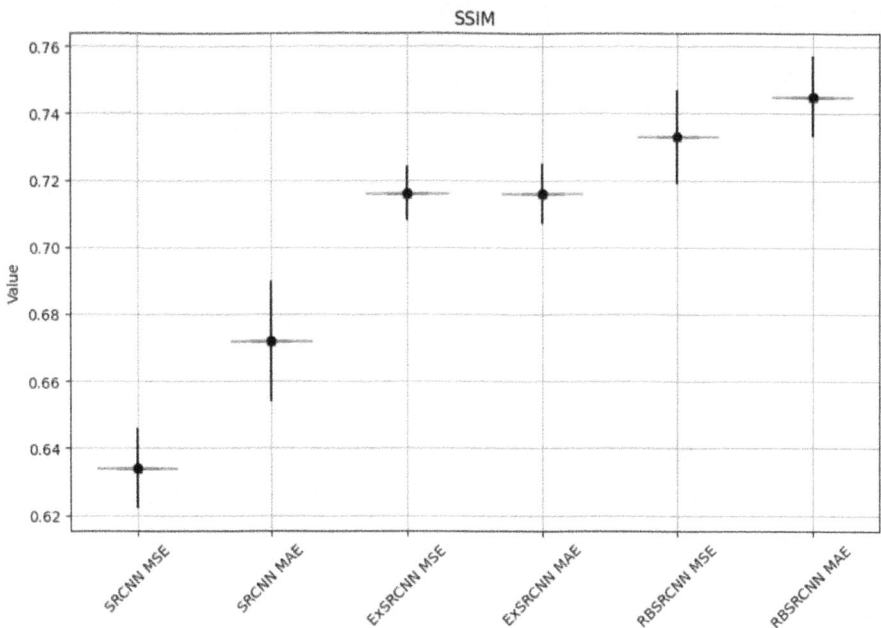

Fig. 7. Graphical view of SSIM for each model with their standard deviation

Table 2. Comparison of model performance in testing

		PSNR	SSIM
SRCNN	MSE	18.599 ± 0.337	0.634 ± 0.012
	MAE	19.714 ± 0.258	0.672 ± 0.018
ExSRCNN	MSE	21.598 ± 0.262	0.716 ± 0.008
	MAE	21.983 ± 0.276	0.716 ± 0.009
RBSRCNN	MSE	24.100 ± 0.307	0.733 ± 0.014
	MAE	**24.786** ± 0.311	**0.745** ± 0.012

Figure 8 shows an example of the SR images provided by the proposed models, where a crop zoom in a region of interest is depicted to verify the performance. All SR images were generated by using the proposed models with MAE loss function. An initial graphical assessment reveals a quantitative loss in anatomical details when transitioning from high-resolution (HR) to low-resolution (LR) images. This is evident in the zoom crop, where a lack of detail and reduced sharpness is observed. While general medical conditions may be discernible, specific diagnoses may prove challenging due to the diminished clarity of features. While specific anatomical details may still appear slightly blurred to the human eye in the images provided by the proposed models, they are closer

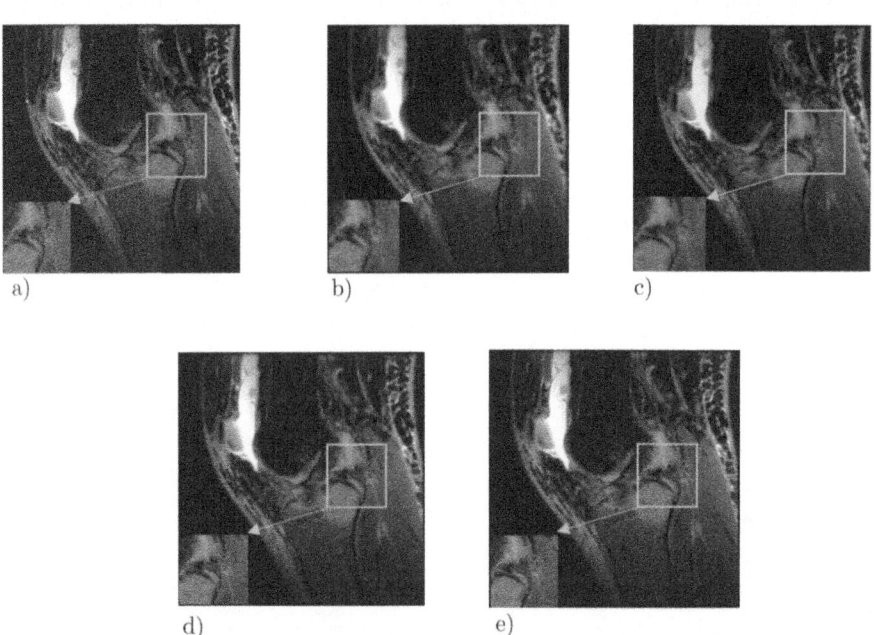

Fig. 8. PD Weighted sagittal MRI. a) Original *HR* image. b) X2 factor *LR* image. c) SRCNN. d) ExSRCNN. e) RBSRCNN

to the original image, with previously invisible damage now becoming visible. The last resultant image provided by the RBSRCNN model is clearer and closely resemble the original HR image, revealing narrower details including potential damage.

5 Conclusions

According to the experiment results, both anatomical structures and injury remained unaltered after performing the proposed superresolution approaches. Although some evaluators (clinicians) still noticed, after observing the HR image, lower quality textures in the muscular anatomy; this does not affect the specific diagnose. However, it could be a problem if we were interested in looking for deep muscle injuries.

In this work, we demonstrate the potential of the proposed models in both research and clinical settings to reduce image acquisition time and imaging costs by acquiring LR images and increasing the image resolution through the proposed models.

References

1. Dong, C., Loy, C.C., He, K., Tang, X.: Image super-resolution using deep convolutional networks. IEEE Trans. Pattern Anal. Mach. Intell. **38**(2), 295–307 (2015)
2. Gao, Y., Li, H., Dong, J., Feng, G.: A deep convolutional network for medical image super-resolution. In: 2017 Chinese Automation Congress (CAC), pp. 5310–5315. IEEE (2017)
3. Liu, H., Han, J., Hou, S., Shao, L., Ruan, Y.: Single image super-resolution using a deep encoder-decoder symmetrical network with iterative back projection. Neurocomputing **282**, 52–59 (2018)
4. Liu, J., Gan, Z., Zhu, X.: Directional bicubic interpolation-a new method of image super-resolution. In: 3rd International Conference on Multimedia Technology (ICMT-13), pp. 463–470. Atlantis Press (2013)
5. Nasrollahi, K., Moeslund, T.B.: Super-resolution: a comprehensive survey. Mach. Vis. Appl. **25**, 1423–1468 (2014)
6. Pham, C.H., Ducournau, A., Fablet, R., Rousseau, F.: Brain MRI super-resolution using deep 3D convolutional networks. In: 2017 IEEE 14th International Symposium on Biomedical Imaging (ISBI 2017), pp. 197–200. IEEE (2017)
7. Qiu, D., Zhang, S., Liu, Y., Zhu, J., Zheng, L.: Super-resolution reconstruction of knee magnetic resonance imaging based on deep learning. Comput. Methods Programs Biomed. **187**, 105059 (2020)
8. Sara, U., Akter, M., Uddin, M.S.: Image quality assessment through FSIM, SSIM, MSE and PSNR-a comparative study. J. Comput. Commun. **7**(3), 8–18 (2019)
9. Serai, S.D.: Basics of magnetic resonance imaging and quantitative parameters t1, t2, t2*, t1rho and diffusion-weighted imaging. Pediatr. Radiol. **52**(2), 217–227 (2022)
10. Standring, S.: Gray's anatomy e-book: the anatomical basis of clinical practice. Elsevier Health Sciences (2021)

11. Thacker, S., Stroup, D., Branche, C., Gilchrist, J., Goodman, R., Kelling, E.P.: Prevention of knee injuries in sports. J. Sports Med. Phys. Fitness **43**, 165–179 (2003)
12. Yi, X., Walia, E., Babyn, P.: Generative adversarial network in medical imaging: a review. Med. Image Anal. **58**, 101552 (2019)

FM-LiteLearn: A Lightweight Brain Tumor Classification Framework Integrating Image Fusion and Multi-teacher Distillation Strategies

Shengbo Tan[1,2], Ying Cai[1,2(✉)], Yang Zhao[3], Junjie Hu[4], Yuanyuan Chen[4], and Chenxi He[1,2]

[1] Key Laboratory of Electronic Information Engineering, Southwest Minzu University, Chengdu, China
`caiying34@yeah.net`
[2] College of Electronic and Information, Southwest Minzu University, Chengdu, China
[3] Australian Centre for AI in Medical Innovation, La Trobe University, Melbourne, Australia
[4] College of Computer Science, Sichuan University, Chengdu, China

Abstract. This paper presents FM-LiteLearn, an efficient and lightweight framework specifically designed for the classification of brain tumors. To address the insufficient diversity and low accuracy in image training samples, the proposed framework comprises three key modules: image fusion, model enhancement, and knowledge distillation. Firstly, we employed an image fusion technique based on Generative Adversarial Networks (GAN), specifically F-DCGAN, which integrates T1-weighted and T2-weighted brain tumor images to obtain more comprehensive tumor feature information. Additionally, we proposed an improved residual network model, T-Resnet18, which incorporates a channel attention mechanism after each residual block to enhance the recognition capability of tumor regions while reducing redundant information. Finally, a multi-teacher knowledge distillation model, MT-KD, was introduced to guide the training of T-Resnet18 using multiple large teacher models, thereby striking a balance between the number of model parameters and performance. This paper presents a novel framework for classifying Astrocytoma, Germ cell tumor, Meningioma, and Neurofibroma types. The algorithm was verified on the BT_NAGMN5 dataset, and the experimental results demonstrate a 9.4% improvement in the accuracy of brain tumor classification. Compared to traditional models and other advanced methods, FM-LiteLearn shows significant advantages in enhancing model generalization capabilities and the accuracy of brain tumor classification. The code is available at https://github.com/goblin327/FM-LiteLearn.

Keywords: brain tumor classification · generative adversarial networks · image fusion · knowledge distillation

© The Author(s), under exclusive license to Springer Nature Switzerland AG 2024
X. Xie et al. (Eds.): AIiH 2024, LNCS 14976, pp. 89–103, 2024.
https://doi.org/10.1007/978-3-031-67285-9_7

1   Introduction

Brain tumors are a common and severe disease that poses a significant threat to human life and health [18,19], with a multitude of types including astrocytomas, germinomas, meningiomas, and neurofibromas. These conditions not only place a heavy physical and psychological burden on patients but also present a serious challenge to clinical physicians [12,13]. Particularly, malignant tumors such as gliomas are characterized by high recurrence rates and high mortality [1], complicating the treatment process. In the field of brain tumor diagnosis, the classification of tumors is a topic of intense interest and considerable challenge. Accurate classification is pivotal for formulating effective treatment strategies and enhancing patient survival rates [2].

MRI is widely regarded as the standard method for diagnosing and predicting the prognosis of brain tumors due to its excellent resolution [14,15], soft tissue contrast, and non-invasive nature [3]. The commonly used MRI imaging sequences include T1-weighted, T1 contrast-enhanced, Fluid-Attenuated Inversion Recovery (FLAIR), and T2-weighted images, each with its distinct focus. FLAIR and T2 images are particularly adept at highlighting areas of edema, while T1 and T1 contrast-enhanced sequences are more concentrated on the core region of the tumor [16,17]. Different MRI sequences provide a diverse range of information about brain tumors and complement each other [4]. Based on these MRI sequences, we utilize a fusion technique to synthesize information from diverse MRI sequences, to generate an enhanced MRI sequence. Concurrently, we integrate a channel attention module into the backbone of our network to sharpen the focus on the lesion areas of brain tumors, thereby facilitating more effective classification of brain tumors.

In recent years, to address the complexity inherent in medical imaging, numerous methods of knowledge distillation have been proposed by researchers [5–9]. This paper aims to develop a training framework grounded in image fusion and multi-teacher knowledge distillation. Specifically, our proposed framework encompasses two distinct stages: Firstly, we introduce an image fusion approach based on Generative Adversarial Networks (GANs) that amalgamates T1 and T2 images to produce a more informative fused image. On top of that, we present an adaptive knowledge distillation (KD) strategy, where our method guides the training of the student model by adaptively aggregating knowledge from multiple teachers.

The main contributions of this paper can be summarized as follows:

1. We propose the F-DCGAN image fusion method, which fuses T1 and T2 images to generate fusion images with multiple features, thereby achieving high generalization and strong robustness in brain tumor classification.
2. We introduce the T-ResNet18 network model, which incorporates a channel attention module to enhance the network's focus on the lesion regions of brain tumors, thereby improving the classification accuracy.
3. We propose the MT-KD knowledge distillation method, which uses multiple high-accuracy network models as teacher models to train lightweight models

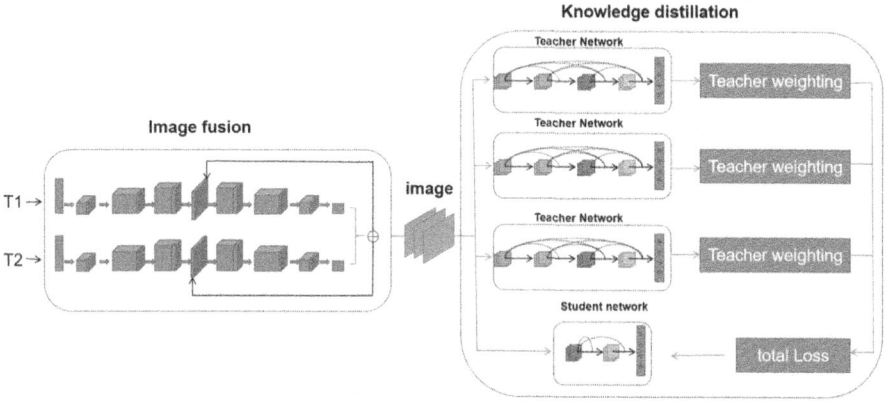

Fig. 1. Framework overview.

with high accuracy and fewer parameters, further improving the classification accuracy.

2   Related Work

Significant advancements have been made in the realm of image processing through the advent of deep learning, particularly in the classification and segmentation of brain MRI images, as well as in the detection and identification of brain tumors. In recent years, a variety of methods have been explored for the classification of brain MRI images. Pashaei et al. [20]. employed Convolutional Neural Networks (CNNs) to extract features from brain images and utilized Kernel Extreme Learning Machine (KELM) for the classification of malignant brain tumors, achieving an accuracy rate of 93.68%. According to Phyae et al. [21], they harnessed multiple Capsule Networks for the classification of brain cancer. By replacing the standard convolutional layers in the Capsule Networks with densely connected convolutional layers, this design elevated the accuracy to 95.03%.

Owing to the complexity and scarcity inherent in medical imaging, a multitude of researchers have, in recent years, shifted their focus to the extraction of richer information from small datasets. Rezaei et al. [23]. leveraged MRI data as input to a generator network, employing Generative Adversarial Networks (GANs) to fabricate novel tumor images, thereby augmenting the dataset. To fortify the robustness of the model, Ahmad et al. [22]. utilized GAN networks to enhance brain tumor imagery during both pre-training and fine-tuning phases. During the pre-training phase, the GANs generated authentic tumor images, which were instrumental in pre-conditioning the deep neural network (DNN).

While these approaches have achieved commendable results, they have also escalated the complexity of the models. Consequently, in our study, we introduce a network architecture designed for training lightweight models on small

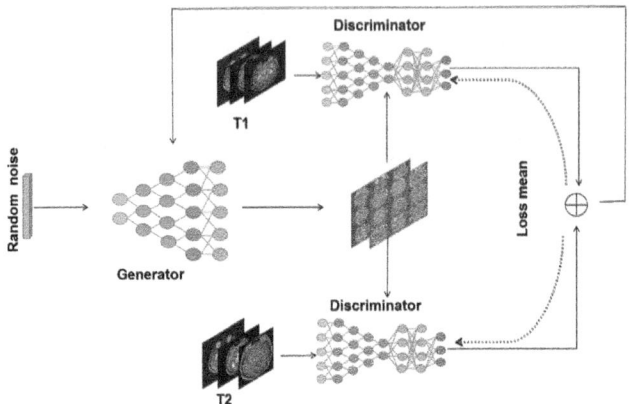

Fig. 2. F-DCGAN model structure.

datasets. Initially, we integrate images of the same anatomical region but of different modalities. Subsequently, we employ an adaptive multi-teacher knowledge distillation technique to effectively cultivate a lightweight network with enhanced generalization capabilities.

3   Method

We propose an efficient and lightweight framework for brain tumor classification. The method consists of three fundamental steps: image fusion, model improvement, and knowledge distillation, as illustrated in Fig. 1. In the following sections, we will elaborate on each of these key components in detail.

3.1   Image Fusion Techniques(F-DCGAN)

Deep Convolutional Generative Adversarial Networks (DCGANs) rely on the robust feature extraction capabilities of Convolutional Neural Networks (CNNs) to ensure the authenticity of the generated data. In this paper, we have adopted the main network structure of the DCGAN and modified the architectures of the generator and discriminator modules to create the F-DCGAN, as shown in Fig. 2.

The DCGAN serves as the foundational framework for model training and validation in this paper. In contrast to traditional Generative Adversarial Networks (GANs), which typically consist of a single generator and discriminator, the F-DCGAN is composed of two symmetrical DCGANs, creating a complex integrated network. These two DCGANs share the same generator but each has its own independent discriminator. By comparing the images generated by the generator with the feature samples produced by the two discriminators and calculating the corresponding loss (as shown in Eq. 1), we continuously refine the network's strategy until the discriminators can no longer distinguish between real and generated data. This iterative optimization process aims to achieve a balanced state for the network, known as Nash equilibrium, at which point the network is not only fully optimized but also capable of accurately estimating the underlying distribution of the data and effectively generating new data samples.

$$\min_{G}\max_{D}V\left(D,G\right)=E_{x}\,Pdata\left(x\right)\ln D\left(x\right)+E_{z}\,P_{z}\left(z\right)\ln\left(1-D\left(G\left(z\right)\right)\right)\quad(1)$$

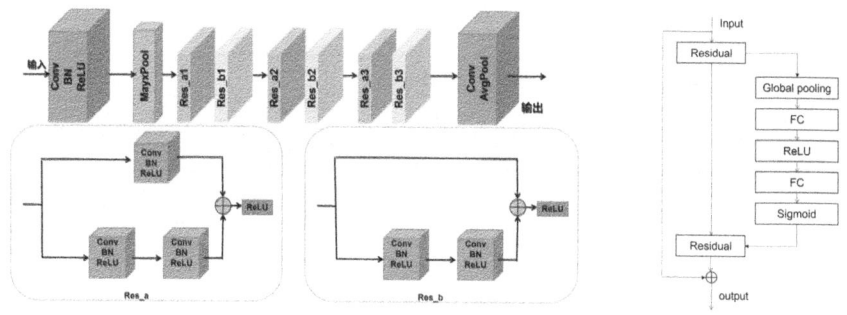

Fig. 3. Network structure of ResNet18(left); Adding SE Attention Mechanism to the Residual Structure of the Network(right).

In the equation, $V(D,G)$ represents the overall loss function to be optimized in the generative adversarial network. Here, z represents a random variable, x represents real data, P_z represents the probability distribution of the generated data, $Pdata$ represents the probability distribution of x, $D(x)$ represents the probability of x being classified as real, and $D(G(z))$ represents the probability of the reconstructed data being classified as real.

3.2   Improvement Based on ResNet18(T-ResNet18)

To achieve high precision and maintain real-time processing capabilities in brain tumor classification tasks, we employ the ResNet18 model as the foundational network architecture. ResNet18 adeptly balances the depth of the network with training efficiency, ensuring sufficient depth while enabling rapid convergence. Furthermore, to address the challenge of identifying small tumor lesions scattered within brain tumor images, we have integrated a Squeeze-and-Excitation (SE) channel attention mechanism into each residual block of the network. This mechanism significantly enhances the network's ability to recognize tumor regions, effectively capturing and extracting key features of various types of brain tumor lesions, as detailed in Fig. 3.

3.3   Multi-teacher Knowledge Distillation(MT-KD)

In this paper, we have made innovative improvements to the multi-teacher knowledge distillation technique. As shown in Fig. 4, the entire distillation architecture is designed to enable lightweight models to learn from multiple teachers who are trained with limited datasets, thereby equipping the student model with the ability to acquire additional information from various teachers. The training steps for the Multi-Teacher Knowledge Distillation (MT-KD) model are as follows:

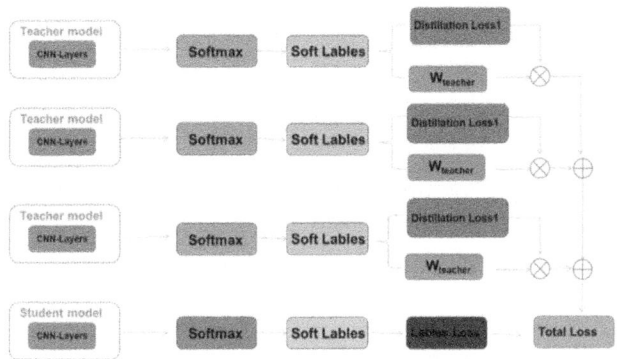

Fig. 4. MT-KD knowledge distillation structure.

The brain tumor image data is fed into the teacher model to yield a probability distribution indicative of tumor classification. To refine the soft labels (q_{SLi}) generated by the teacher model, a temperature scaling technique is employed, leveraging the temperature parameter T. This study pioneers an innovative multi-teacher network selection mechanism, which incorporates a binary mask M_{decide}, to direct the student model's focus towards the most accurate teacher. Subsequently, leveraging the tumor category probability distribution derived from the teacher model, we compute the teacher model's weights to assess its precision.

$$q_{SLi} = \frac{e^{\frac{x_{Ti}}{T}}}{\sum_{i=0}^{n} e^{\frac{x_{Ti}}{T}}} \tag{2}$$

$$M_{decide} = \begin{cases} 1, & if\ (P_{label} = Y_{label}) \\ 0, & Otherwise \end{cases} \tag{3}$$

$$W_{Teacher} = \sum_{k=0}^{m} \frac{\sqrt{\sum_{i=0}^{m} (U_{kn} - A_{ki})}}{m+1} \tag{4}$$

In the equation, P_{label} represents the prediction results of the teacher model, while Y_{label} denotes the true labels. For the k group of data, U_{kn} signifies the predicted value for the correct category, and A_{ki} represents the predicted values for the other categories. The term $m+1$ stands for the total number of categories in each group of data. We employ soft labels and soft prediction results, as well as true labels and hard prediction results, to calculate the soft loss function L_{SOFT} and the hard loss function L_{HARD} using the Kullback-Leibler divergence loss function. The specific formulas are as follows:

$$L_{SOFT} = -\frac{1}{B}\sum_{i=1}^{B}\sum_{j=1}^{C} q_{SLi} \log q_{SPj} \tag{5}$$

$$L_{HARD} = -\frac{1}{B}\sum_{i=1}^{B}\sum_{j=1}^{C} y_{TRUE} \log q_{HPj} \tag{6}$$

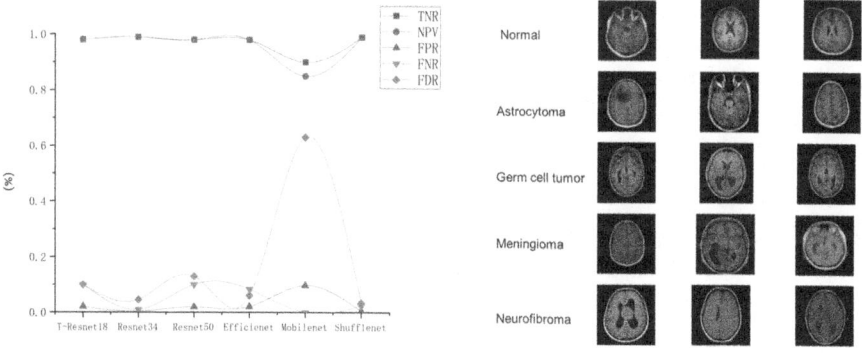

Fig. 5. Comparison chart of other training performance metrics(left); samples from a tumor dataset(right).

In the provided formula, B represents the batch size of the images, and C denotes the number of brain tumor categories. q_{SPj} signifies the soft predictions made by the student model, while y_{TRUE} stands for the corresponding true labels. The hard predictions from the student model are represented by q_{HPj} To balance the contributions of both loss functions, a scaling factor α is introduced to adjust the ratio between them. Consequently, we obtain the hybrid loss function L_{KD}, with the calculation formula as follows:

$$L_{KD} = (1 - \alpha) L_{HARD} + \alpha \sum \left(T^2 L_{SOFT} M_{decide} W_{teacher}\right) \tag{7}$$

The backpropagation of L_{KD} is the key process in which the teacher model imparts implicit knowledge to the student model, significantly improving the student model's classification performance.

4   Experimental Setup

4.1   Datasets

This paper utilized a publicly accessible Magnetic Resonance Imaging (MRI) dataset from the Kaggle repository for model training and evaluation [1]. The dataset encompasses 44 distinct types of brain tumors. To assess the efficacy of our method in dealing with imbalanced datasets, we meticulously selected five brain tumor types from these categories, creating a data subset named BT_NAGMN5[2]. A more detailed description of the dataset can be found in Table 1. This subset includes the following five categories: Normal (201 images in the training set and 50 in the test set), Astrocytoma (141 images in the training set and 35 in the test set), Germ cell tumor (22 images in the training set and 5 in the test set), Meningioma (218 images in the training set and 54 in the test set), and Neurofibroma (104 images in the training set and 26 in the test set). The dataset comprises a total of 856 MRI images of various types of human brains, presented in grayscale and JPEG format (as shown in Fig. 5 on the right). For the training and validation tasks, the dataset was divided such that 80% of the images were used for training, and the remaining 20% were used for testing. [1,2]

Table 1. Dataset details.

Brain tumor categories	original training samples	training samples after data augmentation	original test samples	test samples after data augmentation
Normal	201	201	50	50
Astrocytoma	141	141	35	35
Germ cell tumor	**22**	**86**	**5**	**22**
Meningioma	218	218	54	54
Neurofibroma	104	104	26	26

4.2   Implementation Details

The experimental program was run on a system equipped with an RTX 3070Ti graphics card. The experimental models were implemented using the PyTorch deep learning framework. The Adam optimizer was used as the objective function optimizer. The brain tumor images were cropped to a size of 288×288. Data augmentation techniques were applied to the training set images. The training process consisted of 200 epochs with a batch size of 16. A dynamic learning rate was employed in the training process.

---

[1] https://www.kaggle.com/datasets/fernando2rad/brain-tumor-mri-images-44c.
[2] https://www.kaggle.com/datasets/tbobbbb/btmri44.

4.3   Evaluation Metrics

Accuracy is the most commonly used evaluation metric, which measures the ratio of correctly classified samples to the total number of samples. The formula is as follows:

$$Accuracy = (TP + TN)/(TP + TN + FP + FN) \qquad (8)$$

Recall, also known as sensitivity or true positive rate, is an evaluation metric that focuses on the positive samples in the original dataset. The formula is as follows:

$$Recall = TP/(TP + FN) \qquad (9)$$

TP (True Positives) denotes the count of positive class samples correctly identified, while TN (True Negatives) represents the count of negative class samples accurately recognized. Conversely, FP (False Positives) refers to the instances where negative class samples are incorrectly classified as positive, and FN (False Negatives) indicates the cases where positive class samples are mistakenly categorized as negative. In addition to the aforementioned metrics, this paper also employs the True Negative Rate (TNR), False Positive Rate (FPR), and False Negative Rate (FNR) to further characterize the performance of the model.

Table 2. T-ResNet18 Experimental Results.

Method	ACC(%)	Recall(%)
Resnet18	87.92	74.26
T-Resnet18(Ours)	**89.88**	**76.07**

4.4   Experimental Results

T-Resnet18 Comparative Experiment. Due to the high detail requirement for brain tumor classification, the accuracy of our proposed T-ResNet18 model is 1.96% higher than that of the standard ResNet18(as shown in Table 2). This improvement is attributed to the incorporation of an attention mechanism within the residual blocks of T-ResNet18, which enhances the sensitivity to features of smaller targets, thereby leading to superior results.

F-DCGAN Comparative Experiment. To delve into the specific effects of F-DCGAN image fusion technology on model performance with small-scale datasets, we undertook a meticulous experimental study. At the outset of the experiment, we employed an untreated, original dataset, the details of which are presented in Table 1. Following this, we introduced a dataset that had been enhanced using F-DCGAN technology for comparative analysis, with the specifics of the enhanced dataset detailed in Table 1. In terms of model selection, we included a range of deep learning architectures, such as T-ResNet18 and ResNet50 [10], to perform a comparative analysis of performance. The summarized results of the experiment are displayed in Table 3. Our approach achieved an accuracy rate of 91.28% during the experiment. Compared to the original dataset, the accuracy rates for T-ResNet18 and ResNet50 were improved by 1.4% and 2%, respectively. Moreover, the recall rates for T-ResNet18 and ResNet50 also saw significant enhancements, reaching 13.08% and 17.1%, respectively. These substantial experimental outcomes strongly confirm that, within the context of adversarial neural networks, combining small-scale datasets with F-DCGAN technology can effectively enhance model performance.

Table 3. The training results of the original dataset are compared with the T-DCGAN amplified dataset.

Method	T-Resnet18		Resnet50	
	Acc(%)	Recall(%)	Acc(%)	Recall(%)
Original dataset	89.88	76.07	89.28	70.10
F-DCGAN	91.28	89.15	91.28	87.20

MT-KD Comparative Experiment. We have employed six classic network architectures, namely T-ResNet18, ResNet34, ResNet50, Mobilenet, Efficient-Net, and Shufflenet [11], and applied them to a dataset generated by the synergistic use of F-DCGAN and adversarial neural networks. By evaluating the performance of these networks on classification tasks, we meticulously selected the "teacher" network with the most superior performance. Subsequently, we integrated not only the three distinguished classic networks but also the T-ResNet18 introduced in this paper into the MT-KD (Mean Teacher Knowledge Distillation) method. Ultimately, we assessed the efficacy of the proposed MT-KD framework by comparing the performance of T-ResNet18 before and after the distillation process.

Initially, we conducted training on these six networks utilizing an image fusion technique based on F-DCGAN. The results of the training are depicted in Fig. 5 on the left, Fig. 6, and Table 4. It was observed that the MobileNet network plateaued at an accuracy of approximately 51% after about 50 training epochs, with no significant enhancement achieved thereafter. In contrast, the other five networks all surpassed an accuracy rate of 90%, with T-ResNet34 and ShuffleNet reaching an accuracy rate above 97%. Notably, ShuffleNet exhibited exceptional stability across all parameters throughout the training process. Additionally, upon a comprehensive evaluation of key metrics including recall rate, true negative rate (TNR), and false positive rate (FPR), it was found that

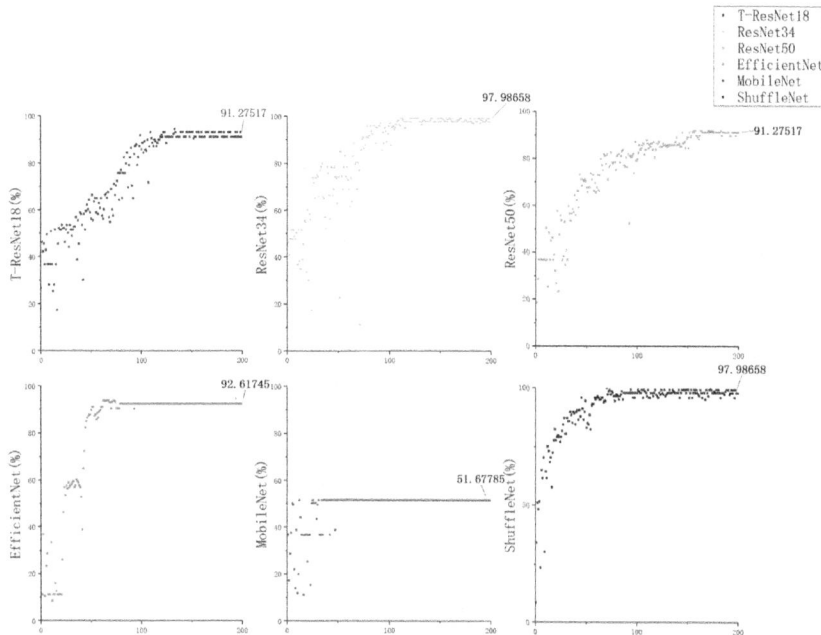

Fig. 6. F-DCGAN amplified dataset training result plot of six classical network models.

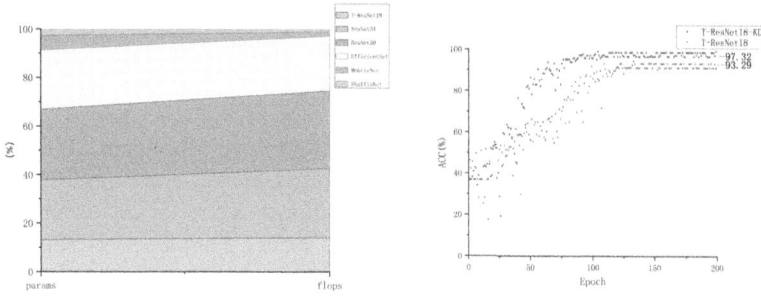

Fig. 7. Comparison chart of parameter quantity and calculation amount area of six classical network models(left);T-Resnet18 results MT-KD knowledge distillation training result graph(right).

ResNet34, EfficientNet, and ShuffleNet all demonstrated superior performance in the task of tumor classification.

Subsequently, we conducted a detailed analysis of the parameter count and computational complexity of these six models to identify three relatively outstanding teacher models. The results are presented in Fig. 7 on the left. Among them, the Shufflenet model offers the optimal combination in terms of param-

Table 4. Training Results of Six Classic Network Models on the Dataset Augmented by F-DCGAN (Underlined models indicate the selected teacher models).

Method	Recall	TNR	NPV	FPR	FNR	FDR	F1	ACC
Resnet34	95.38	0.99	0.99	0.01	0.01	0.05	0.98	97.99
Resnet50	87.20	0.98	0.98	0.02	0.10	0.13	0.92	91.27
Efficienet	93.93	0.98	0.98	0.02	0.08	0.061	0.93	92.62
Mobilenet	36.92	0.90	0.85	0.10	Nan	0.63	0.38	51.68
Shufflenet	96.56	0.99	0.99	0.01	0.02	0.03	0.98	97.99
T-Resnet18(Ours)	89.15	0.98	0.98	0.02	0.10	0.10	0.91	91.28

Table 5. Comparison with related work.

Model	Dataset	Classes	Accuracy
CNN Multi Scale [24]	Nanfang Hospital	3	0.9730
CNN [25]	REMBRANDT	3	0.9613
TL [26]	SARTAJ	3	0.9891
CNN and SVM [27]	Figshare	3	0.9582
Dense Efficient-Net [28]	Figshare	3	0.9997
TL-CNN [29]	Figshare, SARTAJ,BR35H	3	0.9575
LeNet Inspired Model [30]	Figshare,Radiopedia combination	3	0.880
Hybrid GoogLeNet and TL [31]	BR35H	2	0.9910
six TL models [32]	BR35Hand SARTAJ combination	4	0.9712
FM-LiteLearn(Ours)	BT_NAGMN5	5	0.9732

eter count and computational complexity, followed by Mobilenet, T-Resnet18, and Resnet34. Given that Mobilenet exhibited relatively poor performance in training accuracy, and considering that Shufflenet achieved an accuracy rate of 97%, it was decided for this experiment to utilize Shufflenet, Resnet34, and EfficientNet as the teacher networks, with T-Resnet18 serving as the student network.

Ultimately, we employed the Mean Teacher Knowledge Distillation (MT-KD) framework to train the T-ResNet18 network, utilizing Shufflenet, ResNet34, and EfficientNet as the teacher models. Selecting an appropriate temperature parameter and distillation weight can make the probability distribution output by the model more uniform, reducing the over-reliance on specific categories. Such adjustments help the student model to absorb and learn more extensive and general feature representations, thereby enhancing the model's generalization ability. The distillation temperature was set to T=2, and the distillation weight was configured as w=0.3. The experimental outcomes are illustrated in Fig. 7 on the right. Through these experiments, we were able to leverage the MT-KD multi-teacher distillation approach, with Shufflenet, ResNet34, and EfficientNet serving as the teacher models, to train the T-ResNet student model, achieving a 4.03% improvement in the accuracy of the T-ResNet18 model. Consequently, MT-KD knowledge distillation proves to be an extremely beneficial technique that facilitates the transfer of knowledge from complex models to simpler ones, thereby enhancing the accuracy of the latter. It also aids in making the models more efficient and lightweight.

In conclusion, our approach, trained under the FM-LiteLearn framework, has notably outperformed the baseline ResNet18 network, showing a significant 9.4% enhancement in performance. As illustrated in Table 5, our proposed FM-LiteLearn framework has not only matched but also surpassed the performance of existing state-of-the-art methods in brain tumor classification, even without the advantage of a balanced dataset such as BT_NAGMN5. This underscores the effectiveness of our framework post-training. Additionally, the model's compact parameter set contributes to its lightweight nature, offering a swift and efficient solution that is highly promising for clinical use (Table 6).

Table 6. Comparison Based on the BT_NAGMN5 Dataset.

model	dataset	ACC(%)
Resnet18	BT_NAGMN5	89.88
FM-LiteLearn	BT_NAGMN5	**97.32**

5 Conclusion

In this paper, we propose an efficient and rapid classification framework for brain tumor MRI images, named FM-LiteLearn. It is capable of accurately classifying five types of brain tumors—normal tissue, astrocytoma, germinoma, meningioma, neurofibroma, and schwannoma—even under conditions of severe class imbalance. In the experiments, the FM-LiteLearn framework demonstrated an impressive average accuracy rate, achieving 97.31%. The findings indicate that the FM-LiteLearn framework enhances the model's expressive power by integrating T1-weighted and T2-weighted images to create more informative visual representations. Moreover, it employs an innovative Multi-Teacher Knowledge Distillation approach. During the training phase, this method leverages multiple teacher models, with each teacher's contribution being dynamically adjusted. This strategy ensures that the student network can effectively extract valuable features from the teacher networks, significantly improving classification accuracy while reducing computational load. The FM-LiteLearn framework effectively addresses the inherent challenges of complexity and limited data diversity in the classification of brain tumor MRI images.

Acknowledgments. This research has been supported by the Fundamental Research Funds for the Central Universities, Southwest Minzu University (No.3300223136).

References

1. Bidkar, P.S., Kumar, R., Ghosh, A.: SegNet and Salp water optimization-driven deep belief network for segmentation and classification of brain tumor. Gene Expression Patterns **45**, 119248. Elsevier (2022)
2. Ismael, S.A.A., Mohammed, A., Hefny, H.: An enhanced deep learning approach for brain cancer MRI image classification using residual networks. Artif. Intell. Med. **102**, 101779. Elsevier (2020)
3. Mecheter, I., Abbod, M., Amira, A., Zaidi, H.: Deep learning with multiresolution handcrafted features for brain MRI segmentation. Artif. Intell. Med. **131**, 102365. Elsevier (2022)
4. Wadhwa, A., Bhardwaj, A., Verma, V. S.: A review on brain tumor segmentation of MRI images. Mag. Reson. Imaging **61**, 247–259. Elsevier (2019)
5. Hinton, G., Vinyals, O., Dean, J.: Distilling the knowledge in a neural network. arXiv Preprint arXiv:1503.02531 (2015)
6. Xu, P., et al.: Efficient knowledge distillation for Liver CT segmentation using growing assistant network. Phys. Med. Biol. **66**(23), 235005. IOP Publishing (2021)
7. Li, K., Yu, L., Wang, S., Heng, P.-A.: Towards cross-modality medical image segmentation with online mutual knowledge distillation. Proc. AAAI Conf. Artif. Intell. **34**(01), 775–783 (2020)
8. Qi, Y., Zhang, W., Wang, X., You, X., Hu, S., Chen, J.: Efficient knowledge distillation for brain tumor segmentation. Appl. Sci. **12**(23), 11980. MDPI (2022)
9. Chen, L.-C., Papandreou, G., Kokkinos, I., Murphy, K., Yuille, A.L.: DeepLab: semantic image segmentation with deep convolutional nets, atrous convolution, and fully connected CRFs. IEEE Trans. Pattern Anal. Mach. Intell. **40**(4), 834–848. IEEE (2017)
10. Hossain, M.B., Iqbal, S.M.H.S., Islam, M.M., Akhtar, M.N., Sarker, I.H.: Transfer learning with fine-tuned deep CNN ResNet50 model for classifying COVID-19 from chest X-ray images. Inform. Med. Unlocked **30**, 100916. Elsevier (2022)
11. Zhang, X., Zhou, X., Lin, M., Sun, J.: ShuffleNet: an extremely efficient convolutional neural network for mobile devices. In: Proceedings of the IEEE Conference on Computer Vision and Pattern Recognition (CVPR), pp. 6848–6856 (2018)
12. Miglani, A., Madan, H., Kumar, S., Kumar, S.: A literature review on brain tumor detection and segmentation. In: 2021 5th International Conference on Intelligent Computing and Control Systems (ICICCS), pp. 1513–1519. IEEE (2021)
13. Nazir, M., Shakil, S., Khurshid, K.: Role of deep learning in brain tumor detection and classification (2015 to 2020): a review. Comput. Med. Imaging Graph. **91**, 101940. Elsevier (2021)
14. Tiwari, A., Srivastava, S., Pant, M.: Brain tumor segmentation and classification from magnetic resonance images: review of selected methods from 2014 to 2019. Pattern Recogn. Lett. **131**, 244–260. Elsevier (2020)
15. Li, Y., et al.: Whole brain segmentation with full volume neural network. Comput. Med. Imaging Graph. **93**, 101991. Elsevier (2021)
16. Işın, A., Direkoğulları, C., Şah, M.: Review of MRI-based brain tumor image segmentation using deep learning methods. Procedia Comput. Sci. **102**, 317–324. Elsevier (2016)
17. Zhou, T., Ruan, S., Canu, S.: A review: deep learning for medical image segmentation using multi-modality fusion. Array **3**, 100004. Elsevier (2019)
18. Xu, D., Wang, X., Cai, J., Heng, P.-A.: Cross-modality guidance-aided multimodal learning with dual attention for MRI brain tumor grading. arXiv Preprint arXiv:2401.09029 (2024)

19. Liu, Z., et al.: Deep learning based brain tumor segmentation: a survey. Complex Intell. Syst. **9**(1), 1001–1026. Springer (2023). https://doi.org/10.1007/s40747-022-00815-5

20. Pashaei, A., Sajedi, H., Jazayeri, N.: Brain tumor classification via convolutional neural network and extreme learning machines. In: 2018 8th International Conference on Computer and Knowledge Engineering (ICCKE), pp. 314–319. IEEE (2018)

21. Phaye, S.S.R., Sikka, A., Dhall, A., Bathula, D.: Dense and diverse capsule networks: making the capsules learn better. arXiv preprint arXiv:1805.04001 (2018)

22. Ahmad, B., Sun, J., You, Q., Palade, V., Mao, Z.: Brain tumor classification using a combination of variational autoencoders and generative adversarial networks. Biomedicines **10**(2), 223 (2022). MDPI

23. Rezaei, M., Yang, H., Meinel, C.: voxel-GAN: adversarial framework for learning imbalanced brain tumor segmentation. In: Crimi, A., Bakas, S., Kuijf, H., Keyvan, F., Reyes, M., van Walsum, T. (eds.) Brainlesion: Glioma, Multiple Sclerosis, Stroke and Traumatic Brain Injuries: 4th International Workshop, BrainLes 2018, Held in Conjunction with MICCAI 2018, Granada, Spain, September 16, 2018, Revised Selected Papers, Part II, pp. 321–333. Springer International Publishing, Cham (2019). https://doi.org/10.1007/978-3-030-11726-9_29

24. Díaz-Pernas, F.J., Martínez-Zarzuela, M., Antón-Rodríguez, M., González-Ortega, D.: A deep learning approach for brain tumor classification and segmentation using a multiscale convolutional neural network. Healthcare **9**(2), 153 (2021)

25. Sultan, H.H., Salem, N.M., Al-Atabany, W.: Multi-classification of brain tumor images using deep neural network. IEEE Access **7**, 69215–69225 (2019)

26. Ullah, N., et al.: An effective approach to detect and identify brain tumors using transfer learning. Appl. Sci. **12**(11), 5645 (2022)

27. Deepak, S., Ameer, P.M.: Automated categorization of brain tumor from MRI using CNN features and SVM. J. Ambient. Intell. Humaniz. Comput. **12**(8), 8357–8369 (2021)

28. Nayak, D.R., Padhy, N., Mallick, P.K., Zymbler, M., Kumar, S.: Brain tumor classification using dense efficient-net. Axioms **11**(1), 34 (2022)

29. Alanazi, M.F., et al.: Brain tumor/mass classification framework using magnetic-resonance-imaging-based isolated and developed transfer deep-learning model. Sensors **22**(1), 372 (2022)

30. Wahlang, B., et al.: Brain magnetic resonance imaging classification using deep learning architectures with gender and age. Sensors **22**(5), 1766 (2022)

31. Amran, G.A., et al.: Brain tumor classification and detection using hybrid deep tumor network. Electronics **11**(21), 3457 (2022)

32. Gómez-Guzmán, M.A., et al.: Classifying brain tumors on magnetic resonance imaging by using convolutional neural networks. Electronics **12**(4), 955 (2023)

Towards Improving Single-Cell Segmentation in Heterogeneous Configurations of Cardiomyocyte Networks

Fabio Caraffini[1]([✉])[iD], Hassan Eshkiki[1][iD], Mostafa Mohammadpour[2][iD], Nikol Sullo[3][iD], and Christopher H. George[3][iD]

[1] Department of Computer Science, Swansea University, Swansea SA1 8EN, UK
{fabio.caraffini,h.g.eshkiki}@swansea.ac.uk
[2] Department of Computational Perception, Johannes Kepler University, Linz, Austria
mohammadpour@gtec.at
[3] Swansea University Medical School, Faculty of Medicine, Health and Life Sciences, Swansea SA2 8PP, UK
{nikol.sullo,christopher.george}@swansea.ac.uk

Abstract. To explore the formation and deterioration of cellular networks, we develop systems powered by Artificial Intelligence (AI) that accurately distinguish and quantify the differential configuration of cells in those networks (i.e. single cells, multicellular aggregates) as an initial proof-of-concept approach. We use image data acquired from self-organised cardiac cell networks formed in vitro which are difficult to segment using conventional methods. We used two data pre-processing approaches prior to the application of four segmentation algorithms (including two newly generated configurations of the Cellpose algorithm) for a total of eight segmentation pipelines. We demonstrate the effectiveness of a transfer learning capability in improving the accuracy of Cellpose in identifying discrete cells within complex (heterogeneous) cardiac cell network configurations. Our $Cellpose_3^{P1}$ segmentation pipeline displays an F1-Score of 82.34%, a precision of 88.52% and an accuracy of 87.84%. Furthermore, in addition to our new method performing best in its ability to detect discrete cells in each network, it also avoided the problem of erroneously identifying cell boundaries in large multicellular aggregates. This preliminary work shows the feasibility of describing the physical and functional properties of cellular networks using accurate indices of cellular arrangement and heterogeneity.

Keywords: Cell Network · Cardiomyocytes, Segmentation · Cellpose · AI

Supported by the Morgan Advanced Studies Institute, Wales, UK; the National Cardiovascular Research Network (funded by Health and Care Research Wales); the British Heart Foundation.

X. Xie et al. (Eds.): AIiH 2024, LNCS 14976, pp. 104–117, 2024.
https://doi.org/10.1007/978-3-031-67285-9_8

1   Introduction

AI has revolutionised our daily lives by serving as a central component in numerous contexts and fields, including the healthcare industry. There is increasing interest in AI to advance diagnosis, treatment, and patient care [7,28]. Despite the new challenges and issues related to its use in these contexts [28], AI is making significant progress in healthcare applications by detecting patterns in large datasets in a way that humans alone cannot process or process efficiently. Machine Learning algorithms (ML), natural language processing techniques, and computer vision have greatly advanced the extraction of information from large amounts of medical data and help healthcare practitioners in decision-making processes. Typical applications include medical imaging (MRI, X-rays, etc.) [28], drug discovery [17], and electronic health record management [21] to name a few.

In this article, we take a first step toward understanding the formation and deterioration of cellular networks [27] with an AI-driven approach. We focus on cardiac cell networks as an interesting case study since, under experimental conditions in vitro, these networks comprise dynamic configurations of multi-cellular aggregations that arise from physical and functional coupling of individual cells (Fig. 1). At any given point in time, the temporal synchronisation of events across the particular network (e.g., Ca^{2+} signaling) is determined by the organisation and configuration of single cells with distinct boundaries (Fig. 1b, green regions) and those larger structures where it is not possible to define cellular boundaries (Fig. 1b, blue regions). It is therefore important that methods are developed to enable the accurate discrimination and quantification of network regions populated by discrete (boundarised) cells and larger multicellular structures. This initial step is key to understanding the influence and behaviour of cellular configurations in spatially organised cellular networks, which could lead to new knowledge on the link between cardiac cell network deterioration and the progression of cardiovascular disease [12,27]. This is an unexplored domain that is ideally suited for the application of new AI-driven approaches.

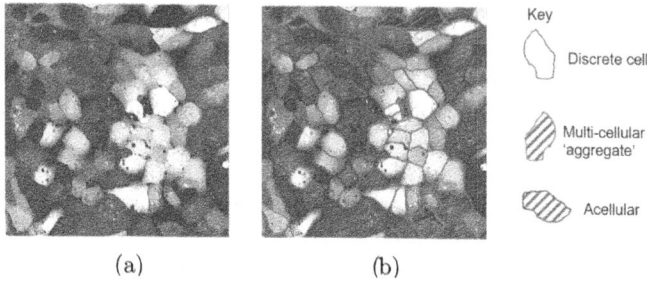

(a)   (b)

Fig. 1. An original greyscaled image (a) and its manually segregated image (b). (Color figure online)

In this proof-of-concept study, we focus on improving the detection of discrete single-cells. The remainder of this paper is structured as follows. Section 2 provides background information on existing cell segmentation systems; Sect. 3 describes the dataset and introduces the methods used to develop and assess the proposed segmentation pipelines to visualise and quantify the physical properties of discrete cells identified; Sect. 4 describes the experimental setup and reports on the validation results; Sect. 5 provides a biological perspective on the information acquired informed by our extensive experience in cardiac cell network research; Sect. 6 concludes this work.

2   Background

The primary goal in 2D cell segmentation is to identify the boundaries that demark cell edges. The expected result is a binary-valued mask showing a region of cells. In traditional computer vision, it is common to apply thresholding to convert a greyscale image to a binary image before segmenting it. This requires setting an intensity value, i.e. the threshold, that discriminates cells from the background by assigning only two possible values to pixels, whether their values are greater or smaller than the threshold. Several variants have been proposed to perform this task optimally, as the wrong choice of threshold value can lead to erroneous identification that introduces analytical artefacts. The Otsu method [18] is an iterative thresholding method that seeks an optimal threshold value by minimising intraclass variance, that is, the weighted variance between foreground and background, and appears to be suitable for white blood cell segmentation [24]. On the contrary, grid search thresholding compares the results of prefixed threshold values with the true label and selects the one that shows the best performance, e.g., in terms of F1-Score [29]. Active contours, see [1], is another 'energy-based' model for cell detection and segmentation that iteratively minimise an energy function while deforming a curve to fit the cell boundary.

In the last decade, Deep Learning (DL) has emerged as a new area of ML that takes advantage of multiple layers of non-linear information processing units for (supervised or unsupervised) feature extraction, pattern analysis, and classification. A Convolutional Neural Network (CNN) is a DL approach suitable for classification problems and image manipulation. Recently, CNNs have been adopted for semantic-based image segmentation tasks by exploiting their classification capabilities to binarily label each pixel of an image and thus segment it [4,5]. Initially, CNNs were used in patch-based methods in biomedical image processing, classifying pixels based on their neighbourhood attributes to address segmentation challenges in, e.g., neural cell imagery. Methods such as the 'multitask learning with a similarity interface' [22] were proposed to make them more suitable for segmentation tasks in microscopy images.

The U-net model proposed in [23] is another DL algorithm that features up- and down-sampling layers and the corresponding skip connections and is well known for its efficiency in segmentation tasks. U-net processes the entire image and directly generates a segmentation map that takes advantage of all contextual information from the image. This method offers advantages over patch-based CNNs. Since its publication, the literature has been populated with variants of

U-net, such as the V-net proposed in [16]. The latter improves upon U-net by including 3D convolution units that make it suitable for 3D segmentation. More complex structures are, e.g., those in [15], where a fully convolutional network is used to enable end-to-end semantic segmentation at the pixel level, and the M-Net model presented in [8], which features a multiscale input layer, a U-shaped convolutional network, a side output layer, and a multi-label loss function. An attentive cell instance segmentation method that uses the joint action of U-net and a single-shot multi-box detector is available in [31], while a versatile algorithm suitable for multiple tasks, including target classification, detection, semantic segmentation, instance segmentation, and recognition of human pose, among others, is known as the mask recurrent-CNN model [14].

Cellpose [26], is a widely used versatile DL algorithm with a U-Net-style architecture and residual blocks for cell and nucleus segmentation that was designed to process various types of images without requiring extensive training data or parameter tuning. Cellpose stands out for its adaptability (even to 3D images without needing specific 3D-labelled data) and ease of use. Cellpose developers trained this model using a variety of images sourced from the Internet from different datasets, including images of red and white blood cells, plasma cells, hanseniaspora, and animal tissue cells, by searching for keywords such as 'cytoplasm', 'cellular microscopy,' and 'fluorescent cells'. This vast training dataset gives Cellpose broad applicability and it is expected to work well even with noise, excessively bright fluorescence, insufficient brightness, or sub-optimal stain quality. For the same reasons, it represents an obvious choice for many healthcare professionals in the analysis of clinical imaging data. However, despite its numerous advantages and rich featureset, Cellpose was developed to detect discrete cellular units clearly demarked by boundaries. As described above and shown explicitly in Fig. 1, these discrete cells are not the only component of physically and functionally coupled cardiac cell networks *in vitro*. The utility of cellular identification tools in this context needs to be rigorously evaluated, and in this preliminary work, we report on our findings to date.

3   Methodology

Conventional ML and complex DL approaches have strengths and weaknesses. The former methods generally exhibit inferior accuracy in segmenting microscopy images with complex backgrounds, especially in the presence of very small, atypically 'bright' elements; they are difficult to design; they face difficulties in handling extensive datasets. However, they have less demand for large training data; they are more explainable and computationally cheaper than the latter. Most CNNs typically require a significantly larger amount of manually-labelled training data and involve more computations than traditional ML approaches [2], all in search of superior performance.

We address the problem of segmenting heterogeneous cell configurations comprising 2D cardiac cell networks *in vitro* which comprise our foundational dataset. We focus on the application of the Cellpose algorithm, recognising it as a state-of-the-art platform for cellular identification/quantification and due to its promising results in semantic segmentation [19,25,26].

We present the results obtained with the three best algorithmic configurations we found. We refer to them as $\mathtt{Cellpose}_i$, with $i \in \{1,2,3\}$, and compare among themselves with another widely used segmentation model. We present two data preparation methods, which we apply to all models under study, thus obtaining eight possible segmentation strategies following the pipeline in Fig. 2. More details are provided in the following sections.

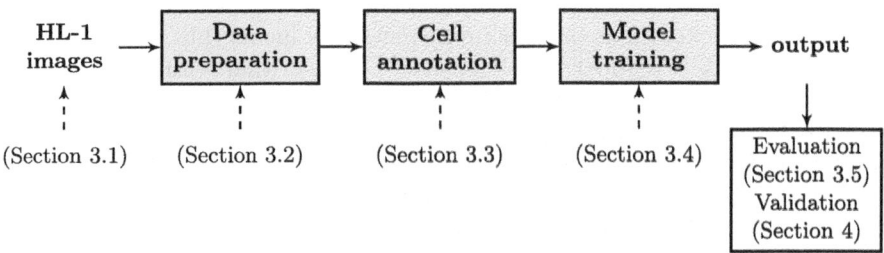

Fig. 2. General segmentation pipeline.

3.1   The HL-1 Cardiac Cell Network Imaging Dataset

HL-1 cardiomyocytes are an immortalised mouse atrial-derived cell line that has been extensively characterised by us [3,6,9,10]. Since HL-1 cells retain a remarkable proliferative capacity, the cellular density and interactions formed by these cells in vitro reflect 'random' self-organised network configurations. We analyse an image dataset comprising 92 HL-1 cell networks in which cells had been loaded with the fluorescent calcium reporter dye, fluo-3. The intense fluorescence of fluo-3 retained inside cells allows for a robust assessment of 'single' cellular boundaries although its distribution across all cells in the network is heterogeneous (Fig. 1a) which can make discrete cellular identification difficult. Each network was visualised using 180 images collected in 60 s (i.e., a frame capture rate of $0.3Hz$). Each image had dimensions of 512×512 pixels and defined a physical area of $61,504 \mu m^2$.

3.2   Data Preparation

To perform segmentation, it is required to produce a composite image from the image stack. We do this by 1) isolating frames for greyscale conversion and, if necessary, preprocessing them to improve the quality of the segmented result (as indicated in the next paragraph); 2) stacking them to compute their average; and 3) scaling the intensities of the average composite image within $0 - 255^1$.

---

[1] This value is imposed by the employed acquisition system.

After trying multiple approaches for Step 1), we empirically found two simple suitable methods that produced satisfactory results. The first approach is to use the greyscaled images and proceed directly to Step 2) (no further processing is needed). In the second method, histogram equalisation is performed on the greyscaled images. This is a technique used in image processing to enhance the contrast of an image by redistributing pixel intensities to cover the entire dynamic range evenly. This process helps to improve the visual appearance of images by making details more visible in both dark and bright areas [30]. Steps 2) and 3) are self-explanatory.

Note that averaging the images is a simple but beneficial approach, which helps filter out noise from (unprocessed) images. As can be seen in Fig. 3a, the unprocessed source experimental images are noisy. However, see Figs. 3b and 3c, the effect of noise is mitigated after averaging the frames.

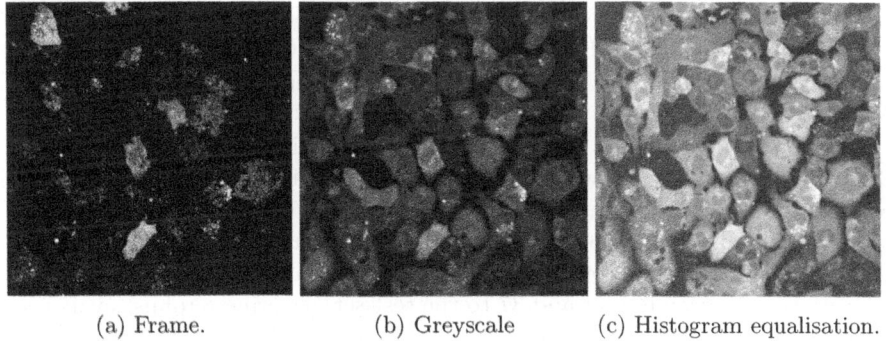

    (a) Frame.   (b) Greyscale   (c) Histogram equalisation.

Fig. 3. Data (image) preparation - an example of a raw single-image frame (a) and its greyscale version without (b) and with (c) histogram equalisation.

For convenience, we refer to the first data preparation pipeline (without equalisation) as p_1 and to the second (with equalisation) as p_2.

3.3 Cell Annotation

The Cellpose Graphical User Interface (GUI) allows drawing Ground-Truth (GT) masks. We used it to label individual cells, as shown in Fig. 4.

In the present work, we focus exclusively on the segmentation/annotation of those cells with a clearly visible boundary (Fig. 1b, green outlines). All 92 composite images previously obtained following the processing described in Sect. 3.2 are annotated, and the corresponding masks are saved for the training process.

3.4 Segmentation Algorithms and Training

We employ Cellpose in three different configurations.

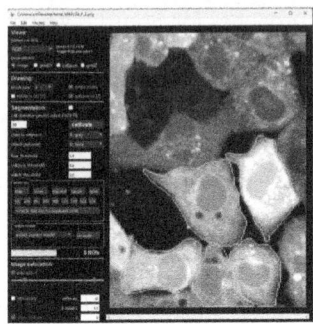

Fig. 4. Using Cellpose GUI to annotate the composite cellular network images.

The first, Cellpose$_1$, simply refers to the built-in pre-trained Cyto2 model available from the CellPose repository [26].

Cellpose$_2$ is instead obtained by retraining the Cellpose architecture from scratch with our dataset. This allows us to see the performance when the model is highly specialised in HL-1 cells.

Cellpose$_3$ is obtained by fine-tuning a pre-trained Cellpose model (i.e., Cellpose$_1$). In summary, we used existing Cyto2 weights to train a new model with our HL-1 data, thus adopting a particular kind of transfer learning [13].

We randomly divide the dataset into training and testing sets using a division ratio of 60/40%. With a total of 92 cell images available, 55 of these images are allocated to the training set and 37 to the test set, ensuring a robust evaluation of the model's performance on unseen data. The algorithms require image masks for training, and we use our annotations for this purpose. Each model is trained for 100 epochs. For optimal training performance and stability, all three versions of Cellpose are empirically optimised with the best configuration featuring a ReLu activation function, a learning rate of 10^{-3}, and a batch size of 8.

We also produce segmentation results with StarDist [25] for comparison. This is another widely used model based on the CNN architecture that detects individual cells by simultaneously generating a distance map and an object probability map. The success of this algorithm is due to the joint use of the maps that enables a precise delineation of cell boundaries for cells with irregular shapes and complex arrangements. StarDist represents cell boundaries using star-convex polygons, offering flexibility in capturing various cellular morphologies. This model also requires annotated data for the training data, typically comprising images paired with manually segmented cell outlines, which facilitates the network's ability to predict cell segmentations accurately. We used a StarDist pre-trained model on a subset of 497 fluorescence microscopy images.

3.5   Evaluation Metrics

We use the five established evaluation metrics described in Table 1, which are calculated in terms of 'pixel-wise' True Positive (TP), False Positive (FP), False Negative (FN), and True Negative (TN), in the context of segmentation [11,20].

Table 1. Performance Metrics in Image Segmentation

Metric	Description	Formula
Accuracy	Proportion of correctly classified samples	$\frac{TP+TN}{TP+TN+FP+FN}$
Precision	Proportion of TP predictions among all positive predictions	$\frac{TP}{TP+FP}$
Recall	Proportion of TP predictions among all actual positives	$\frac{TP}{TP+FN}$
F1-Score	Measure of overlap between predicted and GT regions	$\frac{2\times TP}{2\times TP+FP+FN}$
Intersection over Union (IoU)	Measure of overlap between predicted and GT regions	$\frac{TP}{TP+FP+FN}$

Note that the accuracy metric is often also commonly misused and over-emphasised. F1-Score (also known as Dice similarity) can be of greater significance in segmentation problems, as it allows us to understand alignments with the GT, similarly, for IoU (also known as the Jaccard similarity index).

4   Validation Results

Using the p_1 and p_2 data preparation methods outlined in Sect. 3.2, and applying the four models described in Sect. 3.4, we obtain eight algorithmic setups for the segmentation task. Some graphical results (validation) are shown in Figs. 5 and 6 for the preparation methods p_1 and p_2, respectively.

It can be immediately noticed that the original Cellpose algorithm, i.e., Cellpose$_1$, presents challenges in accurately distinguishing certain cell borders, particularly irregular ones, and when cellular density is visibly higher, leading to difficulties in correctly detecting cells. Furthermore, it occasionally identifies two separate cells instead of a single cell, which adds to its limitations in precise cell detection (Fig. 5b). Cellpose$_2$, see Fig. 5c, shows improved detection capabilities in cases with non-discernible boundaries compared to Cellpose$_1$, but suffers from undersegmentation in certain regions. On visual inspection, Cellpose$_3$ appears to be more accurate than the other Cellpose setups (Fig. 5d) and than StarDist (Fig. 5e), which seems to perform worse than all other models.

Numerically, the segmentation results are validated by the metrics in Table 1 computed throughout the test set, which comprises 37 images. Each evaluation metric is calculated for each cell, and then the average value (avg) and standard deviation (std) are calculated to provide an overall assessment of the performance of the model. Validation results are reported in Table 2, where the best value (i.e., highest avg and smallest std) per model and for each evaluation metric is reported in bold (except for cases with nonsignificant differences). The asterisk shows the algorithmic setup that performs best per metric.

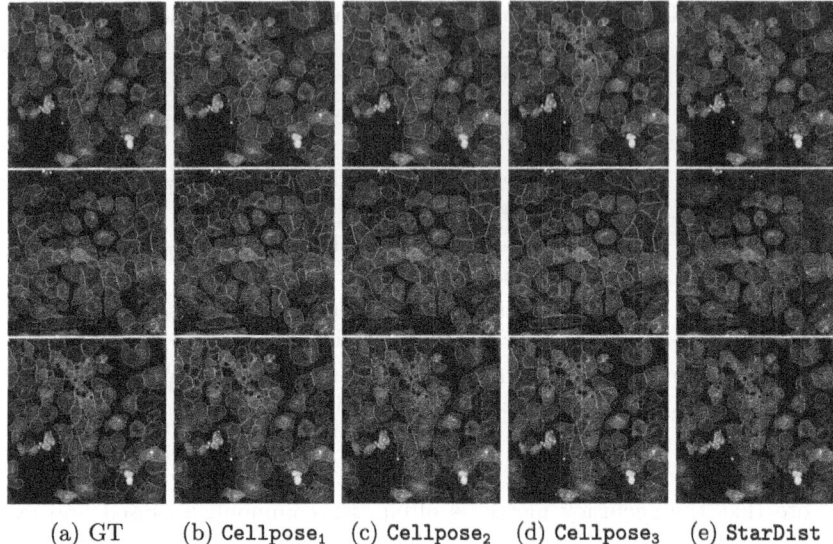

(a) GT   (b) Cellpose$_1$ (c) Cellpose$_2$ (d) Cellpose$_3$ (e) StarDist

Fig. 5. Segmentation results with the p_1 image preparation strategy.

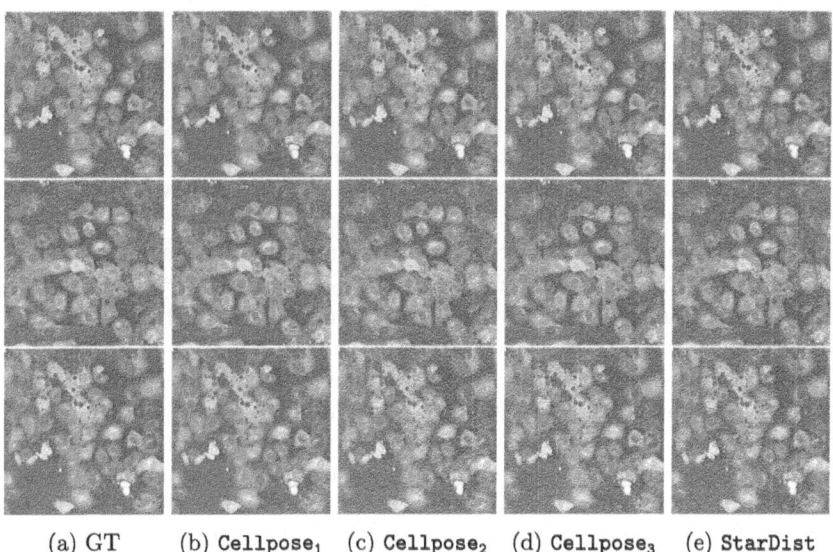

(a) GT   (b) Cellpose$_1$ (c) Cellpose$_2$ (d) Cellpose$_3$ (e) StarDist

Fig. 6. Segmentation results with the p_2 image preparation strategy.

Interestingly, the simpler p_1 data preparation method leads to better performance than p_2 in most cases. Cellpose$_3$ always outperforms the other methods except in terms of recall, where Cellpose$_2$ displays marginally superior performance (of 1.19%). The results for Cellpose$_3$ are satisfactory, with an average

Table 2. Models evaluation results.

Algorithmic setup		Evaluation metrics				
		IoU (%)	F1-Score(%)	Precision(%)	Recall(%)	Accuracy(%)
Cellpose$_1$	p_1	**55.44 ± 22.58**	**67.94 ± 23.67**	71.21 ± 24.60	**72.96 ± 24.12**	**78.34 ± 9.77**
	p_2	49.15 ± 23.10	62.11 ± 24.84	71.24 ± 24.08	63.66 ± 27.80	75.78 ± 10.58
Cellpose$_2$	p_1	**68.43 ± 17.91**	**79.42 ± 17.63**	79.29 ± 19.16	*82.43 ± 17.90	85.53 ± 6.93
	p_2	65.82 ± 18.77	77.40 ± 17.94	**86.05 ± 16.99**	72.38 ± 21.16	84.56 ± 8.16
Cellpose$_3$	p_1	*71.98 ± 16.25	*82.34 ± 14.76	*88.52 ± 9.45	80.24 ± 17.09	*87.84 ± 5.69
	p_2	71.15 ± 16.62	81.79 ± 14.18	88.41 ± 11.88	79.16 ± 16.71	87.21 ± 6.38
StarDist	p_1	**43.75 ± 16.42**	**58.86 ± 17.84**	**81.74 ± 23.46**	50.01 ± 19.80	**73.19 ± 13.48**
	p_2	40.21 ± 20.84	53.94 ± 23.27	67.79 ± 22.57	49.70 ± 26.60	70.62 ± 12.22

precision of 87.84% with p_1 and an average precision of 87.84% with p_2. The IoU and F1-Score are also good, with an average of 71.98% and 82.34%, respectively.

The StarDist algorithm is always outperformed by the three Cellpose configurations, regardless of the preparation of input data. This algorithm displays the best results on round-shaped cells, which is not always the case. In addition, roundness is often a consequence of cell death, which introduces the risk of defining networks by the extent of death. However, the latter appears to be more 'precise' than Cellpose$_1$, as it is StarDist^{p_1} than Cellpose$_2^{p_2}$ (the superscript denotes the data preparation method to simplify notation). Due to the high values of std, it can be argued that StarDist^{p_1} is similar to Cellpose$_1^{p_2}$ in terms of IoU and F1-Score.

Hence, the segmentation pipeline that stands out is Cellpose$_3^{p_1}$, despite histogram equalisation visually resulting in clearer images, and graphical results may also favour p_2 for this reason. This suggests that Cellpose$_3^{p_1}$ detects features that we cannot easily see and which equalisation cannot reveal. It is important to note that the latter enhances contrast when there is a limited range of intensity values. However, in cases where spatial correlation is more significant than intensity, it may result in unrealistic effects that alter the shape of cells.

From the produced segmented images, we extrapolate[2] the area and eccentricity of each identified discrete cell. The first parameter is calculated as the total pixel count within a defined cellular boundary, while the second, indicating cell elongation or roundness, is calculated as the ratio of the best-fit ellipse's focal distance to the cell's shape. These are discussed in the next section.

5   Cellular Network Analysis

Extending some of the qualitative information provided by model validation (Sect. 3.5), we systematically evaluate the quantitative outputs of each model relating to three key metrics (cell number, cell area, and cell eccentricity) in 30 randomly selected networks. We find that StarDist is the algorithm most

---

[2] This is done in Python with measure.regionprops from skimage.

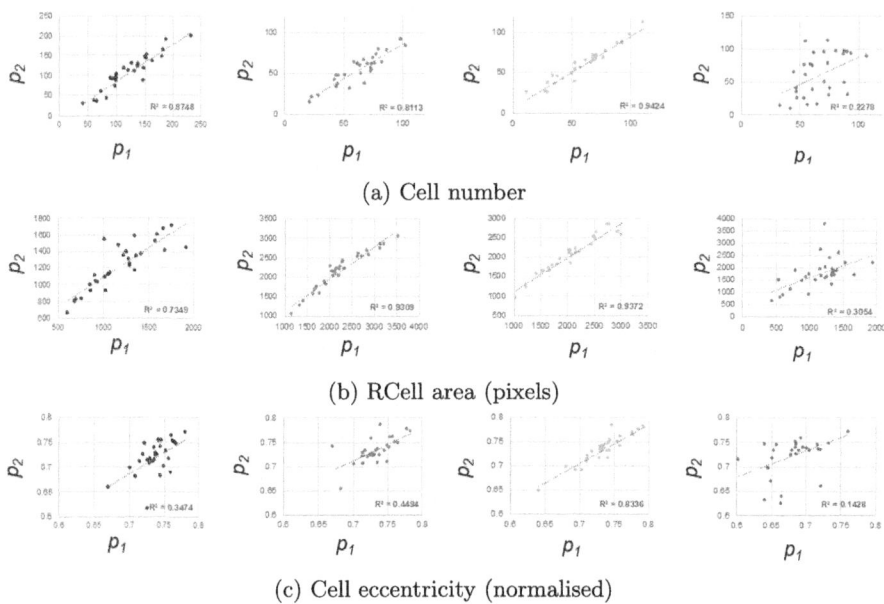

(a) Cell number

(b) RCell area (pixels)

(c) Cell eccentricity (normalised)

Fig. 7. Regression analysis of 30 chosen networks on the effect of P_1 and P_2 for (left to right) $\boxed{\texttt{Cellpose}_1}$, $\boxed{\texttt{Cellpose}_2}$, $\boxed{\texttt{Cellpose}_3}$ and $\boxed{\texttt{StarDist}}$.

influenced by the preprocessing mode and performs poorly on all metrics when p_1 and p_2 were directly compared ($R^2 < 0.35$ in all instances) (Fig. 7).

Cellpose$_2$ and Cellpose$_3$ are much less influenced by the preprocessing mode, and Cellpose$_3$ overall exhibits a better performance ($R^2 > 0.8$ for all metrics). Benchmarking the performance of all methods against Cellpose$_1$, we found that Cellpose$_2$ and Cellpose$_3$ identified many fewer discrete cells (Fig. 8) that are physically larger cells (Fig. 7).

However, upon closer scrutiny of the segmented composite images of each of the 30 networks, we found that while Cellpose$_1$ identifies more 'cells', this algorithm tended to erroneously identify many 'discrete' cells (i.e., nucleated structures) within the multi-cellular aggregates (Fig. 1, blue regions) resulting in the gross over-estimation of the number of discrete cells in the network. Cellpose$_2$ and Cellpose$_3$ does not reproduce this error, and visual inspection of the segmentation done by these methods reveals that their identification of single (discretely boundarised) cells in the network was remarkably accurate. Preliminary data suggest Cellpose$_3$ is the best algorithm for our purpose. The data also show that StarDist identifies numerous elements that are too small to be plausibly considered as cells (i.e., have pixel dimensions < 100; Table 3) and this undesirable feature, together with other limitations (Fig. 7 and 8) highlights that StarDist is not useful for our purposes.

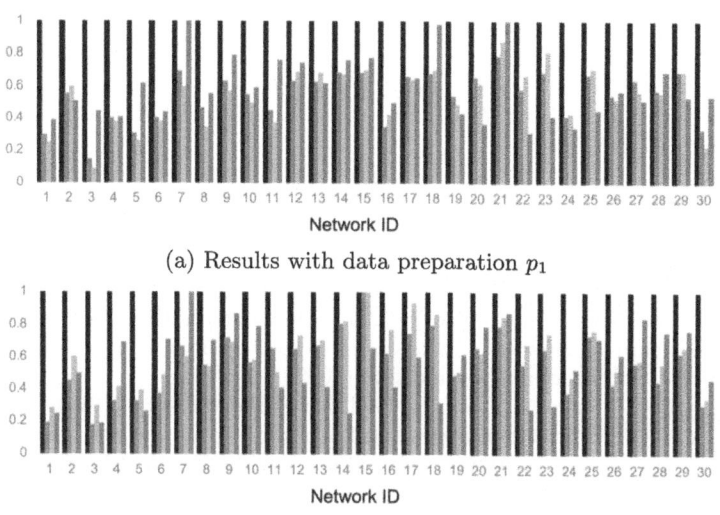

(a) Results with data preparation p_1

(b) Results with data preparation p_2

Fig. 8. Number of discrete cells segmented with $\boxed{\texttt{Cellpose}_1}$, $\boxed{\texttt{Cellpose}_2}$, $\boxed{\texttt{Cellpose}_3}$ and $\boxed{\texttt{StarDist}}$, normalised to $\texttt{Cellpose}_1$.

Table 3. Proportion of segregated non-cellular elements.

Cellpose$_1$		Cellpose$_2$		Cellpose$_3$		StarDist	
p_1	p_2	p_1	p_2	p_1	p_2	p_1	p_2
0.104%	0.213%	0.051%	0.117%	0.052%	0.053%	24.130%	10.597%

6   Conclusion

In this proof-of-concept work, we have shown the utility of a transfer learning algorithm to improve the accuracy of Cellpose to identify discrete cells in complex (heterogeneous) cardiac cell networks. This work should now be extended to the development of parallel methods that can quantify key features that describe the larger multicellular aggregates that are a hallmark feature of in vitro formed cardiac cell networks (e.g., HL-1 and induced pluripotent stem cell-derived cardiomyocyte networks). Pending this outcome, we will then be able to describe cardiac cell networks in terms of 'single cellularity' and 'multicellularity' and begin reconciling these indices with new information on the functional competency of the networks under test (e.g., normal 'healthy' networks or deteriorating 'disease-like' networks).

References

1. Bamford, P., Lovell, B.: Unsupervised cell nucleus segmentation with active contours. Signal Process. **71**(2), 203–213 (1998). https://doi.org/10.1016/S0165-1684(98)00145-5
2. Caicedo, J.C., et al.: Evaluation of deep learning strategies for nucleus segmentation in fluorescence images. Cytometry A **95**(9), 952–965 (2019)
3. George, C.H.: Arrhythmogenic mutation-linked defects in ryanodine receptor autoregulation reveal a novel mechanism of ca < 2+ > release channel dysfunction. Circ. Res. **98**, 88–97 (2006)
4. Ciresan, D., Giusti, A., Gambardella, L., Schmidhuber, J.: Deep neural networks segment neuronal membranes in electron microscopy images. In: Advances in Neural Information Processing Systems **25** (2012)
5. Cireşan, D.C., Giusti, A., Gambardella, L.M., Schmidhuber, J.: Mitosis detection in breast cancer histology images with deep neural networks. In: Mori, K., Sakuma, I., Sato, Y., Barillot, C., Navab, N. (eds.) MICCAI 2013, Part II. LNCS, vol. 8150, pp. 411–418. Springer, Heidelberg (2013). https://doi.org/10.1007/978-3-642-40763-5_51
6. Claycomb, W.C., et al.: Hl-1 cells: a cardiac muscle cell line that contracts and retains phenotypic characteristics of the adult cardiomyocyte. Proc. Natl. Acad. Sci. **95**(6), 2979–2984 (1998)
7. Esteva, A., et al.: Dermatologist-level classification of skin cancer with deep neural networks. Nature **542**(7639), 115–118 (2017)
8. Fu, H., Cheng, J., Xu, Y., Wong, D.W.K., Liu, J., Cao, X.: Joint optic disc and cup segmentation based on multi-label deep network and polar transformation. IEEE Trans. Med. Imaging **37**(7), 1597–1605 (2018)
9. George, C.H., Higgs, G.V., Lai, F.A.: Ryanodine receptor mutations associated with stress-induced ventricular tachycardia mediate increased calcium release in stimulated cardiomyocytes. Circ. Res. **93**(6), 531–540 (2003)
10. George, C.H., et al.: Alternative splicing of ryanodine receptors modulates cardiomyocyte ca2+ signaling and susceptibility to apoptosis. Circ. Res. **100**(6), 874–883 (2007)
11. Ghaznavi, A., Rychtáriková, R., Saberioon, M., Štys, D.: Cell segmentation from telecentric bright-field transmitted light microscopy images using a residual attention U-Net: a case study on Hela line. Comput. Biol. Med. **147**, 105805 (2022)
12. Gintant, G.A., George, C.H.: Introduction to biological complexity as a missing link in drug discovery. Expert Opin. Drug Discov. **13**(8), 753–763 (2018)
13. Hallou, A., Yevick, H.G., Dumitrascu, B., Uhlmann, V.: Deep learning for bioimage analysis in developmental biology. Development **148**(18), dev199616 (2021)
14. He, K., Gkioxari, G., Dollár, P., Girshick, R.: Mask R-CNN. In: Proceedings of the IEEE International Conference on Computer Vision, pp. 2961–2969 (2017)
15. Long, J., Shelhamer, E., Darrell, T.: Fully convolutional networks for semantic segmentation. In: Proceedings of the IEEE Conference on Computer Vision and Pattern Recognition, pp. 3431–3440 (2015)
16. Milletari, F., Navab, N., Ahmadi, S.A.: V-net: fully convolutional neural networks for volumetric medical image segmentation. In: 2016 Fourth International Conference on 3D Vision (3DV), pp. 565–571. IEEE (2016)
17. Mock, M., Edavettal, S., Langmead, C., Russell, A.: Ai can help to speed up drug discovery-but only if we give it the right data. Nature **621**(7979), 467–470 (2023)

18. Otsu, N.: A threshold selection method from gray-level histograms. IEEE Trans. Syst. Man Cybern. **9**(1), 62–66 (1979). https://doi.org/10.1109/TSMC.1979.4310076
19. Pachitariu, M., Stringer, C.: Cellpose 2.0: how to train your own model. Nat. Methods **19**(12), 1634–1641 (2022)
20. Punn, N.S., Agarwal, S.: Modality specific u-net variants for biomedical image segmentation: a survey. Artif. Intell. Rev. **55**(7), 5845–5889 (2022)
21. Rajkomar, A., et al.: Scalable and accurate deep learning with electronic health records. NPJ Digital Medicine **1**(1), 1–10 (2018)
22. Ramesh, N., Tasdizen, T.: Cell segmentation using a similarity interface with a multi-task convolutional neural network. IEEE J. Biomed. Health Inform. **23**(4), 1457–1468 (2018)
23. Ronneberger, O., Fischer, P., Brox, T.: U-net: convolutional networks for biomedical image segmentation. In: Navab, N., Hornegger, J., Wells, W.M., Frangi, A.F. (eds.) MICCAI 2015, Part III. LNCS, vol. 9351, pp. 234–241. Springer, Cham (2015). https://doi.org/10.1007/978-3-319-24574-4_28
24. Salem, N., Sobhy, N.M., El Dosoky, M.: A comparative study of white blood cells segmentation using OTSU threshold and watershed transformation. J. Biomed. Eng. Med. Imaging **3**(3), 15 (2016)
25. Schmidt, U., Weigert, M., Broaddus, C., Myers, G.: Cell detection with star-convex polygons. In: Frangi, A.F., Schnabel, J.A., Davatzikos, C., Alberola-López, C., Fichtinger, G. (eds.) MICCAI 2018, Part II. LNCS, vol. 11071, pp. 265–273. Springer, Cham (2018). https://doi.org/10.1007/978-3-030-00934-2_30
26. Stringer, C., Wang, T., Michaelos, M., Pachitariu, M.: Cellpose: a generalist algorithm for cellular segmentation. Nat. Methods **18**(1), 100–106 (2021)
27. Strogatz, S.H.: Exploring complex networks. Nature **410**(6825), 268–276 (2001)
28. Topol, E.J.: High-performance medicine: the convergence of human and artificial intelligence. Nat. Med. **25**(1), 44–56 (2019)
29. Vicar, T., et al.: Cell segmentation methods for label-free contrast microscopy: review and comprehensive comparison. BMC Bioinform. **20**, 1–25 (2019)
30. Wang, X., Cheng, E., Burnett, I.S.: Improved (stem) cell segmentation with histogram matching image contrast enhancement. In: 2015 IEEE China Summit and International Conference on Signal and Information Processing (ChinaSIP), pp. 816–820. IEEE (2015)
31. Yi, J., Wu, P., Jiang, M., Huang, Q., Hoeppner, D.J., Metaxas, D.N.: Attentive neural cell instance segmentation. Med. Image Anal. **55**, 228–240 (2019)

Texture Feature Analysis
for Classification of Early-Stage Prostate
Cancer in MpMRI

Asmail Muftah[1,2] , S. M. Shermer[3(✉)] , and Frank C. Langbein[1]

[1] School of Computer Science and Informatics, Cardiff University, Cardiff, UK
{MuftahA,LangbeinFC}@cardiff.ac.uk, asmail.muftah@azu.edu.ly
[2] School of Science, Azzaytuna University, Tarhounah, Libya
[3] Faculty of Science and Engineering (Physics), Swansea University, Singleton Park
Campus, Swansea, UK
s.m.shermer@gmail.com

Abstract. Magnetic resonance imaging (MRI) has become a crucial
tool in the diagnosis and staging of prostate cancer, owing to its superior tissue contrast. However, it also creates large volumes of data that
must be assessed by trained experts, a time-consuming and laborious
task. This has prompted the development of machine learning tools for
the automation of Prostate cancer (PCa) risk classification based on
multiple MRI modalities (T2W, ADC, and high-b-value DWI). Understanding and interpreting the predictions made by the models, however,
remains a challenge. We analyze Random Forests (RF) and Support
Vector Machines (SVM), for two complementary datasets, the public
Prostate-X dataset, and an in-house, mostly early-stage PCa dataset to
elucidate the contributions made by first-order statistical features, Haralick texture features, and local binary patterns to the classification. Using
correlation analysis and Shapley impact scores, we find that many of the
features typically used are strongly correlated, and that the majority of
features have negligible impact on the classification. We identify a small
set of features that determine the classification outcome, which may aid
the development of explainable AI approaches.

Keywords: Early-Stage Prostate Cancer · Magnetic Resonance
Imaging · Classification · Machine Learning · Explainable AI

1 Introduction

The early detection of prostate cancer (PCa) typically relies on blood tests such
as the prostate-specific antigen (PSA) test and digital rectal examination (DRE),
followed by transrectal ultrasound (TRUS) biopsy [26]. However, TRUS biopsy
carries the risk of serious complications, including meningitis and sepsis [15].

Supported by Azzaytuna University and the Ministry of Higher Education and Scientific Research, Libya and Supercomputing Wales.

Furthermore, it can lead to the detection of clinically insignificant or indolent cancer, resulting in overdiagnosis and potentially unnecessary treatments [1]. To improve diagnosis and minimize unnecessary biopsies, multiparametric MRI (mpMRI) has become the standard of care in the diagnosis and staging of PCa. The resulting high volume of imaging data generated has in turn stimulated significant research efforts to develop effective machine learning tools to assist radiologists with the segmentation and classification of lesions, and both traditional and deep-learning methods have been applied successfully to the problem of identifying clinically significant lesions (see, e.g., [2,4,7,8,11,14,20,27,29,30]).

Despite the increasing popularity of deep learning approaches, recent work evaluating the performance of convolutional neural networks (CNNs) and transfer learning, as well as traditional machine learning classifiers based on handcrafted features such as first-order statistics, Haralick features [9] and local binary patterns (LBP) [21], suggests that traditional machine learning methods such as Support Vector Machines (SVM) and especially Random Forest (RF) classifiers can perform at least as well as deep learning classifiers or better [3,5,8,13,19,22,23,28]. Machine learning tools based on handcrafted features are also well suited to feature analysis with the aim of explainability. Explainability remains a challenge for machine learning, but recent work, for example, has explored explanable AI to predict cancer based on gene expression [24], and survival rates predicted by synoptic reporting of pathology [10].

In this work, we study explanability in the context of PCa classification based on mpMRI data by exploring the features used by the best-performing traditional machine learning classifiers to understand which are most relevant, and their respective impact on the classification results. The best-performing classifiers trained for classifying rectangular prostate patches into suspicious (positive) and normal (negative) based on first-order statistical features, Haralick texture features and LBP using sequential backward floating feature selection (SBSF) are identified by clustering their performance according to multiple performance metrics (AUC, Accuracy, F1-score, sensitivity and specificity). All classifiers are trained on two complementary datasets, the public ProstateX database, and an in-house dataset of patients with suspected early-stage PCa, as well as a dataset combing these two. Feature correlation and utilization are studied using correlation analysis and Shapley impact scores to reveal a small set of features that consistently explain most of the classification results for both datasets.

2   Datasets

To assess the performance of various machine learning algorithms, two datasets are utilized: the publicly available ProstateX dataset [12] and an in-house collection of anonymized mpMRI data, primarily representing early-stage PCa. The ProstateX dataset comprises 194 negative and 71 positive samples. The in-house dataset comprises 44 negative and 46 positive samples, selected from a cohort of patients who had undergone mpMRI scans at a local clinical imaging unit. Leveraging both datasets enhances the comprehensiveness of our evaluation, provides valuable insights into the applicability of algorithms across diverse patient

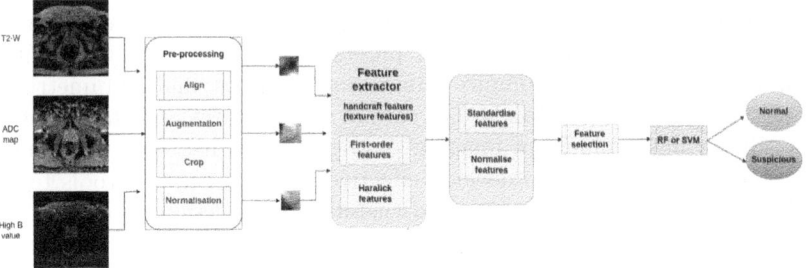

Fig. 1. Traditional machine learning classification pipeline.

cohorts, and facilitates a deeper understanding of their robustness and generalizability in a broader clinical setting.

For both datasets, we incorporate (axial) T2-weighted (T2W) images, apparent diffusion coefficient (ADC) maps, and high-b-value diffusion-weighted images (DWI) generated by the imaging system, as illustrated in Fig. 1. All modalities are registered using the patient coordinate system from the DICOM files, as manual verification suggests that further automated registration is prone to introducing larger errors. The 12-bit intensity values in each modality are rescaled to the range [0, 1]. Given the limited size of the datasets, data augmentation techniques are employed to generate additional samples for each patient in the respective datasets, adding 39 samples per patient. Augmentation methods include rotation, flipping, scaling, elastic deformation, shearing, Gaussian noise, blur, and adjustments to contrast and brightness. Subsequently, PCa lesions are extracted as 2D patches and resized to either 16 × 16 or 32 × 32 based on segmentation masks indicating negative and positive regions for PCa. For the in-house early-stage PCa dataset, classification relies on a set of normal and suspicious regions identified by the reporting radiologist. For the ProstateX dataset, lesion classification is based on the methodology outlined in [6].

3   Methods

In recent work, many configurations for different classifier types were systematically investigated across various parameters for both datasets, including traditional machine learning with handcrafted features and deep learning, pre-trained or trained from scratch. Various configurations for each classifier type were investigated across a range of parameters, and each classifier configuration evaluated according to several standard metrics, including the area under the curve (AUC) of the receiver operating characteristic (ROC), accuracy, F1 score, sensitivity and specificity. In this study we only consider traditional machine learning results as they use explicit features suitable for explanability analysis. The code for the classifiers and the complete training and analysis results are available at [17,18].

First-order statistical features, Haralick texture features, and LBP were calculated for all three MRI modalities used (T2W, ADC, high-b-value DWI), and fed into sequential backward floating feature selection (SBFS) to identify well-performing features and eliminate redundant features, focusing on two of the most frequently used machine learning classifiers, SVM and RF, as illustrated in Fig. 1. This analysis explored different kernel functions and regularization options for SVM, and various hyperparameters for RF, including the number of individual decision trees composing the forest (50, 100, or 150), the maximum depth of each tree (0, 20), minimum samples per leaf (2 or 4) and split (1, 20, or 40) defining the prerequisites for further bifurcations of decision nodes in the tree, as well as preprocessing steps, including intensity standardization, normalization, and combinations of both. Five-fold cross-validation is used to evaluate the effectiveness of the machine learning models and training dataset dependency, resulting in five evaluation scores, reported by their mean and std. deviation across the folds. Based on the results the best traditional machine learning models for each dataset are selected for our feature analysis.

In this work clustering, taking into account all performance metrics, is used to identify the best-performing classifier configurations for further analysis, to understand which features are selected and their relative importance in the classification process. Linear correlation coefficients between feature vectors are calculated to understand the degree of independence of different features. This is especially important due to the large number of features involved and expected redundancy of certain features due strong statistical correlation between certain first-order statistical and texture features, for example.

To elucidate the impact of individual features on the classification results, Shapley values [16], quantifying the average marginal contribution of each feature value to the overall score across all possible combinations, are calculated for all features. This enables us to identify the set of features that contribute the most to the classification, as well as those whose contribution is negligible. In addition to facilitating understanding of how the classifiers make decisions, identification of subsets of relevant features that are consistently used for different datasets by the best-performing classifiers, could be leveraged to reduce the number of features that need to be calculated and develop more efficient algorithms. It may also help to drive approaches towards explainable AI to refer to specific textures and their relations between different modalities in regions of the prostate suspected of being cancerous or not, in traditional as well as deep machine learning.

4 Results

4.1 Best-Performing Machine Learning Classifiers

Figure 2 shows that the best-performing classifiers for both datasets are traditional machine learning classifiers of RF-type when ranked according to AUC. The same also holds for the combined dataset (not shown).

Figure 3 further shows that the performance metrics for the best-performing classifiers for different datasets are strongly correlated with the AUC metric,

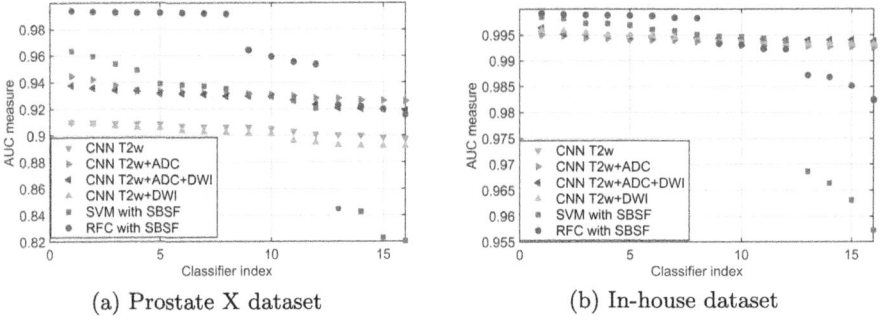

(a) Prostate X dataset   (b) In-house dataset

Fig. 2. AUC metrics of the best classifiers for different types of traditional (RF and SVM with SBSF) and deep learning classifiers (CNNs trained on different combinations of inputs: T2W, T2W+ADC, T2W+ADC+DWI, T2W+DWI) for Prostate-X and in-house datasets show that traditional machine learning classifiers of RF type consistently perform best.

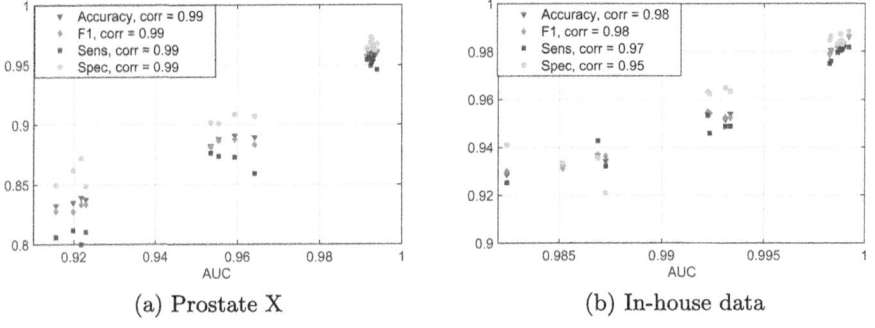

(a) Prostate X   (b) In-house data

Fig. 3. Accuracy, F1-score, sensitivity and specificity are strongly correlated with AUC, supporting use of AUC as the primary metric for ranking classifiers.

justifying use of the former as a primary performance indicator for ranking different classifiers. The figures include results from CNN deep learning classifiers for reference and comparison, which are not further studied here as we wish to identify relevant explicit texture features.

Clustering of the best-performing classifiers by mean AUC, accuracy, F1-score, sensitivity, and specificity shows that, for both the Prostate-X and the in-house dataset, three performance clusters are identified, as shown in Fig. 4. The top-performing cluster for both datasets correspond to identical configurations for the classifiers comprising RF classifiers with 100 trees, no maximum depth, two minimum samples per leaf and one split as prerequisite for further bifurcation. Both patch sizes of 16 and 32 as well as combinations of normalization, standardization or both, are included. It should be noted that the classifiers, although having the same configurations, were trained independently per dataset.

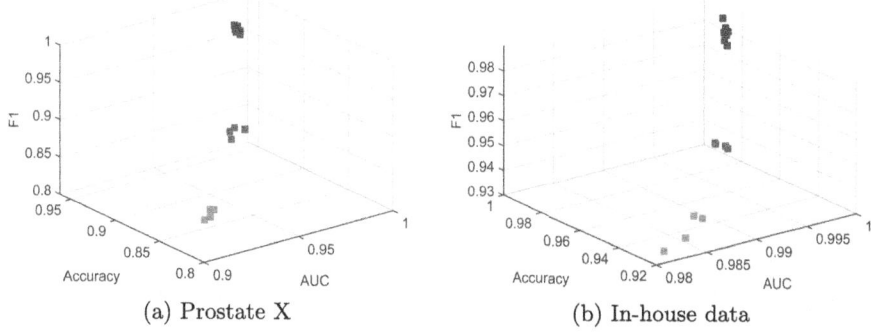

(a) Prostate X   (b) In-house data

Fig. 4. RF classifiers fall into three distinct performance clusters when clustered according to AUC values, accuracy, F1-score, sensitivity and specificity for both datasets (sensitivity and specificity dimensions not shown). The elements in the cluster with the highest performance scores (indicated by blue squares) correspond to identical configurations for both datasets. (Color figure online)

4.2   Feature Value Ranges and Correlations

We study the distributions of feature values for the positive and negative classes. Features are labelled by modality (t2-tra, adc, dwi_c-1400) followed by feature type (mean, std, skewness, kurtosis, Haralick01 to Haralick14, lbp-01 to lbp-35) throughout. Fig. 5 shows the distribution of values for an illustrative example. The feature value ranges for both classes overlap for all datasets, but the ranges are narrower for the positive class, and for this feature, the positive class values are consistently on the lower side. A narrower range of values for the positive class, yet considerable overlap with the negative class, is typical for most features, showing that no single feature is sufficient for classification, as expected. For the other features generally similar behaviour is observed.

Given the large number of features across three different modalities, we expect many features to be correlated. To understand the degree of correlation between features, Fig. 6 shows the feature correlation matrix for the Prostate-X dataset. It can be observed that the first-order statistical means are almost perfectly correlated with the Haralick06 feature values, and there is significant correlation between mean and standard deviation among the first-order order statistical features for the T2W images, while skewness and kurtosis are generally uncorrelated with the other first-order statistical features and most Haralick features. Therefore, it is expected that not all features contribute equally to the classification, and some may be entirely superfluous. The aim of feature selection, as applied via SBFS in training the classifiers, is to eliminate these correlations by removing features that do not significantly change the performance.

4.3   Feature Impact on Model Output: Shapley Values

To gain a better understanding of the impact of individual features on the model output, we calculate the distribution of Shapley values for the features selected by SBFS for the best performing RF model for both datasets. SHAP (SHapley Addictive exPlanations) was chosen over LIME as it is generally more suitable for complex machine learning models. A detailed description and discussion of the methods can be found, e.g., in [25]. The violin and decision tree plots (Fig. 7) show the distribution of the Shapley values for each feature, with color coding indicating the feature values. The plots show that in both cases the model output is almost entirely determined by a small number of around 14 features. For the ProstateX data, 8 of the 14 features that have a non-negligible impact on the model output are first-order statistical features; the remaining six are Haralick texture features (12, 13, 06, 08, 06, 03); no LBP features were used. First-order statistical features clearly dominate, especially T2W mean, as well as skewness (used for all modalities), kurtosis (ADC, DWI) and std (ADC, DWI). It is also noteworthy that features from all three modalities are used (6 T2W, 5 ADC, and 3 DWI). Although fewer DWI features are used, their impact on the overall model output is significant.

For the in-house dataset comprised of mostly early-stage cancer patients, although the shape of the Shapley distributions and the impact of the individual selected features differ, the overall picture in terms of the relevant features is broadly similar, with perhaps a slightly higher contribution of Haralick texture features – about half the features used are first-order statistical, and half are Haralick texture (06, 13, 06, 12, 04, 05, 10) features. Again features from all three modalities are used (6 T2W, 5 ADC, 4 DWI), with skewness and kurtosis playing significant roles in addition to mean and standard deviation (std). It could be argued that one of the LBP features contributes marginally but again, LBP feastures do not appear to play a significant role.

We also considered the performance of classifiers trained on the combined (Prosate-X + in-house) dataset. The Shapley values distributions for the features, shown in Fig. 8, again show that only a few features impact the final result, again dominated by first-order statistical features (10 out of 18) and a

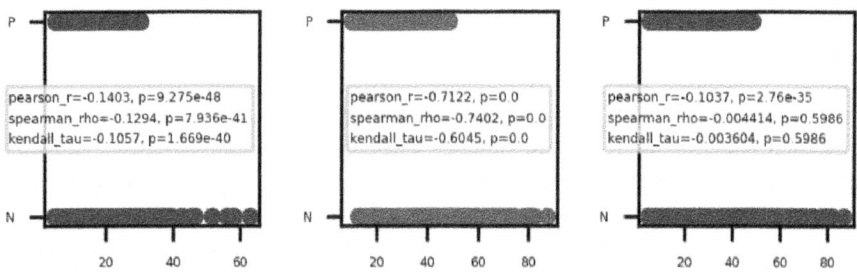

Fig. 5. Feature value ranges for positive and negative patches differ but generally overlap for all datasets, as illustrated here for the mean values of the T2W patches. Left: Prostate-X, middle: in-house dataset, right: combined dataset. Red color indicates strong correlation in terms of Pearson r. (Color figure online)

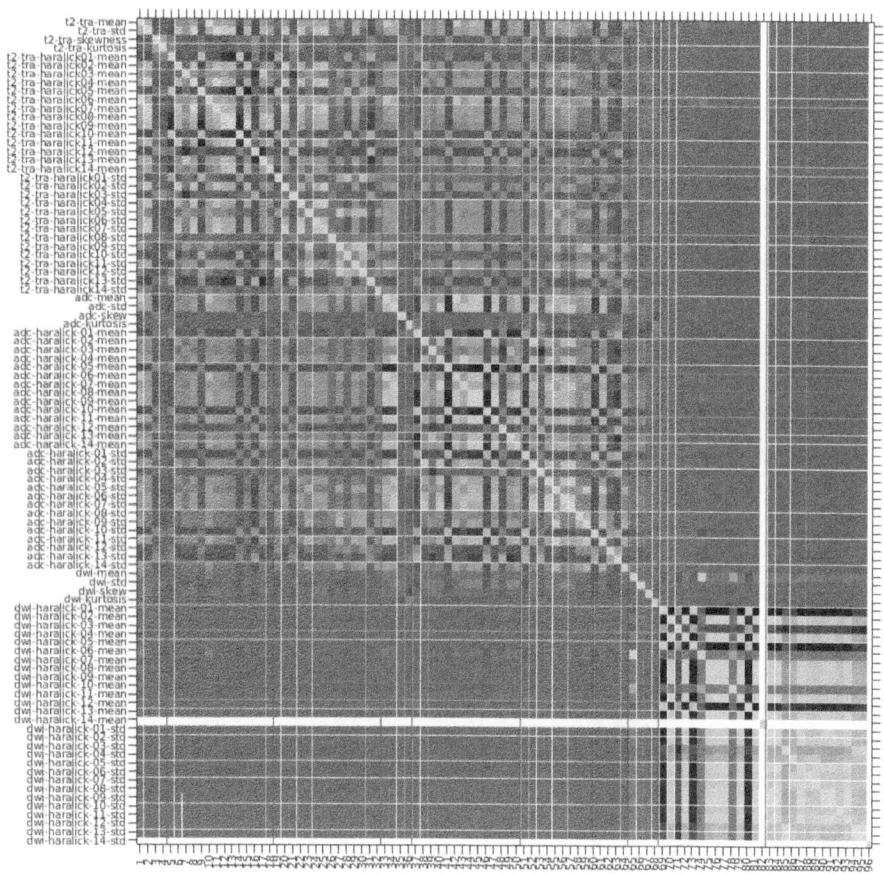

Fig. 6. Feature value correlation matrix for the Prostate-X dataset. The strength of correlation is indicated by the color, with yellow indicating high correlation and blue effectively none. The plot shows that many features are correlated but there are groups of uncorrelated features. The white line corresponds to a feature (for high-b-value DWI) that could not be computed. (Color figure online)

select number of Haralick texture features (11, 13, 08, 13, 06, 01, 03) with negligible contributions from LBPs. Features from all three modalities are used, with T2W mean as well as skewness and kurtosis featuring prominently, and std also being used.

One interesting difference between the Prostate-X (and combined) dataset vs the in-house dataset is that the decision paths are much clearer for the in-house dataset, although part of this could simply be that the dataset is smaller and thus lacks the full co-variance and range of feature values present.

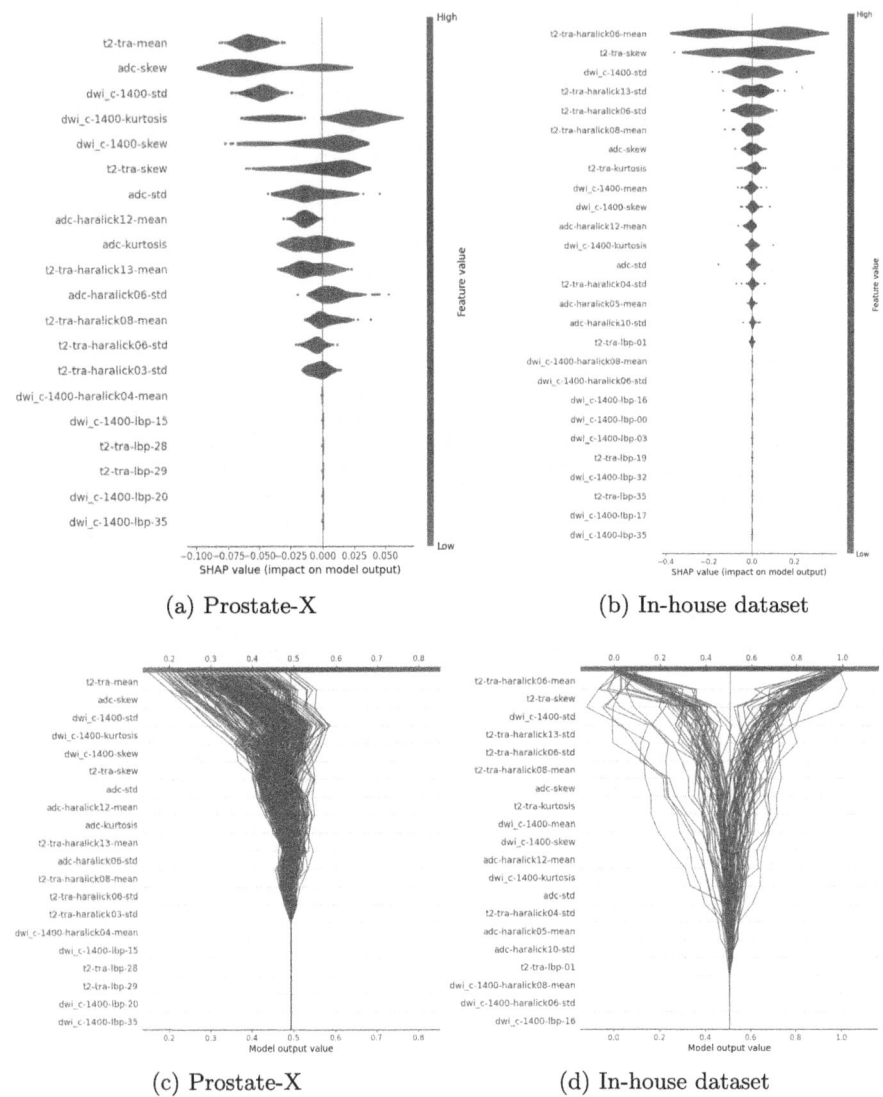

(a) Prostate-X

(b) In-house dataset

(c) Prostate-X

(d) In-house dataset

Fig. 7. Shapley value distributions and decision trees for the best RF classifier with SBSF feature selection for the respective datasets.

4.4   RF Classifiers Trained Without Feature Selection

In the previous section, we considered the impact of various features of the best-performing RF classifier with SBFS feature selection. We also trained an RF classifier of the same type using all features without SBFS. Figure 9 shows the Shapley decision trees, including the most important features for the best RF classifiers without feature selection for both datasets. Figure 10a and 10b show

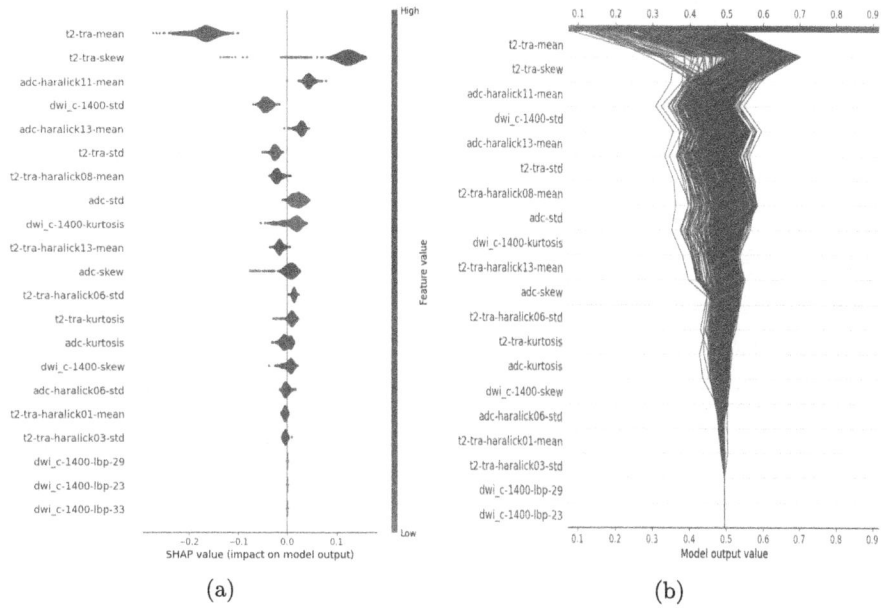

Fig. 8. Violin plots of Shapley value distributions for the combined dataset.

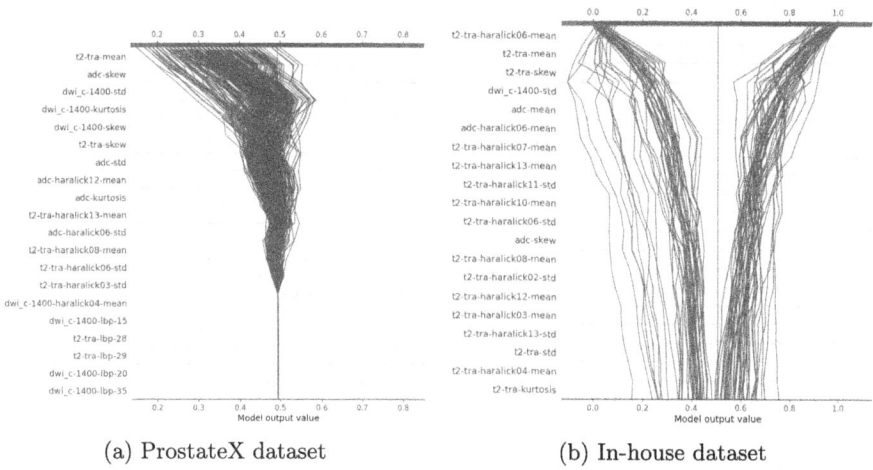

(a) ProstateX dataset

(b) In-house dataset

Fig. 9. Shapley value analysis showing the most significant features used by best RF classifiers, trained using all features without feature selection. The best classifier for both datasets defaulted to an RF classifier with 100 decision trees, no maximum depth, minimum of two samples per leaf.

the Shapley distributions for the top-50 features for the Prostate-X and in-house datasets, respectively. Features omitted due to space constraints have negligible

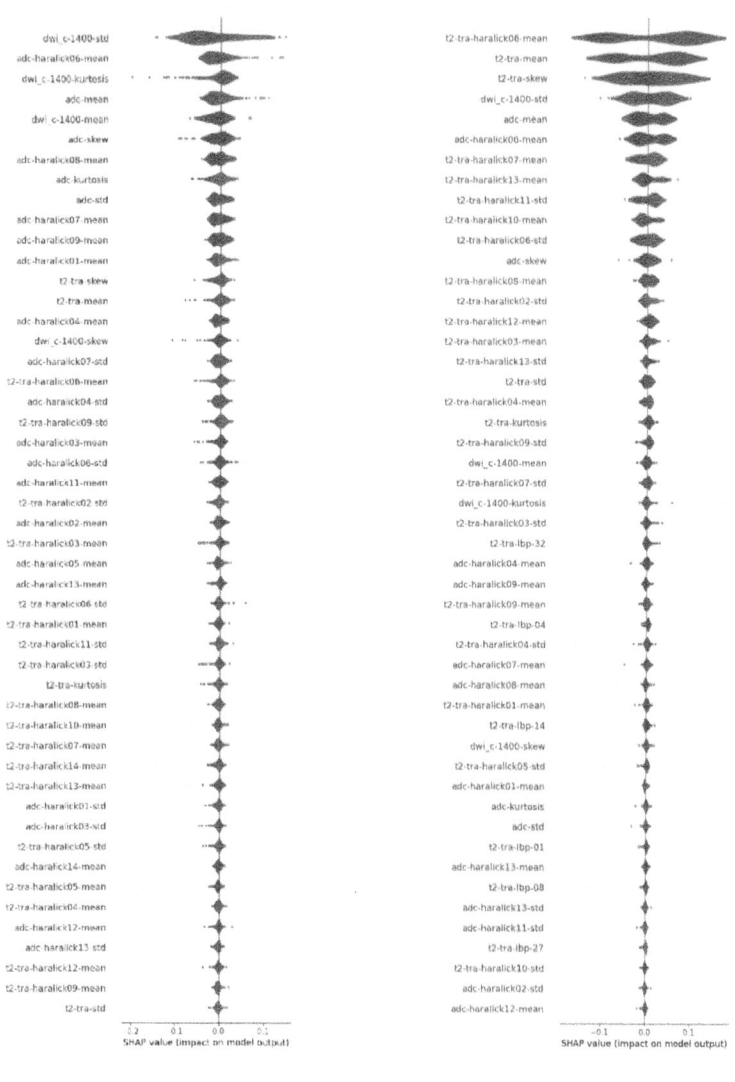

(a) Prostate-X   (b) In-house dataset

Fig. 10. Shapley impact value distributions for best RF Classifier trained using all features without feature selection for both datasets. Only the 50 most significant features are shown. The remaining features are negligible. The color scale indicates feature values ranging from low (blue) to high (red). (Color figure online)

impact. Although slightly more features contribute, most features still have negligible impact; this holds in particular for LBP features. Features derived from all modalities contribute. First order statistical features still play a dominant role but more Haralick features contribute as well. Most importantly, using all features reduces performance of the algorithm compared to best RF algorithm with SBSF.

5 Conclusions

Shapley-value based feature analysis suggests that only a few features determine the classification outcome in most cases, with a dominant role played by first-order statistical features, and a limited number of Haralick texture features. Local binary patterns play no significant role for the best-performing RF classifiers for any of the datasets considered. However, the fact the best algorithms used features from all three modalities suggests that all are contributing valuable information. Also, there is no significant difference for different patch sizes (rescaled from the original size). The fact that the classification results are consistently determined by a small subset of features suggests that many features are redundant, and could be used to design streamlined classification algorithms using fewer features. Despite the limited generalizability of the results, the consistency observed in terms of the relevant features as well as the best classifiers types is encouraging. The much clearer decision trees for the in-house dataset compared to the far more complex split for the Prostate-X dataset require further exploration. It could indicate that classification of early-stage PCa may be clearer, but it may also indicate that larger datasets are needed to cover the covariance. Important next steps are to extend results to larger datasets focused on early-state PCa identification. Despite the traditional machine learning classifiers performing better than their deep learning counterparts, it may be interesting to see which features the deep learning methods use and how they compare to those identified in this analysis, especially as traditional machine learning classifiers may not perform as well on more complex classification tasks on larger datasets. The features identified may also form the basis for specifying specific textures in the various modalities and their relations to identify cancer and explain the decisions.

Acknowledgements. We thank the staff of Swansea University's Clinical Imaging Unit, especially Superintendent Research Radiographer, Anthony Rees, and former clinical director, Dr Rhodri Evans, for providing and annotating the in-house dataset.

References

1. Abraham, N.E., Mendhiratta, N., Taneja, S.S.: Patterns of repeat prostate biopsy in contemporary clinical practice. J. Urol. **193**(4), 1178–1184 (2015)
2. Aldoj, N., Lukas, S., Dewey, M., Penzkofer, T.: Semi-automatic classification of prostate cancer on multi-parametric MR imaging using a multi-channel 3D convolutional neural network. Eur. Radiol. **30**(2), 1243–1253 (2020)
3. Cameron, A., Khalvati, F., Haider, M.A., Wong, A.: Maps: a quantitative radiomics approach for prostate cancer detection. Trans Biomed. Eng. **63**(6), 1145–1156 (2015)

4. Chen, Q., Hu, S., Long, P., Lu, F., Shi, Y., Li, Y.: A transfer learning approach for malignant prostate lesion detection on multiparametric MRI. Technol. Cancer Res. Treatment **18**, 1533033819858363 (2019)

5. Chen, T., et al.: Prostate cancer differentiation and aggressiveness: assessment with a radiomic-based model vs. pi-rads v2. J. Magnet. Resonance Imag. **49**(3), 875–884 (2019)

6. Cuocolo, R., Stanzione, A., Castaldo, A., De Lucia, D.R., Imbriaco, M.: Quality control and whole-gland, zonal and lesion annotations for the prostatex challenge public dataset. Eur. J. Radiol. **138**, 109647 (2021)

7. Deniffel, D., et al.: Using decision curve analysis to benchmark performance of a magnetic resonance imaging-based deep learning model for prostate cancer risk assessment. Eur. Radiol. **30**(12), 6867–6876 (2020)

8. Fehr, D., et al.: Automatic classification of prostate cancer Gleason scores from multiparametric magnetic resonance images. Proc Nat. Acad. Sci. **112**(46), E6265–E6273 (2015)

9. Haralick, R.M., Shanmugam, K., Dinstein, I.H.: Textural features for image classification. Trans Systems, Man, and Cybern. **SMC-3**(6), 610–621 (1973)

10. Janssen, F.M., Aben, K.K., Heesterman, B.L., Voorham, Q.J., Seegers, P.A., Moncada-Torres, A.: Using explainable machine learning to explore the impact of synoptic reporting on prostate cancer. Algorithms **15**(2), 49 (2022)

11. Litjens, G., Debats, O., Barentsz, J., Karssemeijer, N., Huisman, H.: Computer-aided detection of prostate cancer in MRI. Trans Med. Imag. **33**(5), 1083–1092 (2014)

12. Litjens, G., Debats, O., Barentsz, J., Karssemeijer, N., Huisman, H.: ProstateX challenge data. The Cancer Imaging Archive (2017)

13. Liu, B., et al.: Prediction of prostate cancer aggressiveness with a combination of radiomics and machine learning-based analysis of dynamic contrast-enhanced MRI. Clin. Radiol. **74**(11), e1-896 (2019)

14. Liu, X., Langer, D.L., Haider, M.A., Yang, Y., Wernick, M.N., Yetik, I.S.: Prostate cancer segmentation with simultaneous estimation of Markov random field parameters and class. Trans Med. Imag. **28**(6), 906–915 (2009)

15. Loeb, S., et al.: Systematic review of complications of prostate biopsy. Eur. Urol. **64**(6), 876–892 (2013)

16. Lundberg, S.M., Lee, S.I.: A unified approach to interpreting model predictions. In: Proceedings of the 31st International Conference Neural Information Processing Systems, pp. 4768–4777. NIPS'17, Curran Associates Inc., Red Hook, NY, USA (2017)

17. Muftah, A., Langbein, F.C., Shermer, S.: PCaNet Models – Classification, Version 1.0 (2024). https://qyber.black/ca/results-pcanet-models-classification

18. Muftah, A., Langbein, F.C., Shermer, S.: PCaNet Version 1.0 (2024). https://qyber.black/ca/code-pcanet

19. Muftah, A.A.S.: Computer-Aided Diagnosis of Prostate Cancer via Machine Learning using Multiparametric MRI. PhD dissertation, Cardiff University (5 2023)

20. Niaf, E., Rouvière, O., Lartizien, C.: Computer-aided diagnosis for prostate cancer detection in the peripheral zone via multisequence MRI. In: Medical Imaging 2011: Computer-Aided Diagnosis. vol. 7963, pp. 1066–1073. SPIE (2011)

21. Ojala, T., Pietikäinen, M., Mäenpää, T.: Gray scale and rotation invariant texture classification with local binary patterns. In: Computer Vision - ECCV 2000; LNCS. vol. 1842, pp. 404–420. Springer, Berlin, Heidelberg (2000). https://doi.org/10.1007/3-540-45054-8_27

22. Orczyk, C., et al.: Prostate cancer heterogeneity: texture analysis score based on multiple magnetic resonance imaging sequences for detection, stratification and selection of lesions at time of biopsy. BJU Int. **124**(1), 76–86 (2019)

23. Peng, Y., et al.: Quantitative analysis of multiparametric prostate MR images: differentiation between prostate cancer and normal tissue and correlation with Gleason score-a computer-aided diagnosis development study. Radiology **267**(3), 787 (2013)

24. Ramírez-Mena, A., Andrés-León, E., Alvarez-Cubero, M.J., Anguita-Ruiz, A., Martinez-Gonzalez, L.J., Alcala-Fdez, J.: Explainable artificial intelligence to predict and identify prostate cancer tissue by gene expression. Comput. Methods Programs Biomed. **240**, 107719 (2023)

25. Sathyan, A., Weinberg, A.I., Cohen, K.: Interpretable AI for bio-medical applications. Complex Eng. Syst. **2**, 18 (12 2022)

26. Smith, R.A., et al.: Cancer screening in the united states, 2016: a review of current American Cancer Society guidelines and current issues in cancer screening. CA: A Cancer J. Clin. **66**(2), 95–114 (2016)

27. Vos, P.C., Hambrock, T., Hulsbergen-van de Kaa, C.A., Fütterer, J.J., Barentsz, J.O., Huisman, H.J.: Computerized analysis of prostate lesions in the peripheral zone using dynamic contrast enhanced MRI. Medical Physics **35**(3), 888–899 (2008)

28. Wu, M., Krishna, S., Thornhill, R.E., Flood, T.A., McInnes, M.D., Schieda, N.: Transition zone prostate cancer: logistic regression and machine-learning models of quantitative ADC, shape and texture features are highly accurate for diagnosis. J. Magn. Reson. Imag. **50**(3), 940–950 (2019)

29. Yaun, Y., et al.: Prostate cancer classification with multiparametric MRI transfer learning model. Med. Phys. **46**(2), 756–765 (2019)

30. Zhong, X., et al.: Deep transfer learning-based prostate cancer classification using 3 Tesla multi-parametric MRI. Abdominal Radiol. **44**(6), 2030–2039 (2019)

Medical Signal and Image Processing

DELRecon: Depth Electrode Reconstruction Toolbox for Stereo-EEG

Shameer Aslam[1], Qi Chen[2], and Jiaxiang Zhang[1(✉)]

[1] Department of Computer Science, Swansea University, Swansea, UK
{2329852,jiaxiang.zhang}@swansea.ac.uk
[2] School of Psychology, South China Normal University, Guangzhou, China

Abstract. Many focal epilepsy patients resistant to medication are known to respond well to resective surgery. During the presurgical evaluation, stereo-EEG (SEEG) is often used to identify the epileptogenic zone. SEEG monitoring is an invasive procedure where patients are surgically implanted with depth electrodes into the brain. Existing methods for SEEG localization often lead to errors when multiple high-density electrodes are implanted close to each other. This study introduced an open-source MATLAB toolbox, DELRecon, for depth electrode reconstruction from post-implantation CT images. DELRecon included three processing modules: image processing, electrode localization and individual contact labelling. The electrode localization module used iterative clustering to trace each electrode and singular value decomposition to determine the electrode trajectories. The contact labelling module detected and labelled each contact through intensity-based clustering. The toolbox further included user interfaces for manual intervention when necessary. We evaluated DELRecon in a SEEG dataset, including 92 electrodes from 8 patients, totalling 1196 contacts. The toolbox accurately localized over 98% of all contacts. Our results suggested that DELRecon is an efficient solution for automatically localising SEEG electrodes and contacts.

Keywords: Epilepsy · Stereo-EEG · Electrode reconstruction · Singular value decomposition · Clustering

1 Introduction

Focal epilepsy is a chronic disorder which causes seizures, originating from certain regions in the brain described as epileptogenic zone [10]. For pharmacologically intractable patients, respective surgery may be needed to remove epileptogenic zones. The precision of the presurgical evaluation of these patients determines their surgical outcome [19,21]. When non-invasive evaluations are insufficient to formulate a clear surgical plan, the presurgical workup may use stereo-electroencephalogram (SEEG) monitoring to assist, in particular in cases involving deep cortical structures, sulci and subcortical regions [6,9]. For the SEEG procedure, patients are stereotactically implanted with depth SEEG electrodes into suspicious brain regions. Each SEEG electrodes contain multiple contacts to

X. Xie et al. (Eds.): AIiH 2024, LNCS 14976, pp. 135–148, 2024.
https://doi.org/10.1007/978-3-031-67285-9_10

record brain activity, which provides evidence for localizing epileptogenic zones. SEEG data also provides an invaluable resource for researchers to understand brain functions [13].

Analysing SEEG data needs to first localize the 3D coordinates of each contact along each electrode. Some proprietary software can generate SEEG coordinates based on surgical planning [16], which are not available to many researchers. Furthermore, surgical planning may not precisely reflect the final locations of SEEG electrodes. One common approach to localize SEEG electrodes is to combine preoperative MRI and postoperative CT brain images, as SEEG electrode contacts have high Hounsfield values in CT images, and MRI structural images provide anatomical details for localizing SEEG electrodes [4,5].

Computer-aided tools have been proposed to use brain imaging for SEEG electrode localization. Some solutions provide image coregistration and convenient visualization but require manually labelling each electrode and their coordinates [17,20,22]. Others aimed for an automated or semiautomated workflow [1,7,12,18,23].

However, there are several challenges to localising SEEG electrodes from MRI and CT images. First, when two or more electrodes cross each other or are placed within a small vicinity, existing SEEG localization methods based on voxel clustering may not provide correct results [1,7,18,23]. Second, after initializing two contacts in each electrode, some solutions use interpolation and extrapolation to identify all remaining contacts of the electrode [12,15,24]. This method relies on the intercontact distance along the electrode and therefore may be susceptible to accumulating localization errors along the electrodes.

To address these challenges, the current study proposed an open-source Matlab toolbox for Depth Electrode Reconstruction (DELRecon). DELRecon is maximally automated with sufficient user interaction at each level of processing, ensuring accurate contact localization. Its main features include (1) iterative 3D tracking to localise SEEG electrodes crossing each other, within close distance, or in a small brain (e.g., in children); (2) contact localization independent of the intercontact distance; (3) optional GUI-based manual correction when needed; and (4) a final NIfTI image output in the native space, including all electrodes' contacts and their corresponding tissue types.

2   Method

2.1   Toolbox Installation and Requirements

DELRecon is available freely from https://github.com/aslamshameer165/DELRecon. The toolbox is compatible with MATLAB R2021a and later versions. A few external tools are needed, including SPM for image processing (https://www.fil.ion.ucl.ac.uk/spm) and iElectrodes for clustering [2]. The workflow of DELRecon includes three main modules (Fig. 1): (1) image processing, (2) electrode localization, and (3) individual contact labelling. Below we first reported the implementation details of each module and then described the dataset used in Results.

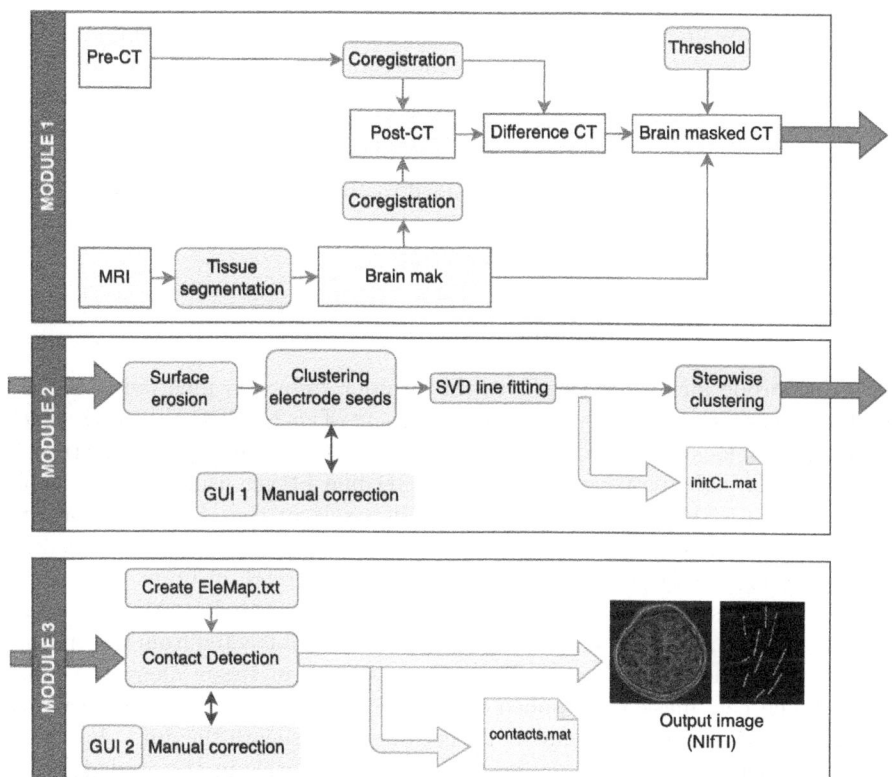

Fig. 1. The processing pipeline of DELRecon. Module 1 performs MRI and CT image processing. Module 2 performs electrode identification and localization. Module 3 identifies individual contacts along each electrode and generates output images.

2.2   Module 1: Image Processing

Module 1 requires minimum user intervention. It uses SPM to process MRI and CT images (Fig. 1, Module 1). This step aims to generate a masked volumetric CT image that retains all voxels associated with SEEG electrodes within the brain. The module requires three input images in the NIfTI format: preoperative structural MRI (e.g., a T1-weighted whole-brain scan), pre-implantation CT (pre-CT) and post-implantation CT (post-CT).

The structural MRI image was first segmented to obtain probability maps of grey matter, white matter and cerebrospinal fluid. These probability maps were combined to construct a brain mask. The brain mask underwent 2 iterations of dilation followed by 2 iterations of erosion using a spherical neighbourhood algorithm to fill any void in the brain mask that may be due to tissue misclassification. Next, post-implantation CT image was referenced to coregister pre-implantation CT and MRI images to avoid any interpolation/extrapolation in electrode voxels when resliced. The estimated co-registration transformation matrix was used to transform the brain mask into the post-implantation CT space. After co-registration, the pre-implantation CT image was subtracted from post-implantation CT and further masked by the brain mask to accentuate the voxels representing electrodes within the brain, because the electrode metal appears with the higher Hounsfield unit on the CT image. The brain-masked difference CT image was optimally thresholded to obtain an electrode image, which retains the voxels with higher Hounsfield units corresponding to the electrodes and has zero-valued voxels otherwise.

2.3   Module 2: Electrode Localization

SEEG electrode localization involves three major steps: (1) identifying a small cluster of voxels that represent the initial segment of each SEEG electrode, which is then used to localize the body of the electrode, (2) determining each electrode's trajectory through iterative refinement of 3D line fitting using singular value decomposition (SVD), and (3) assigning all voxels in the electrode image to their respective electrodes based on electrodes' trajectories (Fig. 1, Module 2).

The initial clustering was performed in a small stretch of brain tissue close to the cortical surface. For this, the brain mask generated in Module 1 was eroded using a spherical neighbourhood method and subtracted from the original brain mask, generating a mask of a narrow stretch of tissue along the brain surface. The new mask was applied to the electrode image to retain the voxels associated with the entry points of all electrodes underneath the dura. A k-mean clustering method is used to assign these non-zero voxels in the eroded region into clusters, with each cluster corresponding to an implanted electrode. At this stage, DELRecon provided a graphic user interface (GUI 1 in Fig. 1) to visualize the initial clustering results and allow manual adjustments if necessary (Fig. 2A). Common misclassifications can be detected and resolved in this interface. For example, users can select a set of voxels to define a new cluster/electrode (when an electrode is missing in the initial clustering result) or to remove a set of voxels (when the initial clustering includes false positives).

After initializing a voxel cluster corresponding to the starting segment of each electrode, trajectories (i.e., orientations in 3D) of all electrodes were calculated iteratively using stepwise clustering (Table 1). In each iteration, for each electrode, we first fitted a 3D line to all voxels already assigned to the electrode's cluster using SVD. Next, we identified 100 unassigned voxels with the smallest distance to any cluster's centre mass and assigned those voxels to the cluster closest to them. The iterations for stepwise clustering ran until either the SVD lines were stable or all the voxels were exhausted. After all the electrode voxels were assigned to their corresponding clusters, SVD fitting was performed again to identify the trajectory of the entire electrode. Finally, each non-zero voxel v in the electrode image was assigned to a cluster c representing a corresponding electrode, based on the minimum value of the following distance metric:

$$c = \mathbf{argmin}_i \left(\beta_1 \cdot d_{\text{SVD},i}(v) + \beta_2 \cdot d_{\text{final},i}(v) + \beta_3 \cdot d_{\text{init},i}(v) \right), \qquad (1)$$

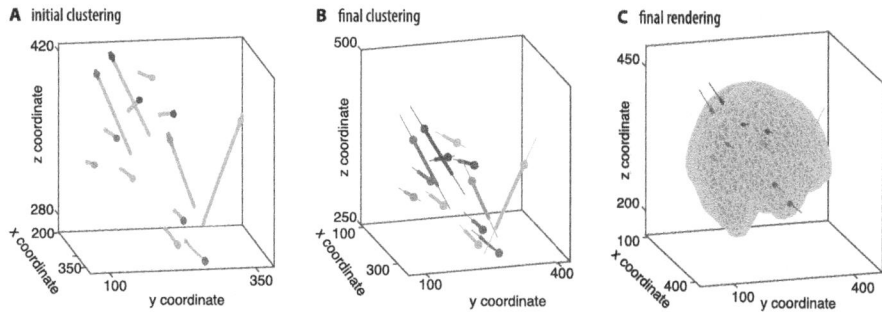

Fig. 2. Electrode localization in a single patient. (A) The GUI for visualizing and manually adjusting the initial clusters of all electrodes. The data points with different colours indicate the initial clusters, corresponding to the initial segments of each electrode. The orange data points indicate unclustered voxels. (B) The final reconstruction of all electrodes after iterative SVD fitting and clustering. (C) The 3D-rendered brain surface for visualizing the reconstructed electrodes, showing in the same viewing angle as in Panel B. (Color figure online)

where i represents the i-th electrode. $d_{\mathrm{SVD},i}$ is the distance between the voxel v and the final SVD line after iterative fitting. $d_{\mathrm{final},i}$ is the Euclidean distance between the voxel v to the centre of the final cluster of electrodes. $d_{\mathrm{init},i}$ is the Euclidean distance between the voxel v to the centre of the initial cluster of the electrode before iterative fitting. By taking into account the three distance measures together, we can effectively assign each voxel to its corresponding electrode. That is, voxels representing an electrode should be (1) close to the electrode's direction, (2) close to the centre of the electrode, and (3) close to the initial segment of the electrode. In practice, reasonable results were obtained by setting the weighting coefficients $\beta_1=20$ and $\beta_2 = \beta_3 = 1$.

Once all the voxels in the electrode images were clustered, the toolbox presented a 3D viewer for visualizing the final electrode trajectory and the electrode clusters (Fig. 2B). The figure provides an opportunity for final sanity checks (Fig. 2C). It also illustrates the unique cluster ID for each identified SEEG electrode, which is required in subsequent analyses.

2.4   Module 3: Individual Contact Labelling

To label individual contacts along SEEG electrodes, DELRecon takes a text file as the input for the process, which specifies the electrode name, its cluster ID (generated in Module 2) and the number of contacts in the electrode (Fig. 1, Module 3). For each electrode, the final fitted SVD lines were used to project all corresponding electrode voxels to a 1D array along the direction of the SVD line (Fig. 3). Contact labelling relied on the fact that adjacent contacts appeared as dense clusters in CT scans with higher Hounsfield values, separated by an insulated space between the contacts, which has lower intensities on the post-implantation CT images. Therefore, by projecting voxel intensity along the 1D

Table 1. Stepwise clustering for electrode localization

Step	Action detail
1. Initialization	Input x: Coordinates of non-clustered electrode voxels
2. Iterative tracking and clustering	a) For each cluster representing each electrode: i. Calculate the centre p of the cluster ii. Apply SVD to the cluster, obtaining the direction vector d b) For each voxel in x: i. Calculate its distance from p along d ii. Label the voxel with the nearest cluster c) Identify the data point which has the largest distance to its corresponding cluster d) Repeat the following steps 20 times: i. Select 100 nearest voxels in x from cluster centres ii. Label each selected voxel with its nearest cluster iii. Redefine clusters with the newly labelled voxels iv. Recalculate the SVD lines for new clusters e) Continue the iteration until: i. The reduced distance of the farthest data point from its cluster is more than 2 units, or ii. All voxels in x have been assigned to a cluster
3. Final Assignment	a) For any remaining voxels in x: Assign the nearest cluster b) Recalculate the final SVD line for each cluster
4. Final Clustering	For each voxel with non-zero values: Assign to the cluster which minimises the distance metric (Eq. 1)

SVD line direction, the centre of each contact has peak intensity compared with that from neighbouring voxels. We performed k-mean clustering to voxels projected to the 1D space, identifying the centroids of clusters that correspond to the locations of contacts along the electrode. A graphical user interface (GUI 2 in Fig. 3) visualizes the contacts' positions and allows correction when necessary. For example, users can change the threshold in the horizontal axis to restrict the length of the electrode, or the threshold in the vertical axis to constrain voxel intensities for clustering. The interface also allows to add or remove contacts during the process.

2.5   Toolbox Outputs

DELRecon generates several outputs. First, after completing contact labelling for all electrodes, the centroids of the contacts were saved in a MATLAB data file 'contacts.mat'. Second, a NIfTI electrode image was generated in the post-implantation CT space, including the position of all contacts in all electrodes.

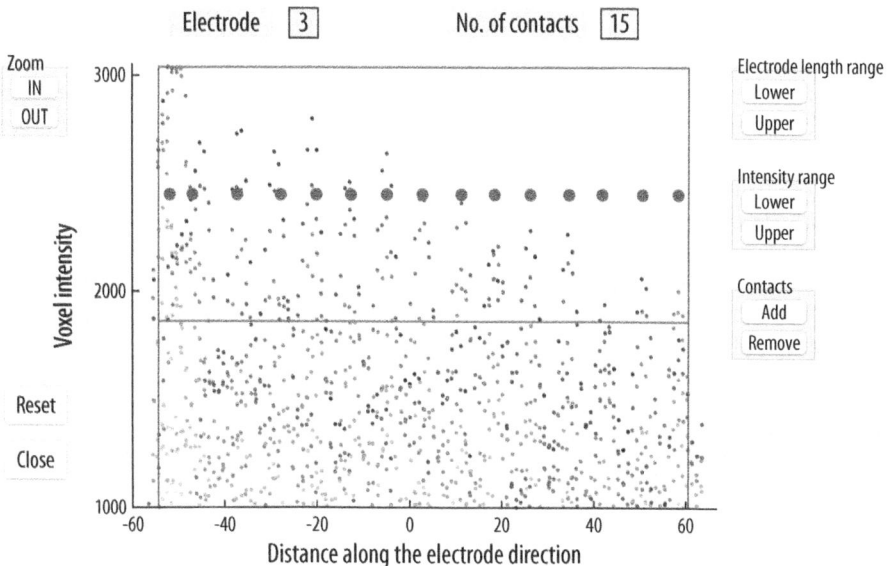

Fig. 3. The GUI for contact labelling. All voxels corresponding to an electrode are projected along the electrode's direction (i.e., the fitted SVD line). After projection, the GUI shows individual voxels' intensity against their distance along the electrode's direction. The grayscale level of the data points corresponds to the distance between the voxel and the electrode's direction. Users can use buttons to manually adjust the cutoff along the electrode's direction (the vertical red lines), the upper and lower thresholds of voxel intensity (the horizontal blue lines), and the number of contacts. After setting those values, 1D k-mean clustering is performed on all chosen voxels to identify the centroid of each electrode's contact (red circles). (Color figure online)

The image can be overlayed onto the patient's MRI image to obtain anatomical labels. The NIfTI electrode image is accompanied by an ITKsnap-compatible label file, which provides information on the contact position and the underlying tissue type (based on the tissue probability maps generated in Module 1). The voxel intensities of each contact in the NIfTI electrode image were coded in a way to directly identify individual electrodes and their associated contact. The first one or two digits of the intensity value represent the electrode's number, and the last two digits of the intensity value represent the contact number of the electrode (e.g., '1105' refers to the 5-th contact in the 11-th electrode). Third, the initial clusters of voxels used for iterative electrode localization in Module 2 were saved in a MATLAB data file 'initCL.mat'.

2.6   Dataset Used for Validation

We tested the toolbox on a data set comprising 8 patients with drug-resistant focal epilepsy who underwent invasive monitoring with stereo-EEG at the 999 Brain Hospital, China (6 males, age range: 4–31 years, mean age: 18.25 years).

Electrode implantation locations were personalized according to imaging and non-invasive EEG data. There were 7 to 15 implanted electrodes per patient and 6 to 16 contacts (i.e. SEEG channels) on each electrode inside the brain. For each patient, a high-resolution whole-brain T1-weighted MRI was acquired before electrode implantation (GE Signa HDx 3T Scanner with a FSPGR sequence; repetition time, 8.8 ms; echo time 3.5 ms; flip angle, 13°; voxel size, 1 × 1 × 1 mm). Two head computed tomography (CT) images were acquired before and after electrode implantation (Philips Brilliance 64 scanner, voxel size, 0.43 × 0.43 × 0.5 mm). This study was approved by the Brain Hospital ethics committee and by the South China Normal University ethics committee. Written informed consent was obtained from all participants.

3   Results

3.1   MRI and CT Image Processing

To test and validate the toolbox, we analyzed 92 SEEG electrodes from 8 patients, which had a total of 1196 contacts. In Module 1 of the toolbox, after MRI tissue segmentation and MRI/CT co-registration, the pre-implantation CT was subtracted from post-implantation CT, followed by brain extraction. Subtracting the pre-implantation CT suppressed all non-electrode voxels, providing an artefact-free electrode image for subsequent analyses (Fig. 4). We set a threshold value of 650 units on the electrode image, under which most non-electrode voxels were excluded. Users can manually change the image threshold.

3.2   Initial SEEG Electrode Clustering

The electrodes' ends close to the brain surface were detected from the electrode image using the image erosion process in Module 2 (Fig. 1). The selected voxels were subjected to a k-mean clustering method to categorise them into individual clusters, each representing the initial segment of an electrode. Four electrodes in two patients were not correctly identified in the initial automated processing (Fig. 5A). These initial errors can be visualized from the GUI (Fig. 5A), and they need to be corrected before further processing. Manual correction can be easily performed in the GUI, which involves removing false positive clusters and adding voxels representing an electrode missed by the clustering algorithm (i.e., false negatives). After correction, the clustering procedure will report and update the results (Fig. 5B).

3.3   Iterative Tracking of SEEG Electrodes

After initial clustering, the SVD line fitting determined the initial direction of each electrode, which was iteratively refined to approximate the true electrode trajectories (Fig. 6). The SVD line refinement was based on the stepwise clustering of the electrode voxels followed by refitting the SVD line based on

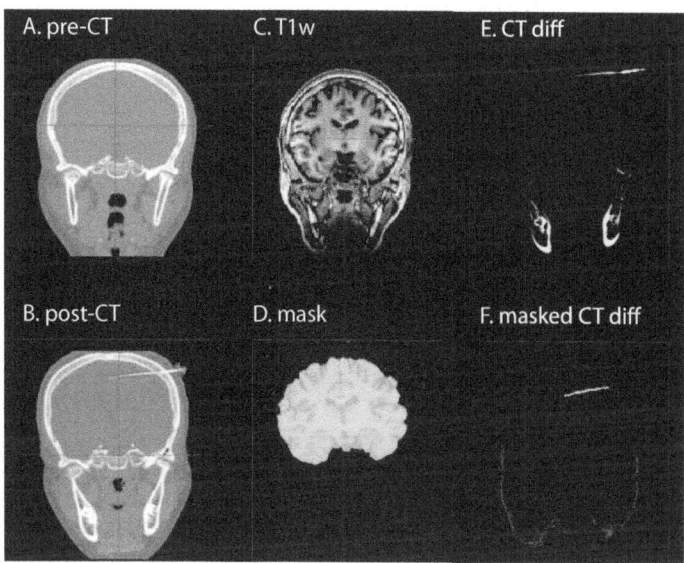

Fig. 4. Input and output images from Module 1. DELRecon takes three images as inputs: (A) a pre-implantation CT image, (B) a post-implantation CT image, and (C) a structural (T1-weighted) MRI image. The toolbox generates a brain mask (D), a different image between post-CT and pre-CT (E). The CT difference image is then masked and thresholded, yielding an electrode image which contains voxels representing SEEG electrodes in the brain (F). The images were from a representative patient.

the updated clusters at each iteration. As demonstrated in Fig. 6, this iterative approach is robust in estimating electrode trajectories in the cases of closely implanted or crossing electrodes. All 92 electrodes in the evaluation dataset were correctly localized.

3.4   Contact Labelling

Contact labelling (Module 3) involves a GUI-based 1D clustering to identify the centroid of each electrode contact along the principal direction of the electrode (Fig. 3). In the GUI, DELRecon sets a range on the electrode's trajectory that represents the length of the electrode, within which the 1D clustering will be conducted. The maximum value of the range was set to exclude the electrode screw from clustering, and the minimum range value was set to accommodate the tip of the electrode. The range can be manually adjusted to accommodate electrodes with different specifications. Furthermore, the 1D clustering procedure only considers voxels whose intensities are within a valid range. Excluding voxels with low intensities assists the clustering method in reducing false positives. Occasionally, a few contacts may be left outside of the brain tissue, DELRecon allows users to change the effective number of contacts from the GUI, which avoids overfitting.

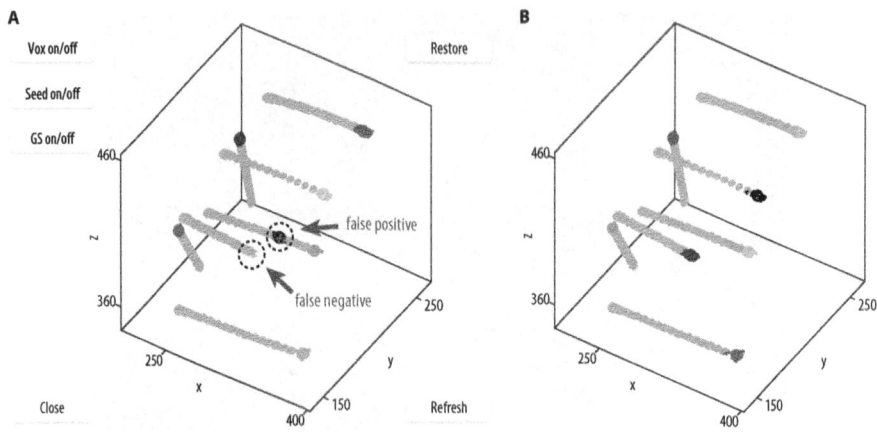

Fig. 5. Manual correction of the initial electrode clustering results. (A) Results from automatic clustering. Each cluster is illustrated in a different colour, which represents the initial segments of an electrode. The orange data points indicate unclustered voxels. The initial voxel clustering yielded a false positive cluster (misclassified a group of voxels as an electrode) and a false negative cluster (missed one electrode). One can remove the false positives and correct the false negatives (by manually assigning a group of voxels to a new cluster). (B) After correction, re-run the clustering method from the GUI. The updated results show that all electrodes were correctly identified. (Color figure online)

3.5   Evaluation

We have evaluated the accuracy and efficacy of DELRecon in electrode localization and contact labelling. We carefully compared outputs from DELRecon and patients' clinical records in the ROSA system [14]. Over 98% (1173 out of 1196) of contacts were accurately localized by DELRecon (Table 2). The 23 mis-

Table 2. Electrode localization and contact labelling results details

Patient	Gender	Age	Elec. no. right hemi	Elec. no. left hemi	Total contacts	Localized contacts
1	F	16	7	0	105	99
2	M	21	0	14	168	165
3	M	27	12	1	176	168
4	F	4	0	9	101	100
5	M	31	0	11	133	132
6	M	18	15	0	202	201
7	M	20	13	0	178	176
8	M	9	10	0	133	132

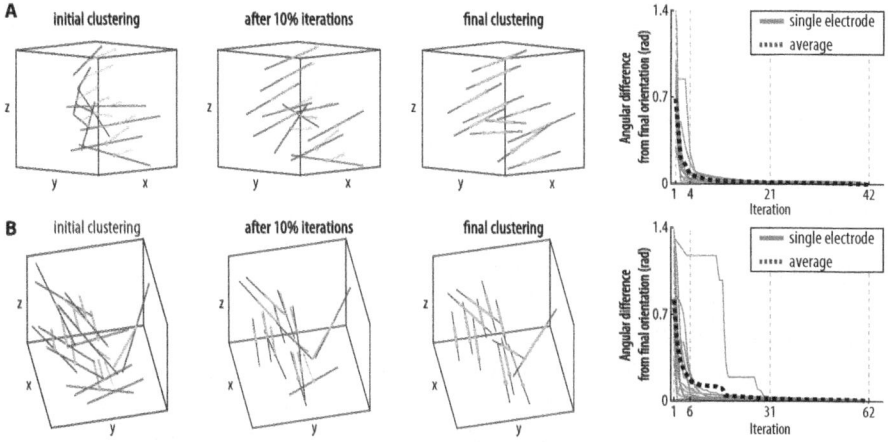

Fig. 6. The iterative tracking of electrodes based on SVD fittings to clustered voxels. (A) and (B) show Module 2 results from two independent patients. In each panel, the first three 3D plots illustrate the estimated directions of all electrodes after the initial clustering, after 10% of the total iterations, and at the final clustering (red lines: estimated direction; green data points: voxels used for clustering and SVD fitting; grey data points: unclustered voxels). In the fourth plot, green lines denote the change in the direction of SVD fittings to individual electrodes after each iteration. The dashed line denotes the average change in the fitted directions across electrodes. (Color figure online)

localized contacts had localization errors larger than 5 voxels. Among those, 17 contacts were from electrodes with oblique trajectories in CT scans. Note that the challenges of localizing contacts in oblique electrodes were reported elsewhere [23].

4   Discussion

DELRecon is an open-source toolbox for efficiently localizing and reconstructing SEEG electrode contacts. The toolbox provided sufficient automation at each processing step while allowing manual intervention for visual inspection and correction. The combination of automated and manual processing enables the toolbox to handle complex SEEG electrode arrangements with high-density contacts. Furthermore, DELRecon outputs a final NIfTI electrode image, containing positional information and the underlying tissue type of each contact and electrode, which can easily be shared, reused, or integrated with other data processing interfaces. The toolbox also generated intermediate outputs describing all the parameters and results to maximise reproducibility.

For both initial electrode segmentation in Module 2 and contact labelling along each electrode in Module 3, DELRecon utilized k-means clustering. It is worth noting that k-means clustering requires *a priori* knowledge about the number of clusters to be identified. In practice, this information is often available from the SEEG implantation plan. Nevertheless, one may consider alternative unsupervised clustering algorithms that can automatically determine the number of cluster centres, e.g., DBSCAN [8,11].

Compared with existing solutions of SEEG electrode localization, DELRecon includes two new features. First, most previous localization solutions also identified the voxels in CT images representing each electrode voxels, either through manually selecting the electrode voxels [2,18], or semi-automatically tracing the electrodes [1,12,15,24], or fully automatically through clustering methods [3,7,23]. These solutions may face challenges when electrodes are close to each other. In DELRecon, the initial segment (i.e., the segment close to the cortical surface) of each electrode was automatically identified via clustering. The identification of the entire electrode and its trajectory was achieved by iterative tracking and stepwise clustering, during which spatial constraints reduce the likelihood of localization error.

Second, recent studies proposed to localize the contacts in SEEG electrodes through interpolation or extrapolation [12,15,24]. However, these methods relied on the precise identification of an initial pair of contacts in each electrode, and reconstruction errors may propagate to other contacts if the initial pair of contacts was incorrectly identified. DELRecon did not rely on the manual initialization of individual contacts. Instead, the toolbox used intensity-based clustering along the primary direction of the electrode to localize individual contacts, which does not depend on electrode architecture or contact density.

It is worth noting a few limitations in the current version of the toolbox. Some existing solutions can reconstruct both SEEG and subdural electrodes [2,12,18,22,23], whereas a few other tools support intracranial signal processing as an extension [3,23]. In contrast, DELRecon is specifically designed for SEEG electrode reconstruction, aiming to address this problem in complicated scenarios. Nevertheless, our scripts are freely available to enable further extensions or to be integrated with other processing pipelines. Same as other toolboxes [1,15], DELRecon currently requires a pre-implantation CT scan to generate the electrode image free from artefacts. Future updates could relax this constraint by introducing a residual removal step to remove non-brain voxels in the post-implantation CT image [2,7].

5   Conclusion

We presented an automated SEEG electrode reconstruction toolbox with adequate manual intervention features for visualization and error correction. The interactive clustering method can handle complex electrode reconstruction problems that may be challenging for other existing tools. Contact localization results were reported in an interpretable NIfTI electrode image along with the contact localization and anatomical details, which could be directly integrated with subsequent analyses. These features will make SEEG electrode reconstruction an easy task for researchers and clinicians.

References

1. Arnulfo, G., Narizzano, M., Cardinale, F., Fato, M.M., Palva, J.M.: Automatic segmentation of deep intracerebral electrodes in computed tomography scans. BMC Bioinform. **16**, 1–12 (2015)
2. Blenkmann, A.O., et al.: ielectrodes: a comprehensive open-source toolbox for depth and subdural grid electrode localization. Front. Neuroinform. **11**, 14 (2017)
3. Cai, F., Wang, K., Zhao, T., Wang, H., Zhou, W., Hong, B.: Brainquake: an open-source python toolbox for the stereoelectroencephalography spatiotemporal analysis. Front. Neuroinform. **15**, 773890 (2022)
4. Cardinale, F., et al.: Stereoelectroencephalography: surgical methodology, safety, and stereotactic application accuracy in 500 procedures. Neurosurgery **72**(3), 353–366 (2013)
5. Cardinale, F., et al.: Cerebral angiography for multimodal surgical planning in epilepsy surgery: description of a new three-dimensional technique and literature review. World Neurosurg. **84**(2), 358–367 (2015)
6. Chauvel, P., Gonzalez-Martinez, J., Bulacio, J.: Presurgical intracranial investigations in epilepsy surgery. Handb. Clin. Neurol. **161**, 45–71 (2019)
7. Ervin, B., et al.: Fast automated stereo-EEG electrode contact identification and labeling ensemble. Stereotact. Funct. Neurosurg. **99**(5), 393–404 (2021)
8. Ester, M., Kriegel, H.P., Sander, J., Xu, X., et al.: A density-based algorithm for discovering clusters in large spatial databases with noise. In: KDD. vol. 96, pp. 226–231 (1996)
9. Iida, K., Otsubo, H.: Stereoelectroencephalography: indication and efficacy. Neurol. Med. Chir. **57**(8), 375–385 (2017)
10. Jehi, L.: The epileptogenic zone: concept and definition. Epilepsy Currents **18**(1), 12–16 (2018)
11. Johnson, S.C.: Hierarchical clustering schemes. Psychometrika **32**(3), 241–254 (1967)
12. Lucas, A., et al.: ieeg-recon: a fast and scalable pipeline for accurate reconstruction of intracranial electrodes and implantable devices. Epilepsia **65**(3), 817–829 (2024)
13. Mercier, M.R., et al.: Advances in human intracranial electroencephalography research, guidelines and good practices. Neuroimage **260**, 119438 (2022)
14. Miller, B.A., Salehi, A., Limbrick, D.D., Smyth, M.D.: Applications of a robotic stereotactic arm for pediatric epilepsy and Neurooncology surgery. J. Neurosurg. Pediatr. **20**(4), 364–370 (2017)
15. Narizzano, M., et al.: Seeg assistant: a 3dslicer extension to support epilepsy surgery. BMC Bioinform. **18**, 1–13 (2017)
16. Nelson, J.H., Brackett, S.L., Oluigbo, C.O., Reddy, S.K.: Robotic stereotactic assistance (rosa) for pediatric epilepsy: a single-center experience of 23 consecutive cases. Children **7**(8), 94 (2020)
17. Princich, J.P., et al.: Rapid and efficient localization of depth electrodes and cortical labeling using free and open source medical software in epilepsy surgery candidates. Front. Neurosci. **7**, 260 (2013)
18. Qin, C., et al.: Automatic and precise localization and cortical labeling of subdural and depth intracranial electrodes. Front. Neuroinform. **11**, 10 (2017)
19. Rathore, C., Radhakrishnan, K.: Concept of epilepsy surgery and presurgical evaluation. Epileptic Disord. **17**(1), 19–31 (2015)
20. Rockhill, A.P., et al.: Intracranial electrode location and analysis in mne-python. J. Open Source Softw. **7**(70) (2022)

21. Rosenow, F., Lüders, H.: Presurgical evaluation of epilepsy. Brain **124**(9), 1683–1700 (2001)
22. Soper, D., et al.: Modular pipeline for reconstruction and localization of implanted intracranial ECOG and SEEG electrodes. PLoS ONE **18**(7), e0287921 (2023)
23. Villalon, S.M., et al.: Epitools, a software suite for presurgical brain mapping in epilepsy: Intracerebral EEG. J. Neurosci. Methods **303**, 7–15 (2018)
24. Wang, Z., Magnotti, J.F., Zhang, X., Beauchamp, M.S.: Yael: Your advanced electrode localizer. Eneuro **10**(10) (2023)

Segmenting Breast Ultrasound Scans Using a Generative Adversarial Network Embedding U-Net

Abraham Etinosa Enobun[1], Uche Henry Anakwenze[1],
Aboozar Taherkhani[1(✉)] , Zacharias Anastassi[1] , Fabio Caraffini[2] ,
and Hassan Eshkiki[2]

[1] School of Computer Science and Informatics, De Montfort University, Leicester, UK
p2688618@my365.dmu.ac.uk,
{aboozar.taherkhani,zacharias.anastassi}@dmu.ac.uk
[2] Department of Computer Science, Swansea University, Swansea SA1 8EN, UK
{fabio.caraffini,h.g.eshkiki}@swansea.ac.uk

Abstract. Breast ultrasound imaging, due to its noninvasive nature and cost-effectiveness, has become an indispensable instrument in the early detection of breast cancer, highlighting the importance of early detection of lesions for timely intervention. In this study, we discuss possible problems deriving from using deep learning techniques on such images and propose novel solutions towards achieving a segmentation tool based on a generative adversarial network architecture. As a proof-of-concept, we build on existing methods to develop our system by modifying a U-Net known as Residual-Dilated-Attention-Gate with the addition of skip modules and dilated convolutional neural networks after the decoder stage. Compared with other state-of-the-art methods in established evaluation metrics, the results indicate that the proposed model achieves the highest accuracy of 98.11%, despite being trained on a limited number of epochs. However, it still requires further tuning and optimisation to enhance precision, ensuring that it is more balanced, robust, and thus competitive with the state-of-the-art.

Keywords: generative adversarial network · U-Net · dilated convolution · breast ultrasound

1 Introduction

Breast cancer has a high global mortality rate. For instance, in China it constitutes 7.82% of the total mortality associated with female malignant tumours, establishing itself as one of the most lethal diseases.

Patients diagnosed with metastatic breast cancer typically face a poor prognosis, characterised by an average 5-year survival rate of approximately 27%. Upon metastasis (cancer that has spread to other parts of the body), the malignancy often progresses to a more severe tumour stage [19]. Although there have

X. Xie et al. (Eds.): AIiH 2024, LNCS 14976, pp. 149–159, 2024.
https://doi.org/10.1007/978-3-031-67285-9_11

been improvements in the methods used to detect breast cancer, patients diagnosed with metastatic breast cancer still tend to have poor outcomes. This poor prognosis is largely due to the fact that cancer is often diagnosed at a later stage, when it is more visible and painful, but also more difficult to treat effectively. This situation underscores the critical need for early detection and diagnosis for timely intervention and risk mitigation. The potential benefits of using AI to aid in these processes are numerous.

The prospective advantages of employing artificial intelligence in these diagnostic and therapeutic processes are numerous, given advances in the manipulation of medical images with AI-driven solutions in the last decades [3,13]. Note that non-invasive breast cancer diagnosis modalities include X-ray, and Magnetic Resonance Imaging (MRI), etc., which results in imagery data. Among these diagnostic modalities, Breast Ultrasound (BUS) imaging, due to its noninvasive nature, absence of ionising radiation, and cost effectiveness, has emerged as an indispensable instrument in the early detection of breast cancer [5].

BUS segmentation facilitates the precise identification and analysis of tumours, thereby increasing diagnostic accuracy. Although segmentation methodologies in various imaging modalities, such as MRI and computed tomography (CT), often employ analogous techniques, BUS segmentation (i.e., the extraction of the tumour region from the image) presents significant challenges. These challenges are primarily attributed to the inherently low quality of ultrasound images, which are marred by speckle noise and low contrast.

In this project, we focus on tumour segmentation in BUS imaging by modifying a GAN to employ U-Net within its architecture. We use dilated convolution to enlarge the receptive field after multiple down-sampling in the encoder and decoder, therefore boosting the classifier's accuracy. In addition, the model uses the residual block which replaces the basic neural units and an attention mechanism.

2   Background and Design Motivations

Segmentation constitutes a pivotal component of image analysis in the context of breast cancer diagnosis, encompassing critical processes such as detection, feature extraction, classification, and treatment. Nevertheless, BUS images are characteristically low-resolution and monochromatic, in contrast to other imaging modalities. Hence, ROIs of malignant regions are often uneven in shape, blurred, and have an indistinct border [9].

Different Deep Learning (DL) methods have been proposed to address the aforementioned challenges in the segmentation of BUS images, from semantic segmentation models such as SegNet [20] to multiple kinds of GANs [8,16,18]. For example, the study in [17] introduces an improved conditional GAN segmentation algorithm to learn tumour features, which employs an atrous convolution layer. To equalise the influence of high-level encoded characteristics, they adopted a channel-wise weighting block. The model undergoes training using a composite loss function comprised of the Structural Similarity Index (SSIM), the

L1-norm, and adversarial loss. An interesting approach proposed in [1] uses the You-Only-Look-Once (YOLO) model [14]. They segment large datasets using full-resolution convolutional networks (FrCN), and a deep convolutional neural network (CNN) determines whether the mass is benign or cancerous. Notably, the DeepLabv3+ semantic segmentation model from [4] is based on an encoder-decoder architecture, wherein the encoder is responsible for extracting both shallow and high-level features, and the decoder integrates these low-level and high-level features to enhance segmentation accuracy. DeepLabv3+ leverages ResNet architectures as its foundational backbone, integrating Atrous Convolution and the Atrous Spatial Pyramid Pooling (ASPP) module. The ASPP module encompasses a global average pooling operation and convolutional layers with varying dilation rates (specifically 1, 6, 12, and 18).

The U-Net model is another widely recognised and favoured approach for mammogram image segmentation. ERU-Net has U-shaped architecture, is designed like an auto-encoder. It contains two pathes, an encoding path (contracting) and a decoding path (expanding). Its capability in training on a relatively limited dataset of annotated images, coupled with the capabilities of high-performance GPU computing, renders it a viable and efficient option for this application [6]. In [10], a novel deeply supervised U-Net model (DS U-Net) integrated with dense conditional random fields (CRFs) is introduced, whereas [23] delineates a Residual-Dilated-Attention-Gate-UNet (RDAU-NET) derived from U-Net. This model substitutes neural units with residual units and incorporates an attention gate (AG) to enhance edge delineation and mitigate network performance degradation issues. These examples show the success and versatility of U-Net.

In this context, we investigate the use of a hybrid system that employs the Wasserstein Generative Adversarial Network [2] to perform the segmentation task. This variant ensures robust convergence and minimises the Wasserstein distance between real and generated data distributions. We used RDA-NET as the generator within the GAN architecture, as shown in Fig. 1. It should be noted that the RDA-NET employed, an improved variant of the fundamental U-Net architecture referenced in [11], incorporates specific modifications to rectify the limitations inherent in the U-Net model and increase the efficacy of the generative framework. The generator aims to produce data with the same distribution as the original to deceive the discriminator, and these generated data will be lesion-segmented maps of Breast Ultrasound Images in our system. With reference to Fig. 1, it can be observed a conventional encoder-decoder architecture. The input is subjected to successive down-sampling stages until it attains a bottleneck layer after which the process is inverted. Within this architecture, information traverses each hierarchical level, encompassing the bottleneck, to effectively capture both high-level and low-level features from the input data. It is ideal to transfer this data directly through the network because many image translation tasks share a significant amount of low-level information between the input and output. To provide the Generator with a way to bypass the bottleneck, we included skip-connections between layers of the same size in the encoder and decoder.

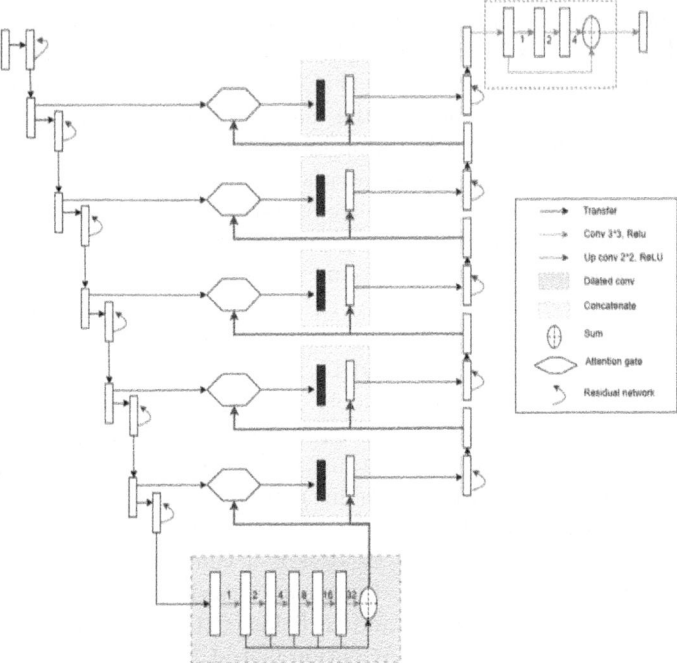

Fig. 1. RDA-U-Net architecture.

We implemented additional changes to the original architecture. Specifically, the original six neural units along the encoder path are replaced with six residual units, employed to prevent accuracy saturation (vanishing gradients) during training. However, smaller feature maps can reduce the accuracy of semantic segmentation. To address this, the outputs of the encoder pipeline are fed into a series of dilated convolution modules. These modules use 3×3 convolution kernels and have dilation ratios of $1, 2, 4, 8, 16$, and 32, respectively. The feature maps from the dilated convolution are summed, forming the output of the dilated convolution which is added to the architecture to broaden the receptive field. The output from this module is directed into the decoder pipeline, which consists of an up-sampling mechanism and five residual networks. Each layer within the decoder facilitates the upsampling process by integrating the intricate feature outputs derived from the decoder with the corresponding semantic information procured from the encoder. In contrast to the traditional U-Net's skip-connection components, we replaced the cropping and copying units with attention-gate modules (one for each residual net in the decoder), thus enabling the model to focus more on the lesion region and less on the unnecessary background.

Note that convolution and pooling in CNNs reduce spatial information, affecting segmentation accuracy. A Fully Convolutional Network (FCN) executes these operations to reduce the spatial dimensions of the image and extract abstract features, subsequently enlarging this output through upsampling. The convolution-pooling phase can be conceptualised as a downsampling operation that may induce information loss, thereby compromising the accuracy of the process and substantially diminishing the transferability of data details.

Since the U-Net encoder is a Fully Connected CNN (FC-CNN), dilated convolutions are used to insert 'holes' (i.e., zeros) into the kernel to achieve a larger receptive field than traditional convolution without a loss of resolution [22]. By design, they are suitable for dense prediction tasks, differing structurally from image classification by computing a label for each pixel. Their use enables us to obtain high-level multiscale contextual information while reducing the number of parameters and computational costs while performing segmentation.

The dilated convolution operator is characterised by a hyperparameter known as the dilation rate, which specifies the extent to which the kernel intervals are expanded[1]. Figure 2 (a) and (b) illustrate the visual field of a 3×3 convolution kernel with $r = 1$ and $r = 2$, respectively. When $r = 2$, the receptive field increases to 7×7 (shown as the orange and blue parts in (b)) compared to traditional convolution ($r = 1$, as shown in the blue part of (a)). Therefore, the dilation process increases the size of the receptive field and compensates for the subsampling.

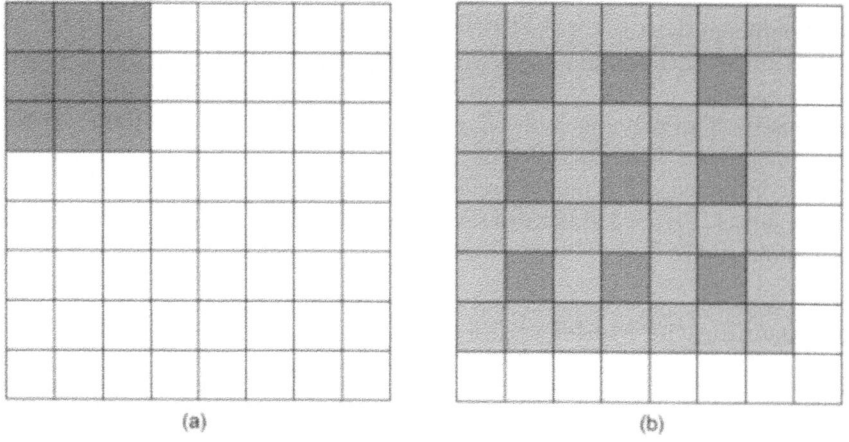

(a)   (b)

Fig. 2. Illustration of receptive field for $r = 1$ and $r = 2$ [23].

In the RDAU-NET model, the feature maps of size 4×4 obtained at the end of the encoder pipeline are fed into a series of dilated convolution modules with $r = 1, 2, 4, 8, 16, 32$ and $N = 3 \times 3$, 7×7, 15×15, 31×31, 63×63 and 127×127 respectively. The outputs of the six convolutions are added, upsampled (by a

---

[1] A dilation rate of 1 results in a classic convolution.

factor of 2), and then fed into the decoder pipeline as shown in Fig. 1. In the dilated convolution module, output feature maps match input sizes but capture information from a wide range of receptive fields, enhancing feature learning.

The proposed system incorporates a greater number of layers to enhance learning capability. Given that this may result in decelerated or halted learning, attributed to the phenomenon known as the 'vanishing gradient', we implement the residual learning correction technique as delineated in [7] to sustain the efficacy of gradient updates throughout the training process. Furthermore, to address common CNN issues like reduced spatial awareness from shared weights and redundant channels in U-Net-like networks [15], we add an attention module in the skip connection and concatenate low-level and high-level features to emphasise relevant channels and suppress irrelevant ones. The inclusion of attention modules in our model is motivated by successful studies, such as the one presented in [12], which integrates an Attention Gate (AG) module into a U-Net framework to facilitate spatial location and subsequent segmentation.

To enhance stability, we have selected a pre-trained model from [11] and used Adam to optimise the loss function with a learning rate of $1 - e4$.

3   Resources and Methods

3.1   Dataset

The experimental dataset is the BUS images in [21], containing a total of 645 low-contrast breast ultrasound images with evenly distributed benign and malignant lesions. Samples in this dataset are partitioned into training, validation, and test subsets. The training and validation subsets comprised 538 and 50 samples, respectively. The test subset included 57 samples, each with corresponding ground truth masks. The model's segmentation performance was evaluated using the test subset. Figure 3 illustrates several sample images along with their ground truth annotations.

3.2   Training the Model

The training procedure is delineated in Algorithm 1. It consists of iteratively alternating training phases for the discriminator and the generator over e epochs until the total allowed number of epochs is reached.

Initially, the discriminator is rendered trainable, whereas the generator remains untrainable. The generator is employed to produce image predictions, enabling the discriminator to classify these images and subsequently update its parameters accordingly. Conversely, the second phase is performed similarly but with an untenable discriminator and a trainable generator. This completes one training iteration and multiple iterations are performed according to the prefixed computation budget (total number of epochs). Following each training iteration, the model undergoes evaluation on the validation dataset. With each successive cycle, the segmentation accuracy in relation to the ground truth is expected

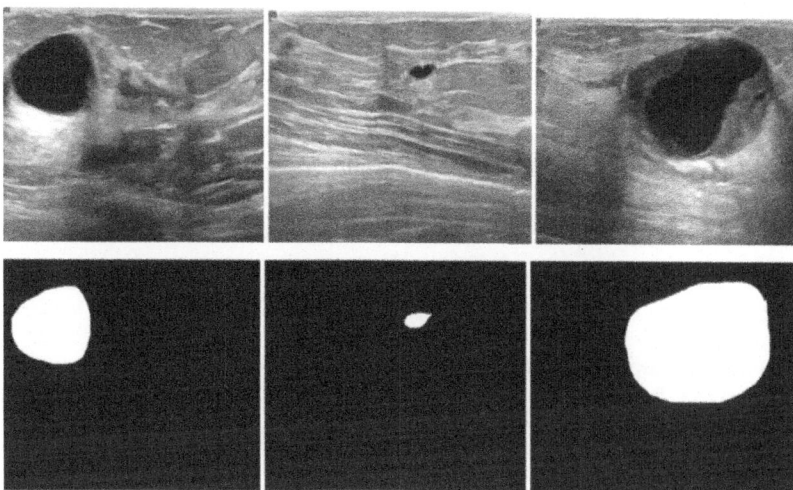

Fig. 3. Sample images from the dataset with their corresponding ground truth directly under

to demonstrate improvement. Optimal performances are achieved when the discriminator's accuracy asymptotically approaches 50%. Indeed, as the generator's performance enhances (i.e., it produces increasingly realistic images), the discriminator's efficacy deteriorates, because it becomes incapable of differentiating between authentic and synthetic data.

Algorithm 1. Training process

1: Fetch X ▷ Training set of BUS images
2: Initialise e ▷ Number of epochs ($e = 50$)
3: Initialise n ▷ Batch size ($n = 32$)
4: $\sigma = \frac{|X|}{n}$ ▷ Steps per epoch
5: **for** e times **do**
6:     **for** σ times **do**
7:         Make the discriminator trainable and the generator untrainable
8:         Use the Generator to predict an image
9:         Prepare batches and train the discriminator
10:     **end for**
11:     **for** σ times **do**
12:         Make the discriminator untrainable and the generator trainable
13:         Train the Generator
14:     **end for**
15: **end for**
16: **return** Trained GAN model

3.3   Experimental Setup

Owing to computational constraints, the experimental phase is conducted with a limitation of 50 epochs to train the model. The results are compared with those derived from state-of-the-art methodologies. Specifically, we have chosen the U-Net, SegNet, and RDAU-NET models for comparative analysis. The input images for all models are standardised to a resolution of 128 × 128, and the segmentation outputs are generated at the same resolution.

3.4   Results

Consistent with the design principles articulated in Sect. 2, we refer to our model as the RDA-NET-GAN. The segmentation outcomes obtained with the setup in Sect. 3.3 are evaluated using established metrics, as detailed in Table 1.

Table 1. Segmentation performance of models across multiple evaluation metrics.

Model	Loss	Acc	Dice	Precision	Sensitivity	Specificity	M-IOU	F1
U-Net	17.95	97.57	82.04	81.85	84.66	98.91	79.83	82.11
SEGNET	18.29	97.52	81.70	81.41	83.95	98.83	79.14	81.71
RDAU-NET	15.30	97.91	84.69	88.58	83.19	99.34	80.67	84.78
RDA-NET-GAN	25.03	98.11	85.84	84.78	75.14	99.07	79.97	66.16

Overall, RDAU-NET appears to offer the most balanced and robust performance across multiple metrics, while RDA-NET-GAN, despite a high accuracy of 98.11, may need further tuning to improve sensitivity and M-IOU. U-Net and SEGNET offer decent performance but are outperformed by RDAU-NET in key areas. The fact that our model improves the accuracy as well as perceived qualitative analysis of the segmented images (show an example of the results in Fig. 4) shows that the idea behind the algorithm is promising, even though it required more investigation to make it competitive with RDAU-NET.

The proposed model has more loss as this is a combined system and the adversarial losses is from the combination of the generator and the discriminator. Below are the outputs while testing the segmentation performance of the proposed model during training.

The suboptimal precision observed for the proposed model can be attributed to the limited number of epochs for which the model was trained, especially in comparison to other models. To a certain degree, this result was foreseeable given the low number of epochs used during the training phase. Strategies to increase the number of epochs without precipitating overfitting will be a focal point of future research activities.

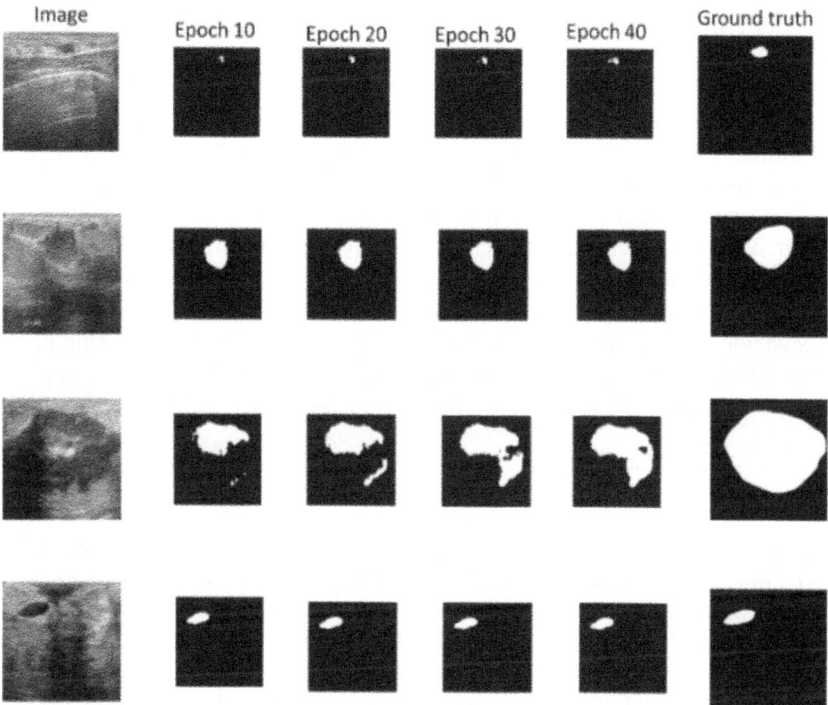

Fig. 4. Segmentation results of the proposed model

4   Conclusion

This study summarises relevant problems and literature gaps in using GAN for segmentation tasks and proposes ways to overcome these problems. When applied to the BUS images at dashed, it shows good visual results and displays the highest accuracy. It can be inferred that the GAN architecture holds significant promise for the segmentation of noisy datasets, and our proof-of-concept study indicates substantial potential for future advancements. Specifically, the incorporation of dilated CNNs after the decoder stage represents a novel methodology for the segmentation of breast lesions. This approach enhances the receptive field, thereby increasing the accuracy compared to directly applying the U-Net architecture. By comparing the model with the state-of-the-art, we are aware that there is room for improvement and that the model is not yet competitive with established methods such as RDAU-NET which is more rosubst and performing across various metrics, while our model performs very poorly in terms of pr precision. This aspect needs to be significantly improved.

During the training phase, the vanishing gradient problem manifested despite the algorithmic design precautions implemented to address the complexities inherent in the deep learning architecture of the proposed method. Therefore, the model requires further optimisation to be more competitive with the state-of-the-art.

It is worth noting that despite the suboptimal precision of the model, this outcome was somehow expected due to the limited number of epochs employed for training. This also demonstrates that acceptable results can still be achieved with a reduced number of training iterations (which can be advantageous in preventing overfitting) and with low-resolution images.

Next, the model will be subjected to additional optimisation to enhance its precision. Furthermore, an extended and more rigorous training phase will be conducted and we will apply this model to various datasets, thereby validating its segmentation capabilities. Additionally, considering that speckle noise is an intrinsic characteristic of ultrasound images, we will examine the impact of filtering techniques to refine our segmentation pipeline.

References

1. Al-antari, M.A., Al-masni, M.A., Choi, M.T., Han, S.M., Kim, T.S.: A fully integrated computer-aided diagnosis system for digital x-ray mammograms via deep learning detection, segmentation, and classification. Int. J. Med. Inform. **117**, 44–54 (2018). https://doi.org/10.1016/j.ijmedinf.2018.06.003, https://www.sciencedirect.com/science/article/pii/S1386505618302880

2. Arjovsky, M., Chintala, S., Bottou, L.: Wasserstein generative adversarial networks. In: International Conference on Machine Learning, pp. 214–223. PMLR (2017)

3. Castiglioni, I., et al.: AI applications to medical images: From machine learning to deep learning. Physica Medica **83**, 9–24 (2021). https://doi.org/10.1016/j.ejmp.2021.02.006, https://www.sciencedirect.com/science/article/pii/S1120179721000946

4. Chen, L.C., Zhu, Y., Papandreou, G., Schroff, F., Adam, H.: Encoder-decoder with atrous separable convolution for semantic image segmentation (2018)

5. Cheng, H., et al.: Automated breast cancer detection and classification using ultrasound images: a survey. Pattern Recogn. **43**(1) (2010). https://doi.org/10.1016/j.patcog.2009.05.012

6. Harrison, P., Michael, E., Ma, H., Li, H., Kulwa, F., Li, J.: Breast cancer segmentation methods: Current status and future potentials. BioMed Res. Int. **2021**, 9962109 (2021). https://doi.org/10.1155/2021/9962109

7. He, K., Zhang, X., Ren, S., Sun, J.: Deep residual learning for image recognition. CoRR abs/1512.03385 (2015). http://arxiv.org/abs/1512.03385

8. Karras, T., Laine, S., Aila, T.: A style-based generator architecture for generative adversarial networks (2019)

9. Kelly, K.M., Dean, J., Comulada, W.S., Lee, S.J.: Breast cancer detection using automated whole breast ultrasound and mammography in radiographically dense breasts. Eur. Radiol. **20**(3), 734–742 (2010). https://doi.org/10.1007/s00330-009-1588-y

10. Rajalakshmi, N. R., Vidhyapriya, R., Elango, N., Ramesh, N.: Deeply supervised U-Net for mass segmentation in digital mammograms. Int. J. Imaging Syst. Technol. **31**, 59–71 (2020). https://api.semanticscholar.org/CorpusID:228916143

11. Negi, A., Raj, A.N.J., Nersisson, R., Zhuang, Z., Murugappan, M.: RDA-UNET-WGAN: an accurate breast ultrasound lesion segmentation using wasserstein generative adversarial networks. Arabian J. Sci. Eng. **45**(8), 6399–6410 (2020). https://doi.org/10.1007/s13369-020-04480-z
12. Oktay, O., et al.: Attention U-Net: learning where to look for the pancreas (2018)
13. Rakic, M., Wong, H.E., Ortiz, J.J.G., Cimini, B., Guttag, J., Dalca, A.V.: Tyche: stochastic in-context learning for medical image segmentation (2024)
14. Redmon, J., Divvala, S.K., Girshick, R.B., Farhadi, A.: You only look once: unified, real-time object detection. CoRR abs/1506.02640 (2015). http://arxiv.org/abs/1506.02640
15. Ronneberger, O., Fischer, P., Brox, T.: U-net: convolutional networks for biomedical image segmentation. CoRR abs/1505.04597 (2015). http://arxiv.org/abs/1505.04597
16. Saffari, N., et al.: Fully automated breast density segmentation and classification using deep learning. Diagnostics (Basel, Switzerland) **10**(11), 988 (2020). https://doi.org/10.3390/diagnostics10110988
17. Singh, V.K., et al.: An efficient solution for breast tumor segmentation and classification in ultrasound images using deep adversarial learning (2019)
18. Singh, V.K., et al.: Breast tumor segmentation and shape classification in mammograms using generative adversarial and convolutional neural network. Expert Syst. Appl. **139**(C) (2020). https://doi.org/10.1016/j.eswa.2019.112855
19. Tashk, A., Hopp, T., Ruiter, N.V.: An innovative practical automatic segmentation of ultrasound computer tomography images acquired from USCT system. Iranian J. Sci. Technol. Trans. Elect. Eng. **43**(2) (2019). https://doi.org/10.1007/s40998-018-0098-9
20. Vianna, P., Farias, R., de Albuquerque Pereira, W.C.: U-net and segnet performances on lesion segmentation of breast ultrasonography images. Res. Biomed. Eng. **37**, 171–179 (2021)
21. Yap, M.H., et al.: Automated breast ultrasound lesions detection using convolutional neural networks. IEEE J. Biomed. Health Inform. **22**(4), 1218–1226 (2017)
22. Yu, F., Koltun, V.: Multi-scale context aggregation by dilated convolutions (2016)
23. Zhuang, Z., Li, N., Joseph Raj, A.N., Mahesh, V.G., Qiu, S.: An RDAU-net model for lesion segmentation in breast ultrasound images. PLoS ONE **14**(8), e0221535 (2019)

Enhancing Predictive Accuracy in Embryo Implantation: The Bonna Algorithm and its Clinical Implications

Gilad Rave[1], Daniel E. Fordham[1], Alex M. Bronstein[2], and David H. Silver[1(✉)]

[1] Rhea Labs, Rhea Fertility, Singapore, Singapore
{gilad.rave,daniel.fordham,david.silver}@rhea-fertility.com
[2] Department of Computer Science, Technion-Israel Institute of Technology, Haifa, Israel
bron@cs.technion.ac.il

Abstract. In the context of in vitro fertilization (IVF), selecting embryos for transfer is critical in determining pregnancy outcomes, with implantation as the essential first milestone for a successful pregnancy. This study introduces the Bonna algorithm, an advanced deep-learning framework engineered to predict embryo implantation probabilities. The algorithm employs a sophisticated integration of machine-learning techniques, utilizing MobileNetV2 for pixel and context embedding, a custom Pix2Pix model for precise segmentation, and a Vision Transformer for additional depth in embedding. MobileNetV2 was chosen for its robust feature extraction capabilities, focusing on textures and edges. The custom Pix2Pix model is adapted for precise segmentation of significant biological features such as the zona pellucida and blastocyst cavity. The Vision Transformer adds a global perspective, capturing complex patterns not apparent in local image segments. Tested on a dataset of images of human blastocysts collected from Ukraine, Israel, and Spain, the Bonna algorithm was rigorously validated through 10-fold cross-validation to ensure its robustness and reliability. It demonstrates superior performance with a mean area under the receiver operating characteristic curve (AUC) of 0.754, significantly outperforming existing models. The study not only advances predictive accuracy in embryo selection but also highlights the algorithm's clinical applicability due to reliable confidence reporting.

Keywords: Embryo Implantation · Deep Learning · Predictive Modeling · Clinical Decision Support · Artificial Intelligence in Reproductive Medicine

1 Introduction

The accurate prediction of embryo implantation probability represents a central challenge in assisted reproductive technology (ART) [1]. As it is the first measurable outcome of success in in-vitro fertilization after embryo transfer, it

X. Xie et al. (Eds.): AIiH 2024, LNCS 14976, pp. 160–171, 2024.
https://doi.org/10.1007/978-3-031-67285-9_12

serves as a proxy measure for the effectiveness of embryo selection [2]. Existing methodologies, while diverse, often fall short in delivering the specificity, objectivity, and reliability required for effective clinical application [3,4]. These range from basic morphological evaluations to intricate predictive modeling that incorporates various biomarkers [5–8]. Techniques such as time-lapse imaging paired with morphokinetic algorithms, although promising, have either not been proven clinically [6] or consistently fail to achieve the necessary precision for clinical settings [5]. Furthermore, while preimplantation genetic testing (PGT) offers extensive data, it also introduces significant ethical and logistical challenges [9].

Addressing this, the Bonna algorithm utilizes a comprehensive suite of deep learning techniques, including the MobileNetV2 convolutional network [10] for efficient image processing, a custom Pix2Pix generative adversarial network [11] for precise embryonic feature segmentation, and Vision Transformers [12] for detailed image analysis. Not only does this amalgamation enhance the algorithm's capability to identify subtle patterns indicative of viability but it also significantly boosts predictive accuracy and reliability beyond traditional methods. Additionally, the Bonna algorithm employs methods to provide confidence scores that correlate with the model's uncertainty, further enhancing its clinical utility in real-life settings [13].

This study rigorously evaluates the Bonna algorithm across datasets from Israel, Spain, Ukraine, and Spain, ensuring robust validation of its capabilities. Recent studies [14] have similarly leveraged multi-center data, underscoring the need for adaptive algorithms due to variations in embryo quality and implantation outcomes. The design of the Bonna algorithm not only addresses these variations but also offers a scalable solution adaptable to diverse clinical environments by using segmentation module (Pix2Pix) to remove optical factors.

By using an ensemble of several machine learning models [15,16], the algorithm capitalizes on their individual strengths in comprehensive image processing and segmentation. This approach provides a nuanced analysis of embryo viability, achieving state-of-the-art predictive performance in reproductive medicine. Ultimately, the Bonna algorithm aims to furnish clinicians with a reliable and personalized decision-support tool, designed to optimize IVF outcomes by selecting embryos with the highest potential for successful implantation.

2   Methodology

2.1   Dataset Collection and Preparation

The dataset for this retrospective cohort study was meticulously assembled from private clinics across three distinct geographical locations: Israel, Spain, Ukraine and France. This strategic selection captures a diverse embryological dataset, which is essential for generalizing model training. The data comprises time-lapse incubator (TLI) video files, specifically from the EmbryoScope and EmbryoScope+ (Vitrolife, Aarhus, Denmark) systems [17], with a resolution of 500 by 500 pixels. For this study, a single frame representing the blastocyst stage—Day 5 of incubation, was extracted from each TLI file at the point of

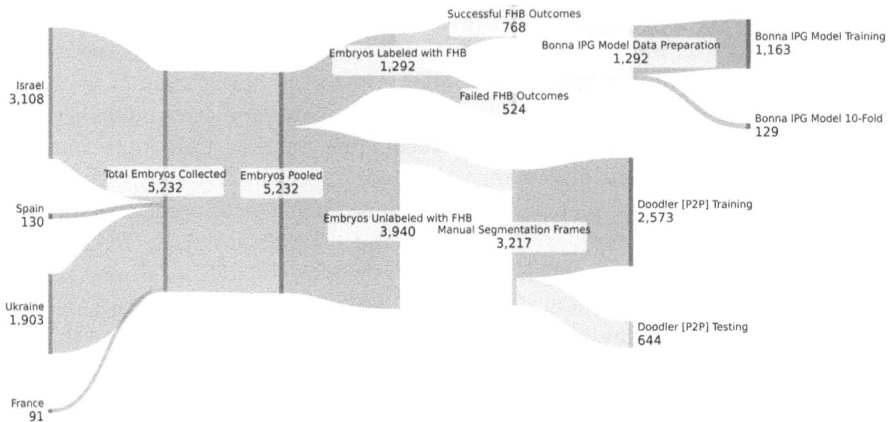

Fig. 1. Sankey diagram illustrating the comprehensive data flow of embryos from initial collection at various international sites through to the final stages of modeling. This includes steps such as categorization by Fetal Heartbeat (FHB) status, division into training and testing datasets, and processing through the Bonna IPG and DoodlerP2P (our custom Pix2Pix) models, highlighting the data preparation and utilization strategy employed.

embryo transfer. The dataset includes a total of 5,141 embryos derived from numerous patients who underwent ovarian stimulation cycles between 2012 and 2019. The demographic and embryological data specifics are as follows: Israel (3,108 embryos), Spain (130), Ukraine: (1,903), and France (91). This dataset was carefully stratified into categories based on the critical inclusion criterion of known implantation data (KID), defined here as the ultrasound evidence of a fetal heartbeat (FHB) [18] between 5 to 8 weeks post-transfer. This marker is pivotal not only for assessing embryo viability but also as a definitive test for implantation success, thereby indicating pregnancy [19].

2.2   Data Processing and Flow

Labeling and Stratification. A total of 1,292 embryos had Known Implantation Data (KID), with 741 embryos (57%) with positive Fetal Heartbeat (FHB) outcomes (successful implantation), and 551 embryos (43%) with negative Fetal Heartbeat (FHB) outcomes (failed implantation) (Fig. 1).

Demographics Summary of KID Embryos. Due to data de-identification, the exact number of patients in the study was unknown. Ethnicity, the reason for IVF, obstetric history, past medical history, or other medical classifiers were not available. 1,138 (88%) of the 1,292 embryos had associated maternal age at the time of embryo collection, ranging from 20 to 47 years (mean 34 years). These demographics were noted for contextual background and were not directly used in the model training or at inference time.

Model Preparation and Training. The embryos were segregated into successful and unsuccessful groups based on FHB outcomes for targeted Bonna IPG (Implantation Probability Grade) model training. From the remaining 3,851 embryos that did not have FHB labeling, we selected 3,217 frames at random, from different development stages, for the manual segmentation training essential for the DoodleP2P model's initial training phase. This structured and detailed preparation of the dataset ensured that both the Bonna IPG and DoodleP2P models were trained on robust and highly representative data, thereby enhancing the reliability and accuracy of the implantation predictions.

2.3   Model Architecture and Implementation.

The Bonna algorithm is based on the power of multiple advanced deep-learning models to optimize the prediction of embryo implantation outcomes. This section outlines the specific architecture and implementation details.

Architecture. As schematically summarized in Fig. 2, Bonna includes three primary components, each chosen for its specific capabilities in image analysis and feature extraction:

MobileNetV2 [10]: Known for its efficient parameterization, MobileNetV2 was selected primarily for its robust capability in capturing contextual embeddings from embryo images. This model processes the input images to extract lightweight yet informative features that include textures and edges, which are critical for the initial stages of image analysis.

DoodleP2P (customized Pix2Pix) [11]: This generative adversarial network (GAN) is used for segmenting the embryo images. It isolates significant biological features such as the zona pellucida and blastocyst cavity, which are essential for assessing embryo quality. The output of the DoodleP2P model is a three-channel mask, with each channel representing different biological parts: the zona pellucida, the cells, and the blastocyst cavity. These channels provide a pseudo-coloring of the embryo, helping to highlight and differentiate critical structures.

Vision Transformer (ViT) [12]: The Vision Transformer complements the feature set by adding a global perspective to the analysis [20]. It processes the segmented images to capture complex patterns that are not readily apparent in local image segments, such as spatial relationships and integrative morphological features, which are important for a comprehensive evaluation.

Implementation. The implementation of the Bonna algorithm involved several important steps designed to maximize the predictive performance.

Pre-processing. comprised normalization of all input images to standard scales to reduce model sensitivity to light and color variations [21], and augmentation with rotation, scaling, and flipping employed to enrich the dataset and ensure that the model is robust to various orientations and sizes of embryos [22].

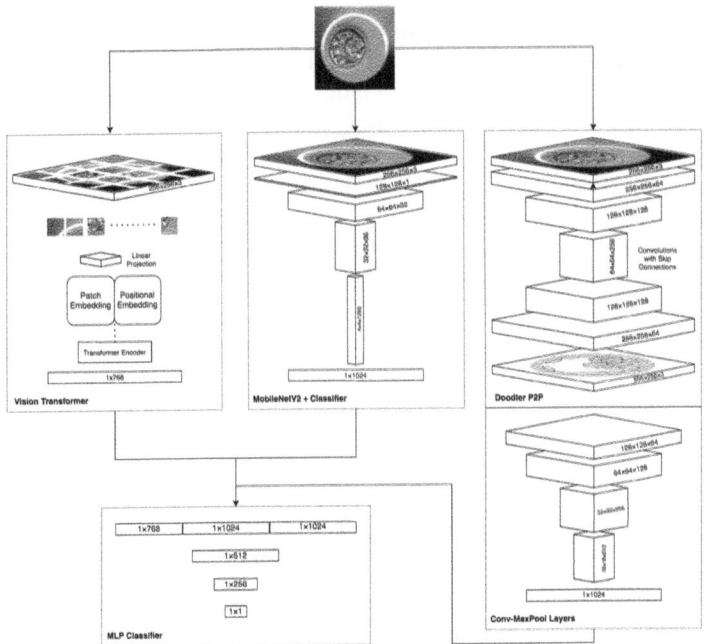

Fig. 2. Flowchart of the Bonna algorithm detailing the orchestrated integration of MobileNetV2 for feature extraction, DoodlerP2P for precise embryo segmentation, and Vision Transformer for enhanced pattern recognition. This schematic illustrates how these models synergistically contribute to the robust prediction of embryo implantation probabilities.

Feature extraction comprised MobileNetV2 and ViT features in tandem concatenated into a feature vector containing both local contextual as well as global morphological characteristics.

Segmentation and embedding relied on the DoodleP2P model to segment out critical areas within the embryo images [23]. The three-channel mask output by DoodleP2P, representing different biological parts, was used to train a custom convolutional neural network (CNN) that further refines the embeddings by focusing on these key features.

Classification: The final prediction was made using a multi-layer perceptron (MLP) classifier [24], which integrates the embeddings into its architecture to classify the likelihood of implantation. The classifier categorizes embryos into two primary outcomes: 'Likely to implant' and 'Unlikely to implant'. These categories are determined based on the presence or absence of a fetal heartbeat (FHB), which is the clinical endpoint of interest in this study. The MLP was trained using the standard cross-entropy loss, which measures the performance of the classification model whose output is a probability value between 0 and 1.

Inference Phase and Prediction Stability. The inference phase is essential for estimating the posterior probability of the Implantation Probability Grade (IPG) based on the images, which is critical to the Bonna algorithm's effectiveness. To enhance the robustness and reliability of predictions, the algorithm employs a "jitter" process involving multiple simulations and augmentations. This approach helps mitigate variability and stabilize the prediction outcomes.

At inference time, each embryo image first undergoes augmentation by 16 random transformations including rotations, translations, scaling, and flips. These augmentations accommodate different positional and morphological nuances of embryos as encountered in clinical settings [25].

Each of the 16 augmented images is then processed with 16 dropout simulations. This regularization technique mimics the effect of model averaging and helps stabilize the predictions by randomly omitting subsets of features or neurons [26].

This "jitter" process generates a total of 256 inputs per embryo, using which the predictive score distribution is obtained.

The standard deviation (STD) of the predicted score is used to assess the prediction confidence, quantified using the negative logarithm of the standard deviation, $-\log(\text{STD})$, with higher values denoting greater prediction confidence.

The empirical confidence intervals calculated from the score distribution are directly linked to the algorithm's performance, which we quantitatively assessed using the Area Under the Curve (AUC) of the Receiver Operating Characteristic (ROC) [27]. In the scenario of embryo selection, which fundamentally involves ranking each embryo in a cohort based on likelihood of success, the AUC is an invaluable metric. It provides a statistical measure of the model's ability to accurately rank embryos, estimating the probability that a viable embryo (positive instance) is scored higher than a non-viable one (negative instance). This capability to correctly prioritize embryos is critical for effective selection and significantly influences clinical outcomes. High AUC values indicate superior discrimination ability of the model, pivotal in clinical settings where the implications of false positives or negatives are substantial. Thus, by minimizing score variability and maximizing prediction confidence, the Bonna algorithm not only achieves high precision but also ensures dependable consistency across its predictions, reinforcing its suitability for high-stakes clinical decision-making.

3   Results

This section summarizes the tools and methodologies employed to evaluate the performance of the Bonna algorithm, focusing on comparative analysis with existing models through Receiver Operating Characteristic (ROC) curves and Area Under the Curve (AUC) metrics.

3.1   Model Performance Evaluation

The performance of the Bonna algorithm was systematically evaluated against a range of existing models, with a particular focus on those utilized for the embryo implantation prediction task. The evaluation criteria centered around the AUC metric, which provides an aggregate measure of performance across all possible classification thresholds. The ROC curve and AUC comparison chart highlight the effectiveness and superiority of our model.

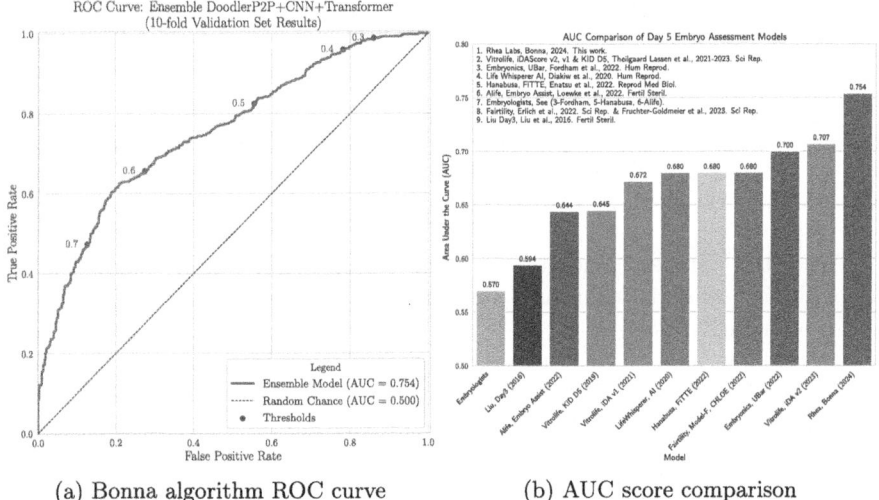

(a) Bonna algorithm ROC curve   (b) AUC score comparison

Fig. 3. (a) ROC plot depicting the sensitivity (true positive rate) and specificity (1−false positive rate) of the Bonna algorithm's predictions, providing insights into its diagnostic ability. (b) Mean AUC scores of the Bonna algorithm compared with those attained by contemporary embryo selection models [6, 14, 28–32], underscoring its superior predictive capabilities.

The ROC curve (Fig. 3) plots the true positive rate (sensitivity) against the false positive rate (1-specificity) at various threshold settings.

The Area Under the ROC Curve (AUC) score provides a useful quantitative measure of the sensitivity-specificity tradeoff. An AUC of 1 represents perfect prediction, while an AUC of 0.5 suggests no discriminative power on a balanced test set. The Bonna algorithm's AUC of 0.754 reflects high competency in distinguishing between classes (successful vs. unsuccessful implantation), far exceeding the typical benchmarks set by existing models.

3.2 Confidence and Predictive Accuracy

A standout result from our study is the pronounced correlation between prediction confidence and AUC scores, which notably underscores the Bonna algorithm's precision. Our analysis involves setting various confidence cutoff percentiles and observing their impact on the AUC scores. The results are compelling, particularly at higher confidence levels.

The framework used in the Bonna algorithm allows us to set empirical confidence thresholds, which helps categorize predictions according to their likelihood of accuracy. By increasing the confidence cutoff percentile, we selectively evaluate predictions that the model deems to be more certain by binning the confidence score into quantile levels, as depicted in Fig. 4.

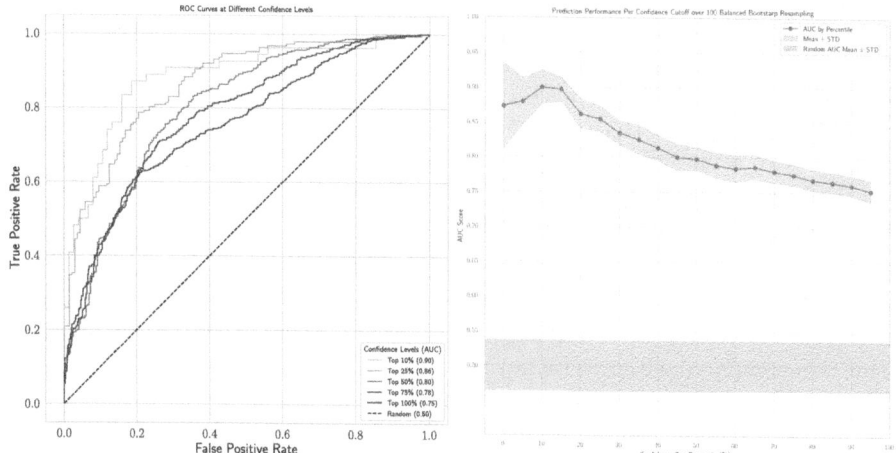

(a) ROC Curves for different confidence threshold percentiles

(b) AUC with Confidence Intervals

Fig. 4. Graph of AUC scores as a function of confidence percentile cutoffs for the Bonna algorithm. (a) Demonstrates exceptional predictive accuracy particularly at higher confidence levels, with AUC peaking at 0.9 at the 10th percentile. (b) The trend suggests that the higher the confidence percentile cutoff, the more reliable the predictions. The shaded areas are confidence intervals from bootstrapped sampling of the dataset 100 times.

This strong correlation between prediction confidence and AUC scores not only validates the Bonna algorithm's robust predictive capabilities but also enhances its clinical applicability. By implementing a model with high precision at elevated confidence levels, clinicians can make more informed decisions, potentially leading to improved IVF outcomes. This reliability is crucial for clinical settings where decision accuracy is paramount, and the Bonna algorithm stands out as a particularly dependable tool in such high-stakes environments.

4   Discussion and Conclusion

The Bonna algorithm has established a profound correlation between high confidence predictions and AUC scores, achieving a peak AUC of 0.9 at the 10th and 15th confidence percentiles. These findings are of considerable clinical relevance.

The algorithm's capability to deliver accurate predictions on embryo implantation based on high-confidence intervals and acknowledge cases in which the prediction is less accurate offers a reliable tool for clinicians practicing assisted reproductive technology (ART). This advancement facilitates enhanced personalization in treatment strategies, potentially optimizing patient outcomes and improving resource management.

Study Highlights. This study's methodology integrates a combination of deep learning techniques, including MobileNetV2 for efficient image processing, the customized DoodleP2P for precise feature segmentation, and a Vision Transformer for advanced pattern recognition. This integration achieves state-of-the-art predictive accuracy. The rigorous validation of the algorithm, involving 10-fold cross-validation and robust testing procedures such as image augmentation and dropout at the inference stage, further underscores the model's reliability and robustness.

Comparison to Competing Models. The performance of the Bonna algorithm was compared with several key models in the domain. Firstly, although not tested on identical datasets, the predictive performance of the Bonna algorithm demonstrates notable superiority over traditional embryologists' assessments and when compared to the iDAScore v2 [14], which is recognized as best-in-class for this task.

It is worth noting that although some methodologies claim very high AUC scores [5, 33] of 0.93 & 0.98 respectively, they suffer from methodological flaws including non-transferred embryos as negatives or using human scores as ground-truth labels. These practices not only introduce selection bias but also inaccurately inflate performance metrics. Such high AUC scores are generally achieved in simpler tasks and do not reflect the complex nature of predicting successful embryo implantation, which also depends significantly on transfer skill and maternal factors.

Clinical Implications of the Confidence Score. Providing confidence scores significantly enhances the Bonna algorithm's reliability and confidence in clinical predictions of embryo implantation. This method uses the variability among 256 outcomes per embryo, derived from multiple dropout simulations and image augmentations, to calculate prediction certainty. This is quantified through the negative logarithm of the standard deviation $-log(\text{STD})$, where higher values denote greater confidence. The clinical utility of conformal prediction improves the precision and reliability of medical decisions by aligning the confidence measure with the Area Under the Curve (AUC).

Clinical Integration and Future Directions. The remarkable performance achieved by the Bonna algorithm allows its application in clinical settings, where its high predictive accuracy and certainty can significantly aid in informed decision-making processes. This tool's integration into clinical practice promises to refine how decisions are made in ART, with a solid potential to enhance the efficacy of embryo selection and implantation strategies.

The Bonna algorithm is, however, limited by its reliance on retrospective data and the specificity of its current applications. Prospective studies are essential to establish its real-time effectiveness and adaptability across various IVF clinics worldwide and should include a broader demographic of patients. While expanding outcome measures to include live births could provide a more comprehensive success metric, this introduces complexity as such measures integrate broader, non-embryonic factors like maternal health, which are beyond the predictive scope of embryo imagery. Furthermore, the algorithm's broader acceptance and utility would benefit from improvements in explainability [34], helping clinicians understand decision processes. However, explainability can come at a cost [35].

Future Research. Future research should focus on refining prediction confidence techniques to enhance reliability and accuracy, further integrating the algorithm into clinical practice. Additionally, applying the principles and techniques developed for the Bonna algorithm to other areas of medical imaging could significantly expand its impact and utility across different medical fields. This expansion not only broadens the clinical applications but also fosters innovative approaches in predictive modeling and patient care optimization.

Competing Interests. The developed algorithm has potential for future commercial applications by an entity employing the authors.

References

1. Mastenbroek, S., et al.: Embryo selection in IVF. Hum. Reprod. **26**(5), 964–966 (2011). https://doi.org/10.1093/humrep/der050
2. Maheshwari, A., McLernon, D., Bhattacharya, S.: Cumulative live birth rate: time for a consensus? Hum. Reprod. **30**(12), 2703–2707 (2015). https://doi.org/10.1093/humrep/dev263
3. Van den Abbeel, E., et al.: Association between blastocyst morphology and outcome of single-blastocyst transfer. Reprod. Biomed. Online **27**(4), 353–361 (2013). https://doi.org/10.1016/j.rbmo.2013.07.006. Epub 2013 Jul 18. PMID: 23953585
4. Alpha Scientists in Reproductive Medicine and ESHRE Special Interest Group of Embryology. The Istanbul consensus workshop on embryo assessment: proceedings of an expert meeting. Hum. Reprod. **26**(6), 1270–1283 (2011). https://doi.org/10.1093/humrep/der037
5. Khosravi, P., Kazemi, E., Zhan, Q., et al.: Deep learning enables robust assessment and selection of human blastocysts after in vitro fertilization. NPJ Digit. Med. **2**, 21 (2019). https://doi.org/10.1038/s41746-019-0096-y
6. Fordham, D.E., et al.: Embryologist agreement when assessing blastocyst implantation probability: is data-driven prediction the solution to embryo assessment subjectivity? Hum. Reprod. **37**(10), 2275–2290 (2022). https://doi.org/10.1093/humrep/deac171

7. Gardner, D.K., et al.: Blastocyst score affects implantation and pregnancy outcome: towards a single blastocyst transfer. Fertil. Steril. **73**(6), 1155–1158 (2000). https://doi.org/10.1016/S0015-0282(00)00518-5

8. Hernández-Vargas, P., Muñoz, M., Domínguez, F.: Identifying biomarkers for predicting successful embryo implantation: applying single to multi-omics to improve reproductive outcomes. Hum. Reprod. Update **26**(2), 264–301 (2020). https://doi.org/10.1093/humupd/dmz042

9. Munné, S., et al.: Preimplantation genetic testing for aneuploidy versus morphology as selection criteria for single frozen-thawed embryo transfer in good-prognosis patients: a multicenter randomized clinical trial. Fertil. Steril. **112**(6), 1071–1079.e7 (2019). https://doi.org/10.1016/j.fertnstert.2019.07.1346

10. Sandler, M., et al.: Mobilenetv2: inverted residuals and linear bottlenecks. In: Proceedings of the IEEE Conference on Computer Vision and Pattern Recognition (CVPR) (2018)

11. Isola, P., et al.: Image-to-image translation with conditional adversarial networks. In: Proceedings of the IEEE Conference on Computer Vision and Pattern Recognition (CVPR) (2017). https://arxiv.org/abs/1611.07004

12. Dosovitskiy, A., et al.: An image is worth 16x16 words: transformers for image recognition at scale. In: ICLR (2021). https://openreview.net/forum?id=YicbFdNTTy

13. Shafer, G., Vovk, V.: A tutorial on conformal prediction. J. Mach. Learn. Res. **9**, 371–421 (2008). http://jmlr.org/papers/v9/shafer08a.html

14. Theilgaard Lassen, J., et al.: Development and validation of deep learning based embryo selection across multiple days of transfer. Sci. Rep. **13**(1), 4235 (2023). https://doi.org/10.1038/s41598-023-31136-3

15. Dietterich, T.G.: Ensemble methods in machine learning. In: Kittler, J., Roli, F. (eds.) MCS 2000. LNCS, vol. 1857, pp. 1–15. Springer, Heidelberg (2000). https://doi.org/10.1007/3-540-45014-9_1

16. Zhou, Z.H.: Ensemble Methods: Foundations and Algorithms. Chapman and Hall/CRC (2012). https://www.crcpress.com/Ensemble-Methods-Foundations-and-Algorithms/Zhou/p/book/9781439830031

17. Montag, M., Kajhøj, T.Q., Agerholm, I.E.: Description of time-lapse systems: embryoscope™. In: Meseguer, M. (ed.) Time-Lapse Microscopy in In-Vitro Fertilization. chapter 11, pp. 11–30. Cambridge University Press, Cambridge (2016)

18. Zegers-Hochschild, F., et al.: The international glossary on infertility and fertility care, 2017. Fertil. Steril. **108**(3), 393–406 (2017). https://doi.org/10.1016/j.fertnstert.2017.06.005

19. Sayed, S., et al.: Time-lapse imaging derived morphokinetic variables reveal association with implantation and live birth following in vitro fertilization: a retrospective study using data from transferred human embryos. PLoS ONE **15**(11), e0242377 (2020). https://doi.org/10.1371/journal.pone.0242377

20. Maurício, J., Domingues, I., Bernardino, J.: Comparing vision transformers and convolutional neural networks for image classification: a literature review. Appl. Sci. **13**, 5521 (2023). https://doi.org/10.3390/app13095521

21. Singh, D., Singh, B.: Investigating the impact of data normalization on classification performance. Appl. Soft Comput. **97**(Part B), 105524 (2020). https://doi.org/10.1016/j.asoc.2019.105524

22. Shorten, C., Khoshgoftaar, T.M.: A survey on image data augmentation for deep learning. J. Big Data **6**, 60 (2019). https://doi.org/10.1186/s40537-019-0197-0

23. Garcia-Garcia, A., et al.: A review on deep learning techniques applied to semantic segmentation. arXiv preprint arXiv:1704.06857 (2017). https://arxiv.org/abs/1704.06857

24. Haykin, S.: Neural Networks: A Comprehensive Foundation. Prentice Hall PTR (1994)

25. Börnfors, F., Klint, E.: Data Augmentation to Increase Multi-Site Robustness for Convolutional Neural Networks - A case study on MRI segmentation of target and organs at risk for prostate cancer (2019). ISSN 1404-6342. Student Paper

26. Gal, Y., Ghahramani, Z.: Dropout as a Bayesian approximation: representing model uncertainty in deep learning. In: Proceedings of the 33rd International Conference on Machine Learning - vol. 48, pp. 1050–1059, New York, NY, USA (2016). JMLR.org

27. Hajian-Tilaki, K.: Receiver operating characteristic (roc) curve analysis for medical diagnostic test evaluation. Caspian J. Int. Med. **4**(2), 627–635 (2013). PMID: 24009950; PMCID: PMC3755824

28. Liu, Y., et al.: Time-lapse deselection model for human day 3 in vitro fertilization embryos: the combination of qualitative and quantitative measures of embryo growth. Fertil. Steril. **105**(3), 656–662.e1 (2016). https://doi.org/10.1016/j.fertnstert.2015.11.003. Epub 2015 Nov 23

29. Loewke, K., et al.: Characterization of an artificial intelligence model for ranking static images of blastocyst stage embryos. Fertil. Steril. **117**(3), 528–535 (2022). https://doi.org/10.1016/j.fertnstert.2021.11.022

30. Enatsu, N., et al.: A novel system based on artificial intelligence for predicting blastocyst viability and visualizing the explanation. Reprod. Med. Biol. **21**(1), e12443 (2022). https://doi.org/10.1002/rmb2.12443

31. Erlich, I., et al.: Pseudo contrastive labeling for predicting IVF embryo developmental potential. Sci. Rep. **12**, 2488 (2022). https://doi.org/10.1038/s41598-022-06336-y

32. Diakiw, S.M., et al.: Development of an artificial intelligence model for predicting the likelihood of human embryo euploidy based on blastocyst images from multiple imaging systems during IVF. Hum. Reprod. **37**(8), 1746–1759 (2022). https://doi.org/10.1093/humrep/deac131

33. Tran, D., et al.: Deep learning as a predictive tool for fetal heart pregnancy following time-lapse incubation and blastocyst transfer. Hum. Reprod. **34**(6), 1011–1018 (2019). https://doi.org/10.1093/humrep/dez064

34. Weiss, T., et al.: Interpretable deep-learning unveils structure-property relationships in polybenzenoid hydrocarbons. ChemRxiv (2022). This content is a preprint and has not been peer-reviewed

35. Bronstein, M.: The road to biology 2.0 will pass through black box data. Towards Data Science (2024). https://towardsdatascience.com/the-road-to-biology-2-0-will-pass-through-black-box-data-bbd00fabf959. Accessed 15 Apr 2024

Bacterial Behaviour Analysis Through Image Segmentation Using Deep Learning Approaches

Afroza Rahman[1]([✉]), Miraz Rahman[2], and Md Atiqur Rahman Ahad[1]

[1] University of East London, London, UK
afroza.cs102@gmail.com, mahad@uel.ac.uk
[2] King's College London, London, UK
k.miraz.rahman@kcl.ac.uk

Abstract. Antimicrobial Resistance (AMR) refers to the ability of microorganisms to resist the effects of certain medicines. Medicines that were previously known effective against diseases caused by different types of microorganisms are now incompetent towards the same treatment because of AMR, which also increases the risk of severe illness. By understanding AMR and the potential factors that lead to it, we can see how microorganism behaviour analysis has become a great tool. The limitation of human visual capabilities requires automated image-based solutions to analyse bacterial behaviour effectively. In this paper, we exploit growth stage-based multiple images of bacteria, i.e. *E. coli* (*Escherichia coli*) to Analyse bacterial behaviours to get valuable insight. We have used the Deep Learning algorithms to get segmented images for each of the growth stages. Our objective is to use U-net and StarDist to get bacterial behavioural features and compare their performances in terms of Ground Truth and predicted segmented masks. For both the Ground Truth and predicted segmented mask, we have determined total bacterial cell count, average bacteria volume, central distance from the image center, total area, average aspect, average solidity, average extent, average orientation, average Local Binary Patterns (LBP) and features of Gray-Level Co-occurrence Matrix (GLCM) such as contrast, dissimilarity, homogeneity, energy, and Angular Second Moment for each of the images. Also, we have analysed area change and movement from one frame to another frame, which represents bacterial growth over specific periods. Analysing these features will allow the researcher to identify the best-performing model for each of the calculating features of bacteria. Comparing these features between the actual mask and predicted segmented mask can help to identify valuable insights regarding bacterial behaviour which can be useful to identify factors that contribute towards AMR.

Keywords: Bacterial Behaviour Analysis · Image Segmentation · Deep Learning · Antimicrobial Resistance · AMR

© The Author(s), under exclusive license to Springer Nature Switzerland AG 2024
X. Xie et al. (Eds.): AIiH 2024, LNCS 14976, pp. 172–185, 2024.
https://doi.org/10.1007/978-3-031-67285-9_13

1   Introduction

Analysis of microorganism images allows healthcare specialists to diagnose infectious diseases caused by bacteria, fungi, or another microorganism [1]. However, microorganism image analysis is a critical approach because of the cell complexity and structure of microorganisms [2]. Microorganisms play a vital role in our ecological systems. It is estimated that there are nearly 10 million microorganisms can be found in a single drop of water [3]. Bacteria, fungi, parasites, and viruses are essential for the sustainability of our environment [4].

Some microorganisms such as viruses, bacteria, fungi, and others can spread diseases to humans and living animals. These can cause minor infections, severe infections, and even death. In the year 2019, there were 7.7 million people died due to various bacterial infections which refers to the 13.6% of people or 1 in every 8 people in the world on the other hand bacterial human pathogens are increasing very rapidly every year [5].

AMR is a natural phenomenon that happens when microorganisms are exposed to antibiotic drugs [6]. AMR is now considered a global health emergency which makes treatment more and more difficult and requires an urgent global response [7]. Therefore, it is necessary to study AMR and develop new antibiotics through global investments [8]. In this case, AI-based models to analyse behaviours of bacteria can help to identify valuable insight regarding AMR and allow the researcher to fight AMR. It is predicted that AMR could lead 10 million people to death by the year 2050, which is alarming news [9]. We need to identify other root causes of AMR such as overdose and misuse of antibiotics and techniques to control AMR [10, 11].

To study AMR, analysis of bacterial images can be a great tool. Microscopic images of bacteria can be used to identify features and behaviours of bacteria. However, bacterial original images can be misleading in terms of noise generation. Therefore, actual mask image is an excellent alternative to use for analysis. On the other hand, generating an actual mask for each image is not only time-consuming but also costly. Therefore, Deep Learning (DL)-based models can be used to get predicted masks quickly and efficiently. Then those predicted mask images can be used to identify valuable patterns and insights of bacterial behaviours.

Analysing microscopic Images also needs a large number of datasets which is expensive and time-consuming. It is necessary to extract important features from images from small datasets to understand the nature of bacteria and the process of resistance towards available drugs. So that researchers can focus more on advancing the existing antibiotics rather than collecting and evaluating microscopic images. To make their work easier and focused on solving AMR-based challenges we are using Deep Learning based models to do image analysis focusing behaviour analysis of bacterial pathogens.

Figure 1 shows the overview of our explored work. In this study, we have used DL models such as U-Net and StarDist to generate predicted masks from datasets having both original images and actual masks for training and testing.

We have trained our U-Net model using original images and actual masks. After that, we tested and measured accuracy over predicted masks.

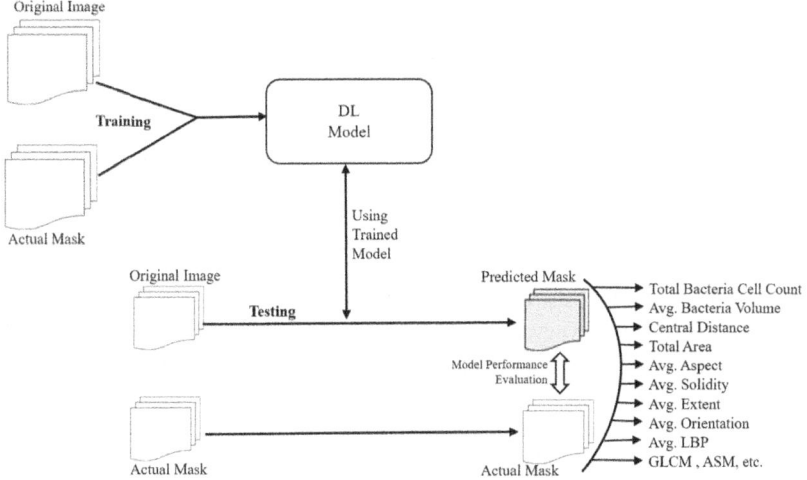

Fig. 1. Overview of our methodology.

Then we have identified some valuable properties of bacteria such as total bacterial cell count, average bacteria volume, central distance from the image center, total area, average aspect, average solidity, average extent, average orientation, average Local Binary Patterns and features of Gray-Level Co-occurrence Matrix such as contrast, dissimilarity, homogeneity, energy, and Angular Second Moment for each of the actual images and predicted images generated from U-Net and StarDist. We have also examined the area changes and movement from one frame of the actual mask and predicted mask to another immediate frame of the actual mask and predicted mask within a specific time duration.

This paper is divided as follows. Section 2 discusses a literature review focusing on both recent and previous works related to bacterial behaviours using AI techniques. Section 3 shows data description and terminologies. Section 4 explains our methodology and Sect. 5 discusses result analysis. Finally, Sect. 6 concludes the paper focusing conclusion and future work.

2   Literature Review

In this section, we aim to discuss both recent works and previous works related to bacterial image segmentation, and bacterial behaviours observations focusing on AMR and AI.

In [12], authors focused more on increasing the accuracy of the result of segmentation extending the StarDist algorithm. It also compared the results of classical image processing models and deep learning models for segmentation models. However, it was more focused on single-cell segmentation and it is hard to use in 3D images. They did not analyse the behaviour of the bacteria.

In [13], the authors used DL approaches for Medical Modality Image Segmentation. They have reviewed how Convolutional Neural Networks (CNN), Recurrent Networks, Attention Models, and Generative Adversarial Networks (GANs) can be used to perform medical modality image segmentation. However, we did not find any attention towards microscopy image analysis, particularly for microorganisms. Besides, they did not mention any approach to identify image features using these models. In this work, we used various approaches to identify key bacterial behaviours from segmented images after using U-Net and StarDist.

On the other hand, in [14], authors proposed classification methods for phase contrast time-lapse microscopy images using DL to classify four species of bacteria which are (*E. faecalis, E. coli, K. pneumoniae, and P. aeruginosa*), which are relevant to human health. They achieved more than 98% accuracy. But, we did not find any specific comparison among models and which models work better in terms of which type of bacterial behaviours identification. In this work, we have done a vital comparison between two models that are U-Net and StarDist demonstrating their performances in every specific case.

In [15], authors proposed a method using CNN in transmission electron microscope images to identify drug-resistant cells which leads to AMR. They used Pearson's Correlation Coefficient, to investigate the genes which are associated with morphological features.

However, we did not find any explanation for finding bacterial behaviours such as total aspect, total bacteria volume, and others as well as which approach is suitable to identify specific bacterial behaviours.

From [16], we got motivation for this work. We have used a subject of their dataset. The authors proposed DeepBacs for multitask bacterial image analysis using Dl approaches. They showed image segmentation using various techniques, worked on artificial labeling, denoising, enhanced image resolution, and more. But, we did not find any specific approach for determining bacterial behaviours such as central distance from the image centre, average solidity, average extent, and more. In this work, we have analysed various bacterial behaviours which may provide valuable insights towards bacterial study and AMR.

In [17], authors expressed their opinions about monitoring and investigating microorganisms using AI. The authors showed how researchers can use DL methods to study the classification, detection, segmentation, and quantification of microorganisms. However, we found a clear gap regarding analysing microorganisms' behaviours such as bacterial behaviours and movements in microscopic image segmentation. In this paper, we analysed bacterial movement from frame to frame in specific periods, which may help medicine researchers to examine effects of antibiotics on bacteria that are antimicrobial on microorganisms.

3   Data Description and Terminologies

3.1   Data Description

In this study we have exploited Brightfield Images of *E. coli* bacteria from Deep-Bacs open-source Dataset [16]. The dataset is a subset of a large dataset that contains different bacteria images in various conditions. We have divided the dataset into three fragments. Each fragment contains several growth-based time series image data of *E. coli* bacteria. The bacteria cell type is *E. coli* MG1655 wild type strain (CGSC #6300) Here, we have total two types of image data in the dataset which are actual image data and actual mask data. Using our selected models we have generated predicted segmented mask data.

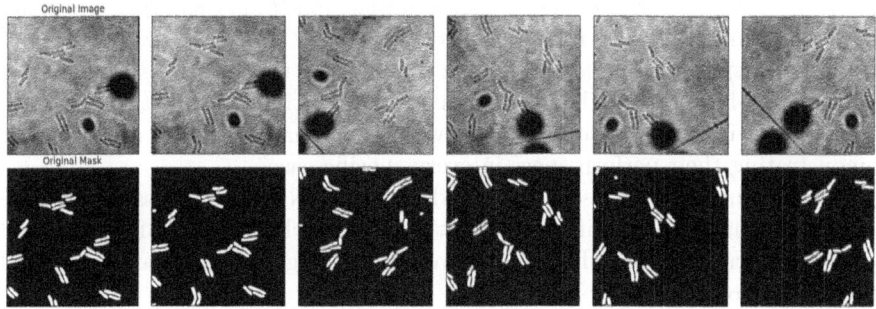

Fig. 2. Several sample image of original images alongside their respective ground truth masks.

The microscopy image data is in 2D, which are recorded at 1 min interval. To capture image data the device was used, the Nikon Eclipse Ti-E, which equipped with an Apo TIRF 1.49NA 100x oil immersion objective. Here image size is 1024×1024 (79 nm/pixel), 19/14 individual frames. The generated file format is 8-bit '.tif'. The raw image data were captured in 16-bit mode where image size was 512×512. Figure 2 shows some of the original images and their corresponded actual masks or ground truth from dataset.

3.2   Explored Attributes of Bacteria

Total Bacteria Count: To calculate the total bacteria number in an image we need to follow some steps which include segmentation, contour detection, and counting. We used the adaptive thresholding method for image segmentation and then did Contour detection using OpenCV which uses the Suzuki-Abe algorithm to find contouring in binary images after that we counted the number of contourings considering them as a single bacteria. To enhance the understanding of the behaviour of microbial organisms community total number of bacteria vital parameters for image Analysis. The equation used for Adaptive Thresholding,

$$T(x,y) = \text{mean or Gaussian mean of } I_{\text{local}}(x,y) - C \tag{1}$$

$$I_{\text{segmented}}(x,y) = \begin{cases} 255 & \text{if } I(x,y) > T(x,y) \\ 0 & \text{otherwise} \end{cases} \tag{2}$$

where, $T(x,y)$ is the threshold applied to each pixel (x,y), calculated as the Gaussian-weighted or simple mean of the surrounding pixel values, $\mu(x,y)$, minus a constant C to fine-tune the segmentation.

Average Bacteria Volume: From the contouring, the Bacteria volume is calculated. It assumes that the bacterium is perfectly circulated. The most important reason to calculate this parameter is to Analyse and monitor growth patterns for individual bacteria as in microscopy images it is very hard to accurately differentiate the colony of bacteria. It will be crucial if the AI models are not able to identify it precisely.

Total Area: To calculate the Total Area, which refers to the shape analyzing feature we need three important properties of geometric which are Circularity (understanding the morphological behavior of bacteria cell), Eccentricity (how the bacteria is forming to compare its shape reformation from its original shape which will be very useful to understand Antimicrobial Resistance cell that where is the difference from normal cell) and Convexity (Analyse the physical features and health of bacteria cell).

Centralization Distance from Image Center: Distance of the center of the image to the bacterial centroid. Helps to understand the movement and clustering behaviour of bacteria. To understand the dynamics of colony formation of bacteria and how and using which process bacteria become resistant to antibiotics.

Average Aspect Ratio: This ratio represents the average of all detected bacteria in the image. During bacterial infections, some bacteria change their shape. To understand is stages of pathogenic bacterial infection Aspect Ratio is required.

Average Extent: Collecting data to take microscopic images some bacteria can be seen in irregular shapes due to stress or in the process of dying. To Analyse the behaviour of bacteria it is very necessary to understand which are important descriptors for Bacteria morphology.

Average Orientation: It helps to understand the interaction between bacterium, how it responses toward the environment it is surrounded by and most importantly analyse the development direction of bacterial tissue.

Local Binary Pattern (LBP): It is used to extract the important features from an image [18]. It generates accurate grouping result for different bacterial types in automatic image processing program.

Frame to Frame Area and Movement Change: This Analysis play an major role to find out insight about antimicrobial cure. By this exploration of changes we can also monitor the bacterial growth stages according to AMR.

GLCM Features: GLCM is used for image analysis to understand the texture feature in the image and extract it. Contrast, Dissimilarity, Homogeneity, Energy, and ASM are the statistical measures that we extract from GLCM. *Contrast*: It is defined as,

$$\text{Contrast} = \sum_{i,j=0}^{L-1} P(i,j) \times (i-j)^2 \tag{3}$$

where, $P(i,j)$ is the GLCM, L is the number of gray levels, and (i,j) represent pixel intensities.
Homogeneity and Energy: The Homogeneity is defined as,

$$\text{Homogeneity} = \sum_{i,j=0}^{levels-1} \frac{P(i,j)}{1+(i-j)^2} \tag{4}$$

where, $P(i,j)$ is the element at the ith row and j^{th} column of the GLCM, and *levels* represents the number of intensity levels in the image. The Energy is defined as,

$$\text{Energy} = \sum_{i,j=0}^{levels-1} P(i,j)^2 \tag{5}$$

To analyse bacterial phenotype behaviour, to understand structural patterns GLCM is important. Contrast is used for determining imbalances in bacterial cell walls, while Dissimilarity measures the differences in the pathological state of bacteria. Homogeneity helps cluster different types of bacteria. Energy focuses on regular or normal bacteria that do not exhibit any irregularities, particularly those influencing AMR, analyzing these can reveal which features protect the bacterial cell wall that antibiotics cannot breach. Finally, ASM is employed to study the density of bacterial colonies and identify areas where active bacteria growth is observed.

4   Methodology

We divided our methodology into two parts. In the first part, we generated a predicted mask using U-Net [19] and StarDist [20] from original bacterial images and ground truth masks. We have separated the test input original images and their ground truth masks into three divisions which contain continuous frames in specific time delays. In the training part, we used a complete training dataset containing both original and ground truth bacterial images. After training our U-Net model and StarDist, we tested our model using three-division original image data. Here, U-Net and StarDist models generated predicted mask images for each of the original corresponding images. Then we determined the accuracy of the U-Net model and StarDist by comparing generated predicted masks and their actual masks. Figure 3 shows the flow chart of the first part, which is generating predicted masks using U-Net and StarDist.

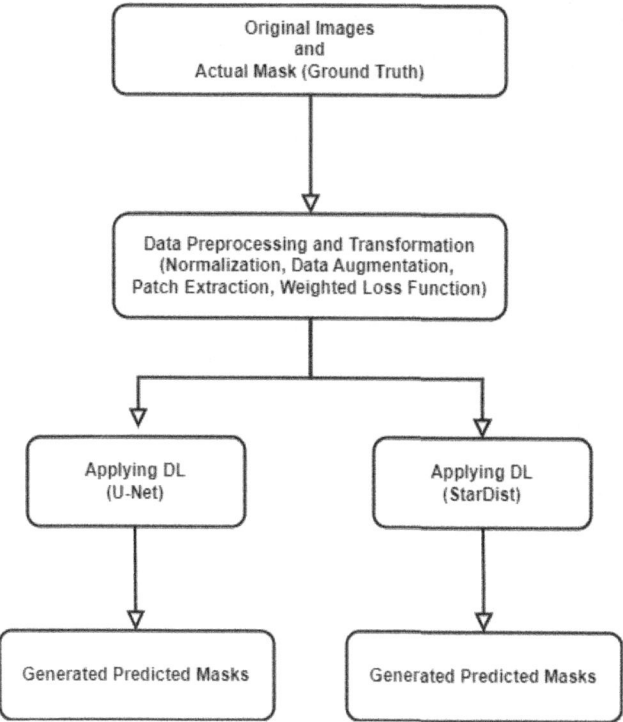

Fig. 3. Flow chart of the first part: generation of predicted masks using U-Net and StarDist.

In the second part of our work, we used all the generated predicted mask images and their corresponding actual mask images to determine bacterial behaviours and features. For each of the actual masks, we calculated all the mentioned bacterial behaviours. Also, for each of the generated predicted masks, we calculated all the mentioned bacterial behaviours.

Table 1. Detailed Workflow of Bacterial Behaviour Analysis, Segmentation, and Temporal Growth Dynamics.

Stage	Description
Input	Image Data: Series of grayscale images containing bacterial colonies.
Output	Bacterial Behaviour Metrics: Cell count, average volume, distance from image center, total area, texture features
	Temporal Growth Metrics: Changes in area and centroid movements between consecutive frames.
Part 1: Image Processing and Segmentation	
Data Preprocessing and Transformation	Normalize images, apply data augmentation, extract image patches, and use weighted loss functions for training data
Deep Learning (DL) Models	Utilize U-Net and StarDist architectures for segmenting bacterial colonies in the images
Bacterial Segmentation	Generate predicted masks from the DL models.
Part 2: Bacterial Behaviour Analysis	
Feature Extraction	Detect contours, calculate cell count, volume, centroid distance, and shape descriptors (aspect ratio, solidity, extent, orientation). Apply LBP for texture and compute GLCM features (contrast, dissimilarity, homogeneity, energy, ASM)
Data Aggregation	Average the extracted features across all bacteria within an image to provide a summary statistic per frame.
Part 3: Temporal Growth Dynamics	
Frame-to-Frame Analysis	Calculate area change and centroid movements between frames to assess bacterial growth dynamics
Visualization	Generate visual outputs to display original and processed images with highlighted bacterial contours and centroids

Then we compared and checked similarities and differences in behaviours between outputs from actual masks and generated predicted masks. Manually creating actual masks from original bacterial images is both time-consuming and costly. Therefore, our comparison may justify using generated masks instead of actual masks for bacterial behaviours analysis. Figure 4 shows the flow chart of second part which is determining bacterial behaviours from actual masks and generated predicted masks. Table 1 shows the Detailed Workflow of Bacterial Behaviour Analysis, Segmentation, and Temporal Growth Dynamics.

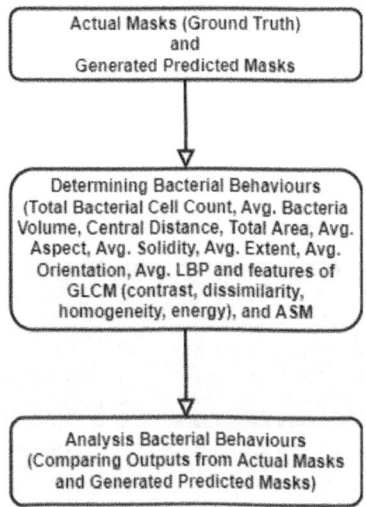

Fig. 4. Flow chart of second part: determining bacterial behaviours from actual masks and generated predicted masks.

5   Result and Analysis

In this section, we discussed the performance of U-Net and StarDist approaches in our work. Here Fig. 5 shows some actual image and their corresponding ground truth images. Besides it also shows generated predicted masks using U-Net and generated predicted masks using StarDist.

Table 2 shows the performance metrics of DL models that is U-Net and StarDist in this case. For each of the divisions (D1, D2, D3, D4 and D5) the table shows Intersection over Union (IoU), Dice, Accuracy, Precision, recall, F1 Score, Matthews correlation coefficient (MCC), Sensitivity, Specificity, Area Under the Curve - Receiver Operating Characteristic (AUC-ROC), and Area Under the Curve - Precision-Recall (AUC-PR). According to Table 2, we can notice that U-Net consistently shows better performance in all metrics, especially in IoU, Dice, Accuracy, Recall, F1 Score, MCC, and AUC-ROC, While StarDist has better Specificity and high Precision. However, Stardist lower scores in IoU, Dice, Recall, F1 Score, and AUC measures indicate that it is less effective at segmenting compared to U-Net from our selected dataset.

Table 3 represents that StarDist perform better to calculate Central Distances, Avg. Aspect ratio, and Avg. Solidity than U-Net. U-Net outperforms better in Total Bacteria Count, Avg. Bacteria Volume, and Avg. Orientation. Even if StarDist does not generate good result for Total bacteria count like U-Net, it is good at spotting bacteria until it get strong similarities between Ground Truth and Predicted Masks. Other features generate almost similar result for both models. Here, average LBP is 0.10 for Ground Truth, U-Net and StarDist.

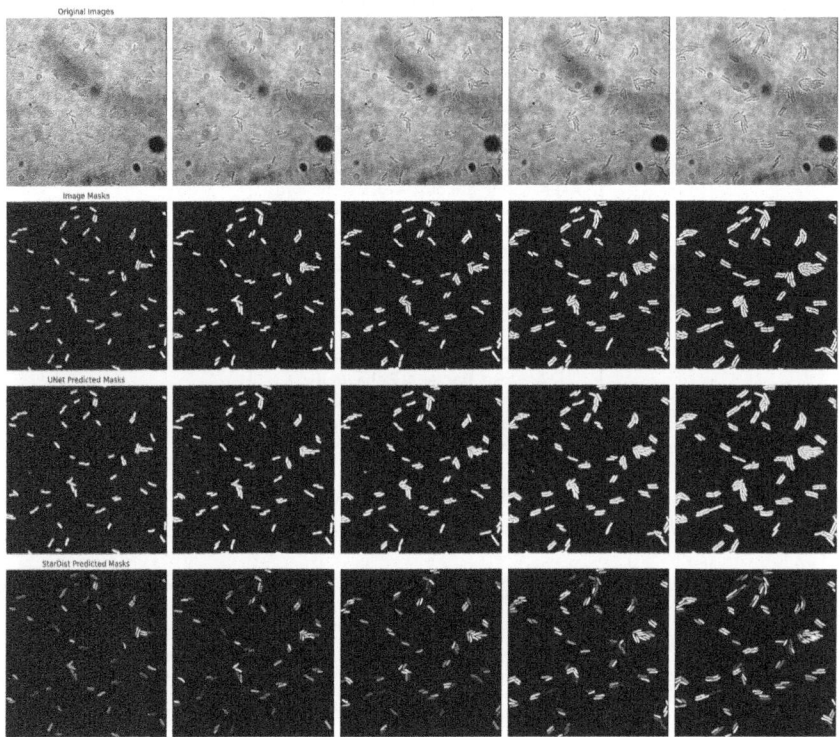

Fig. 5. Predicted Masks for U-net and Stardist

Table 2. Performance Metrics of DL Models

DL Model	IoU	Dice	Accuracy	Precision	Recall	F1 Score	MCC	Sensitivity	Specificity	AUC-ROC	AUC-PR
U-Net (D1)	0.85	0.92	0.99	0.87	0.98	0.92	0.92	0.98	0.99	0.99	0.92
U-Net (D2)	0.78	0.87	0.99	0.89	0.86	0.87	0.87	0.86	1.0	0.93	0.88
U-Net (D3)	0.84	0.91	0.99	0.88	0.95	0.91	0.91	0.95	0.99	0.97	0.92
StarDist (D1)	0.45	0.62	0.97	0.95	0.46	0.62	0.65	0.46	1.0	0.73	0.72
StarDist (D2)	0.29	0.43	0.98	0.94	0.29	0.43	0.51	0.29	1.0	0.64	0.63
StarDist (D3)	0.46	0.62	0.97	0.95	0.47	0.62	0.65	0.47	1.0	0.73	0.72
Avg. U-Net	0.82	0.90	0.99	0.88	0.93	0.90	0.90	0.93	0.99	0.96	0.91
Avg. StarDist	0.40	0.56	0.97	0.95	0.41	0.56	0.60	0.41	1.00	0.70	0.69

Table 3. Comparison of Bacterial Behaviour for Frames 1-5.

Type	Frame	Total Bacterial	Avg. Bacteria Volume	Central Distance	Total Area	Avg. Aspect	Avg. Solidity	Avg. Extent	Avg. Orientation
Ground Truth	1	43	1504.43	29.91	64690.50	0.63	0.92	0.90	46.31
	2	44	1810.74	47.41	79672.50	0.58	0.90	0.91	48.24
	3	40	2392.96	41.09	95718.50	0.56	0.88	0.88	54.88
	4	41	2876.85	47.95	117951.00	0.56	0.87	0.87	56.49
	5	39	3791.56	67.66	147871.00	0.49	0.84	nan	53.24
U-Net	1	48	1461.14	33.08	69711.00	0.43	0.74	0.90	57.00
	2	49	1706.69	25.41	83536.50	0.39	0.71	0.91	58.37
	3	49	1961.80	33.20	100314.50	0.38	0.72	0.89	59.20
	4	63	1787.39	111.43	116945.00	0.38	0.70	0.88	55.95
	5	97	1468.16	26.77	146129.50	0.38	0.72	0.88	58.97
StarDist	1	78	653.37	45.35	50962.50	0.55	0.85	0.91	41.93
	2	79	808.13	146.90	63842.50	0.51	0.83	0.92	48.97
	3	85	890.91	41.68	75727.00	0.49	0.82	0.90	52.76
	4	63	1600.79	52.03	100850.00	0.48	0.82	0.88	56.62
	5	63	1975.81	52.89	124476.00	0.46	0.84	0.88	53.38

Table 4. Comparison Area Change and Movement for U-net and Stardist.

Area Change and Movement	Ground Truth	U-Net	StarDist
Frame 1 to Frame 2	(14982.00, 253.17)	(13825.50, 317.08)	(12880.00, 439.70)
Frame 2 to Frame 3	(16046.00, 340.24)	(16778.00, 341.95)	(11884.50, 448.11)
Frame 3 to Frame 4	(22232.50, 244.30)	(16630.50, 343.72)	(25123.00, 336.89)
Frame 4 to Frame 5	(29920.00, 222.79)	(29184.50, 423.46)	(23626.00, 378.94)

According to Table 4, StarDist generated better result for movement between frames. On the other hand, U-Net shows better performance in Area Change between frames. Here, we used only U-Net and StarDist in this work. We selected U-Net because it excels at detailed localization for creating accurate masks. On the other hand, StarDist's shape-based optimization is ideal for distinguishing overlapping bacteria.

6 Conclusion

Studying bacterial behaviours from microscopic images using AI can save both time and effort. Also, medicine specialists could get valuable insights regarding bacterial behaviours from any datasets within a short time after using DL approaches, which eventually will allow them to develop new medicines to fight AMR. Finding to stop and delay AMR could save millions of lives worldwide.

This research work focused to identify bacterial behaviours from microscopic images from both actual mask images and predicted mask images after using U-Net and StarDist. We identified some of the vital bacterial behaviours such as average bacteria volume, central distance from the image center, total area, average aspect, average solidity, average extent, average orientation, and LBP. Also, we determined other features of GLCM such as contrast, dissimilarity, homogeneity, energy, and ASM for each of the actual mask images and predicted mask images. This analysis may provide valuable insight to researchers to identify patterns and ways of experimenting with new antibiotics. Also, we also analysed bacterial area changes and movement from one frame to another considering certain periods. This may help medicine specialists to identify the optimal point for administering antibiotics. Moreover, we provided comparisons between U-Net and StarDist, focusing on which approach performs better for specific behavior identification.

In our future work, we aim to increase dataset and data variability i.e. we will work with other types of microorganisms. Also, we aim to use other approaches such as V-Net, SegNet, and LinkNet and demonstrate a large comparison for more precise recommendations. Finally, we will increase the number of way to study bacterial behaviours and analyse how these behaviours contribute towards Antimicrobial Resistance (AMR).

References

1. Treebupachatsakul, T., Poomrittigul, S.: Microorganism image recognition based on deep learning application. In: 2020 International Conference on Electronics, Information, and Communication (ICEIC), Barcelona, Spain, pp. 1–5 (2020)
2. Balomenos, A.D., Stefanou, V., Manolakos, E.S.: Bacterial image analysis and single-cell analytics to decipher the behavior of large microbial communities. In: 2018 25th IEEE International Conference on Image Processing (ICIP), Athens, Greece, pp. 2436–2440 (2018)
3. Fuerst, J.A.: Microorganisms-A Journal and a Unifying Concept for the Science of Microbiology (2014)
4. Parmar, S., Daki, S., Bhattacharya, S., Shrivastav, A.: Chapter 8 - Microorganism: an ecofriendly tool for waste management and environmental safety. In: Shah, M.P., Rodriguez-Couto, S., Thapar, R. (eds.) Development in Wastewater Treatment Research and Processes, pp. 175–193. Elsevier, Kapoor (2022)
5. The Lancet. https://www.thelancet.com/journals/lancet/article/PIIS0140-6736(22)02185-7
6. Prestinaci, F., Pezzotti, P., Pantosti, A.: Antimicrobial resistance: a global multifaceted phenomenon. Pathog Glob Health **109**(7), 309–18 (2015)
7. Toner, E., Adalja, A., Gronvall, G.K., Cicero, A., Inglesby, T.V.: Antimicrobial resistance is a global health emergency. Health Secur. **13**(3), 153-5 (2015)
8. Cook, M.A., Wright, G.D.: The past, present, and future of antibiotics. Science Translational Medicine (2022)
9. Al-Tawfiq, J.A., Ebrahim, S.H., Memish, Z.A.: Preventing Antimicrobial Resistance Together: Reflections on AMR Week 2023. J. Epidemiol. Glob Health (2024)
10. Cirkovic, I., Švabić-Vlahović, M.: Nosocomial antibiotic strain resistance. Galen Medical Journal (2022)

11. Yadav, A., Singh, A., Singh, A., Yadav, A., Singh, S.: Segmentation of Microscopy images using Multi-Scale Retinex with Chromacity Preservation and Otsu Thresholding (2023)
12. Jelli, E., et al.: Single-cell segmentation in bacterial biofilms with an optimized deep learning method enables tracking of cell lineages and measurements of growth rates. Molecular Microbiol. **119**(6), 659–676 (2023)
13. Lavanya, K., Vijay Devi, P.: Various approaches in deep learning for medical modality image segmentation. In: 2023 International Conference on Advances in Electronics, Communication, Computing and Intelligent Information Systems (ICAECIS), pp. 470–479
14. Hallström, E., Kandavalli, V., Ranefall, P., Elf, J., Wählby, C.: Label-free deep learning-based species classification of bacteria imaged by phase-contrast microscopy. bioRxiv
15. Hayashi-Nishino, M., Nishino, K., Aoki, K.: Identification of bacterial drug-resistant cells by the convolutional neural network in transmission electron microscope images. Front. Microbiol. **13** (2022)
16. Spahn, C., Gómez-de-Mariscal, E., Laine, R.F., et al.: DeepBacs for multi-task bacterial image analysis using open-source deep learning approaches. Commun. Biol. **5**, 688 (2022)
17. Zhang, Y., Jiang, H., Ye, T., Juhas, M.: Deep learning for imaging and detection of microorganisms. Trends Microbiol. **29**(7), 569–572 (2021)
18. Ojala, T., Pietikäinen, M., Harwood, D.: Performance evaluation of texture measures with classification based on Kullback discrimination of distributions. In: Proceedings of the 12th IAPR International Conference on Pattern Recognition (ICPR 1994), vol. 1, pp. 582–585 (1994)
19. Ronneberger, O., Fischer, P., Brox, T.: U-Net: Convolutional Networks for Biomedical Image Segmentation (2015)
20. Schmidt, U., Weigert, M., Broaddus, C., Myers, G.: Cell detection with star-convex polygons. In: Lecture Notes in Computer Science. Springer International Publishing, pp. 265–273 (2018)

Assisted Living Technology

Innovations in Mosquito Identification: Integrating Deep Learning with Citizen Science

Mulaedza Mathoho, Dustin van der Haar$^{(\boxtimes)}$ ⓘ, and Hima Vadapalli ⓘ

Academy of Computer Science and Software Engineering, University of
Johannesburg, Cnr University Road and Kingsway Avenue, Auckland Park,
Johannesburg 2092, Gauteng, South Africa
{dvanderhaar,himav}@uj.ac.za

Abstract. In response to the escalating global threat of mosquito-borne diseases, this research introduces an innovative application of deep learning techniques to address the critical need for precise mosquito identification. Utilising a diverse dataset generously contributed by citizen scientists, this study aims to utilize existing advanced computer vision models capable of accurately detecting and classifying mosquitoes. The model underwent extensive training and evaluation, demonstrating remarkable accuracy and generalization capabilities. Evaluation metrics were employed to assess the model's performance comprehensively, including precision, recall, F1 score, accuracy, specificity and ROC AUC. The results showcase the model's effectiveness in accurately identifying and classifying mosquitoes across various taxonomic categories and environmental conditions. By leveraging cutting-edge AI technology and engaging citizen scientists, this initiative represents a significant step forward in revolutionizing mosquito surveillance and combating the spread of mosquito-borne diseases.

Keywords: Deep learning · Mosquito identification · Citizen science

1 Introduction

The escalating prevalence of mosquito-borne illnesses emphasizes the necessity of devising sophisticated mosquito detection and classification tools. Conventional methods are often manual and time-consuming, necessitating a more efficacious and scalable solution. To that end, using advanced tools that can accurately and efficiently detect and classify mosquitoes is crucial to curtailing the spread of these diseases [13]. Using deep learning plays a crucial role in this research involving citizen science and capturing real-world images of mosquitoes through mobile devices. This innovative approach enhances data diversity while promoting public engagement in addressing the imperative public health challenges associated with mosquito-borne diseases [12].

X. Xie et al. (Eds.): AIiH 2024, LNCS 14976, pp. 189–202, 2024.
https://doi.org/10.1007/978-3-031-67285-9_14

Based on statistics, the death toll caused by malaria is staggering, surpassing 400,000 annually. It is unacceptable that most of these fatalities are innocent children under the age of 5 [14]. Although malaria is a preventable disease, it continues to claim the lives of 619,000 people and infect over 247 million annually across 84 countries [14]. It's unacceptable that nearly 3.2 billion people are at risk of contracting this disease. It's time to take action and end this global health crisis. It is imperative to decrease this number in the present world, and prompt steps must be taken. To combat this global concern, the Mosquito Identification Challenge [1] has partnered with the Mosquito Alert citizen science project to revolutionize mosquito surveillance. Thanks to advanced computer vision techniques and AI-powered solutions, this initiative involves citizens in disease prevention and streamlines the meticulous task of mosquito identification. This proposal presents a comprehensive approach to addressing this urgent public health issue, offering a powerful solution to protect communities from the dangers of mosquito-borne illnesses [2]. The main aim is to revolutionize public health through advanced AI technology, particularly in identifying mosquitoes. This is evident in the Mosquito Identification Challenge.

Mosquitoes carry deadly diseases such as malaria, dengue fever, and Zika virus [12]. Traditional methods of detecting and classifying mosquitoes have limitations that hinder their effectiveness [13]. These methods rely heavily on manual labour, which can be time-consuming and impractical for large-scale surveillance. Furthermore, the distribution of mosquito classes in real-world scenarios is often unbalanced, with some classes being more prevalent than others. This creates a significant challenge for developing accurate classification models that handle diverse scenarios. Researchers are exploring new approaches to address these challenges, including machine learning algorithms and computer vision techniques. These methods have shown promise in detecting and classifying mosquitoes accurately, even in complex scenarios. By leveraging these advanced technologies, we can improve our ability to monitor and control mosquito populations and reduce the transmission of deadly diseases [1,13].

Convolutional Neural Networks (CNNs) have impressive abilities in classification tasks, including the classification of mosquito images. However, their effectiveness is heavily reliant on datasets with balanced class distributions. The imbalanced distribution of mosquito species is a major obstacle in achieving accurate classification across various scenarios.

Citizen science initiatives that use mobile applications for mosquito data collection are a valuable source of data. However, manual identification and analysis processes limit these initiatives' scalability and efficiency. There is a pressing need for automated solutions to streamline the identification process and handle the increasing volume of data generated through citizen science [8].

The Mosquito Identification Challenge sets itself apart by acknowledging and addressing the multifaceted nature of the problems in mosquito surveillance. The skewed class distribution within the dataset poses a substantial hurdle, demanding novel strategies for precise detection and classification across diverse conditions, closely mirroring the complexities of real-world scenarios [1].

2   Similar Works

The potential of deep learning and computer vision techniques for mosquito surveillance and classification is growing interest among researchers. Several research initiatives have explored these advanced methods with promising results-notably, Goodwin et al., [7] proposed a CNN architecture specifically tailored for mosquito species identification using image datasets collected from trap cameras deployed in diverse environmental settings. Their study demonstrated promising results in accurately classifying mosquitoes based on species, contributing valuable insights into automated surveillance methods for mosquitoborne diseases.

Similarly, Ahmad [3] investigated transfer learning techniques to adapt pretrained CNN models for mosquito detection in various environmental conditions. Their approach leveraged pre-existing knowledge from large-scale image datasets, enhancing the model's ability to generalize to different habitats and lighting conditions commonly encountered in mosquito surveillance efforts.

Furthermore, McFeeters [9] conducted a study on integrating remote sensing data with machine learning algorithms to create spatial models of mosquito habitats. The study combined various data sources, such as satellite imagery, meteorological data, and mosquito presence records, to predict mosquitoes' abundance and distribution patterns. The study aimed to provide insights into effective mosquito control strategies and disease prevention measures.

In addition to these studies, there have been advancements in citizen science initiatives, which have made it possible to collect large-scale datasets of mosquito images from volunteers worldwide. These initiatives, such as the Mosquito Alert citizen science project, engage citizens in mosquito surveillance efforts, allowing for the collection of real-world data on mosquito presence and distribution [4].

While these research endeavours have made significant strides in advancing the field of mosquito surveillance, challenges remain in developing robust and scalable models capable of accurately identifying mosquitoes across diverse environmental conditions and taxonomic categories. By building upon the existing body of work and integrating innovative approaches such as citizen science participation and advanced machine learning techniques, our research aims to address these challenges and contribute to developing effective mosquito surveillance systems for public health interventions.

3   Method

In response to the challenges above, the present study proposes a novel approach that integrates deep learning methodologies with citizen science participation towards improving mosquito identification and surveillance. Advanced computer vision models detect and classify mosquitoes from diverse datasets collected through mobile applications. Our method enables the precise identification and classification of mosquitoes, providing a valuable tool for developing effective mosquito control strategies. Citizen science participation ensures large-scale data collection and contributes to the overall accuracy of the methodology. These findings significantly affect public health, particularly in regions with prevalent mosquito-borne diseases.

3.1   Dataset Properties

The dataset used in this study comprises 10,700 images captured from real-life situations, depicting the complex ecosystem where mosquitoes flourish [1]. These images were not artificially selected but were contributed by citizen scientists who used their mobile devices to capture them. Therefore, the dataset is an authentic representation of various scenarios in the ecosystem [1]. The dataset was split into three subsets for training, validation, and testing purposes. The split ratio was set to 80-10-10, where 80% of the data was allocated to the training set, 10% to the validation set, and the remaining 10% to the test set. This ratio was chosen to ensure that each subset had enough data to represent the dataset and support model training, hyperparameter tuning, and final evaluation [11].

3.1.1   Image Contexts

The dataset contains images of mosquitoes in different habitats, ranging from urban to rural environments. These images cover a wide range of situations where mosquito surveillance is necessary. Including diverse environments ensures that our model can generalize well and be effective in real-world scenarios [6].

3.1.2   Mosquito Morphology Variation

Mosquitoes are species that display a wide range of morphological diversity. The dataset has been intentionally designed to capture this variation, featuring mosquitoes in various body positions and sizes. This deliberate inclusion ensures the model is trained to identify and classify mosquitoes across various anatomical variations. This contributes to its robustness and ability to handle real-world complexities [1].

3.1.3   Lighting Conditions

Another critical facet of the dataset is its representation of varying lighting conditions. Mosquitoes can be active at any time of the day and in any lighting conditions. Therefore, the dataset of mosquito images includes pictures taken in various lighting scenarios such as daylight, dusk, and nighttime. This variation in lighting conditions challenges the model to accurately identify mosquitoes under different luminance levels. Overall, the dataset is designed to improve the accuracy of mosquito detection models by presenting them with a range of challenging scenarios [1].

3.1.4 Annotated Expertly by Entomologists

The dataset results from the meticulous annotation performed by expert ento-mologists, ensuring the accuracy and reliability of the labelled data. Each image comes with precise bounding box coordinates, which denote the spatial location of the mosquitoes within the image. The associated class labels indicate the tax-onomic categorization, encompassing six distinct classes: Aedes aegypti, Aedes albopictus, Anopheles, Culex, Culiseta, and the Aedes japonicus/Aedes koreicus species complex [1].

This dataset is of immense value to society and academia, providing an exten-sive and accurate collection of labelled data for research and development pur-poses. The careful annotation process performed by expert entomologists ensures the quality of the data, making it a reliable resource for any research project requiring labelled mosquito images. The dataset's comprehensiveness and accu-racy make it a valuable tool for developing and testing machine learning algo-rithms, providing an efficient means of training classification models.

3.1.5 Unbalanced Class Distribution

One of the main challenges in the dataset is the uneven distribution of mosquito classes. This is similar to the real-world scenario where certain species or gen-era of mosquitoes are more common than others. Therefore, it is important to address this imbalance while developing an accurate classification model that can classify mosquitoes correctly across varying frequencies of occurrence [11].

3.2 Data Preprocessing

To achieve the model's best performance, preprocessing techniques, such as resiz-ing and normalization, were applied to the images. After that, the data was encapsulated into a customized dataset class to make the loading process smooth and easy. This also helps map string labels to numerical labels without any hassle [13].

3.3 Model Architecture

Our deep learning model has been constructed utilizing the ResNet-18 archi-tecture, a well-renowned framework for image classification tasks, as shown in Fig. 1. By leveraging the features of a pre-trained ResNet-18 model, we have replaced its final fully connected layer with a layer tailored to our specific task. This new layer encompasses six output nodes, each corresponding to one of the six mosquito classes [16].

Through this process, we have developed a more efficient and effective model for mosquito classification. By utilizing the ResNet-18 architecture as a founda-tion, we have drawn upon its highly-regarded capabilities for image classification while also customizing the model to meet our specific needs. This approach has allowed us to build a deep learning model that can accurately classify mosquitoes in a more streamlined and effective manner [16].

3.4   Training and Evaluation

Periodic evaluations are done on a test dataset to assess the model's performance. Precision, recall, and F1 scores are utilized to conduct a comprehensive evaluation.

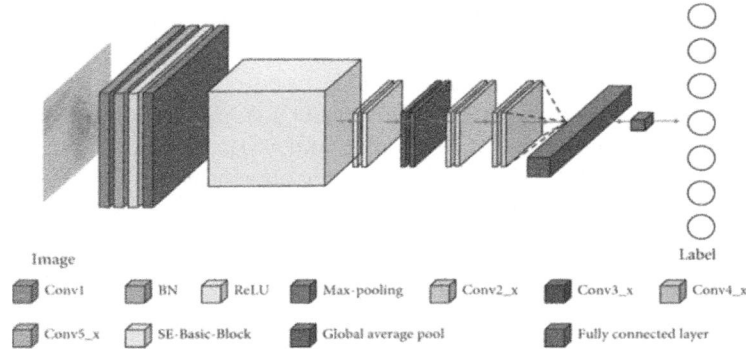

Fig. 1. RESNet-18 Architecture

4   Results

The outcomes of our extensive evaluation have cast light on the effectiveness of the deep learning model we developed for mosquito detection and classification.

4.1   Accuracy and Generalization

The training and test accuracy is depicted in the Fig. 2 below, which highlights the model's capacity to understand and adjust to the intricacies of the dataset. Significantly, the accuracy reaches a high and stable level, which suggests that the model has learned to apply its knowledge to new and unknown examples [2,16].

4.2   Loss Analysis

In this section, we delve into the behaviour of the loss throughout the training process depicted in Fig. 3 and its implications for model performance and generalization.

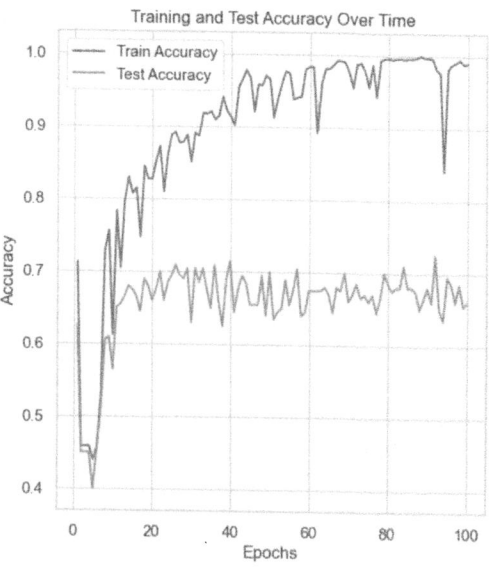

Fig. 2. Train and Validation Accuracy

4.2.1   Training Loss Dynamics

Analyzing the loss function's trajectory throughout the training phase provides valuable insights into the model's learning process. The training dataset was subjected to iterative processing, during which the loss function consistently decreased across epochs. This suggests the model effectively minimized the discrepancy between predicted and actual values. This decreasing trend in the loss function highlights the efficacy of the learning process and the model's ability to adapt to the training data [16].

4.2.2   Validation Loss Evalution

The loss function consistently decreased throughout the training phase, indicating that the model was learning from the training data. However, after the 50th epoch, the validation loss unexpectedly increased. This increase suggests that the model may have been overfitting the data. Monitoring the model's performance on unseen data is important to ensure it can generalize well. The test set, separate from the training and validation sets, is reserved for final evaluation. This ensures that the model's performance is assessed without bias [16].

4.2.3   Early Stopping Technique

We employed the early stopping technique after the 50th epoch to address the risk of overfitting. This technique involves monitoring the validation loss during training and halting the training process when the validation loss begins to increase. Implementing early stopping aimed to prevent the model from becoming overly specialized to the training data, thereby improving its ability to generalize to new and unseen instances [15].

4.2.4   Implications and Considerations

The model's generalization capabilities necessitate careful consideration of the unexpected increase in test loss beyond the 50th epoch. The anomalous surge in test loss challenges the model's ability to perform well on new data. The complexity of a dataset or the inherent difficulty of the mosquito identification task may contribute to the challenges encountered when identifying mosquitos. Careful monitoring of loss dynamics and implementing strategies to reduce overfitting are essential to ensure optimal model performance. One such strategy successfully employed is early stopping, which balances the model's complexity with its generalisation performance. By striking a balance between these two factors, early stopping can help to ensure that the model remains effective while minimizing the risk of overfitting [16].

Analyzing the trajectory of the loss function can provide valuable insights into the learning dynamics of the model and its ability to generalize to diverse scenarios. It is crucial to understand these nuances to optimize the model's performance and ensure its effectiveness in real-world applications.

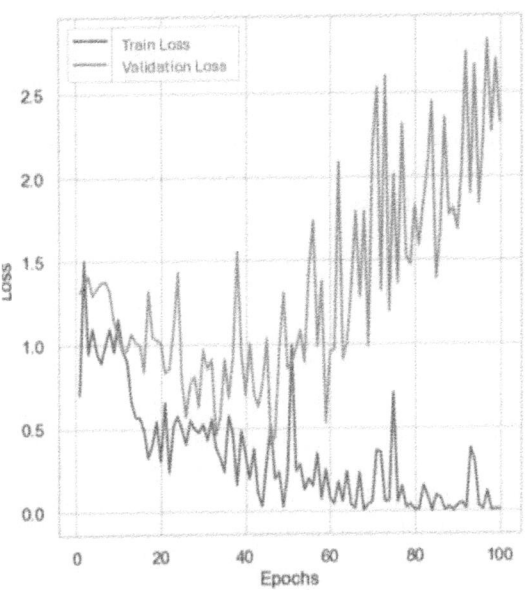

Fig. 3. Train and Validation Loss

4.3   Evaluation Metrics

A range of evaluation metrics was utilized to comprehensively assess the model's performance. These metrics offer insights into various aspects of the model's behaviour and effectiveness in classifying mosquitoes accurately across different taxonomic categories.

4.3.1   Precision

Precision measures the proportion of true positive predictions among all positive predictions made by the model. In the context of mosquito classification, precision indicates the model's ability to correctly identify mosquitoes of a specific species without misclassifying others. The model achieved a Precision score of 0.86 on the test data, meaning that, out of all the instances where the model predicted the mosquito species, 86% of those predictions were correct, thus implying that there are relatively few false positives.

4.3.2   Recall

Recall, also known as sensitivity, quantifies the proportion of true positive predictions the model captures relative to all actual positive instances in the dataset. In mosquito surveillance, recall reflects the model's capacity to detect mosquitoes of a particular species, including instances the model may miss. The model achieved a Recall score of 0.87 on test data, meaning that, out of all the actual mosquitoes present in the dataset, the model correctly identified 87% of them.

4.3.3   F1 Score

The F1 score is the harmonic mean of precision and recall, providing a balanced measure of the model's performance in precision and recall. It considers false positives and negatives and is particularly useful for evaluating classification models in imbalanced datasets, such as those encountered in mosquito surveillance. The model reported an F1 Score of 0.8650 on test data. The model shows a great balance between precision and recall, which is crucial for such a model where correctly identifying species (precision) and capturing most of the species present (recall) are important.

4.3.4   Accuracy

Accuracy represents the proportion of correctly classified instances out of the total number of instances in the dataset. While accuracy provides a general measure of the model's correctness, it may be influenced by the class distribution. It should be interpreted with other metrics, especially in imbalanced datasets. The model was able to achieve an accuracy score of 89% on test data. Combined with the previously mentioned F1 score of 0.8650, this model demonstrates strong performance, balancing precision, recall, and overall accuracy, making it a strong candidate for practical application in the field and helping inform decisions with significant public health implications.

4.3.5   Specificity

Specificity measures the proportion of true negative predictions among all negative predictions made by the model. It indicates the model's ability to correctly identify instances that do not belong to a specific class, thus complementing measures of sensitivity and precision. The mode achieved a specificity rate of 80% on test data. This shows that the model more effectively identifies the different mosquito species.

4.3.6   Area Under the Receiver Operating Characteristic Curve (ROC AUC)

The ROC AUC is a widely used metric for evaluating the performance of binary classification models. It quantifies the model's ability to distinguish between positive and negative instances across various threshold values. While originally designed for binary classification tasks, the ROC AUC can be adapted for multi-class classification by considering each class against the rest. The model achieved an accuracy of 89% on test data, demonstrating its strong discriminatory power and ability to distinguish between different mosquito species.

4.4   Robustness Across Scenarios

The robustness of the model across various scenarios is a crucial aspect of the results. The model's ability to accurately detect and classify mosquitoes in different body positions, sizes, and lighting conditions demonstrates its adaptability to the complexities of real-world environments. This level of resilience is a testament to the model's potential to significantly contribute to mosquito surveillance efforts in a range of ecological settings. Overall, the results suggest that the model has the potential to become an essential tool in mosquito surveillance programs, providing reliable and accurate data that can inform decision-making processes and help mitigate the spread of mosquito-borne diseases.

5   Comparison with Existing Literature

In a significant study conducted by Wilke et al. [18], CNNs were used for the identification of mosquito species from images. The focus was on classifying mosquitoes from a dataset consisting of images taken under controlled conditions. Our approach builds upon this study by utilizing a more diverse dataset containing real images captured by citizen contributors in various contexts. The diversity in the data presents additional challenges, such as varying lighting conditions and body positions, which our model effectively addresses through robust data augmentation techniques and advanced CNN architectures. In an earlier study, Sáez et al. [17] successfully tackled class imbalance in mosquito datasets using oversampling and synthetic data generation techniques. Building on this foundation, our approach integrates these techniques with additional strategies, such as focal loss and class-weighted loss functions, to further enhance the model's ability to handle the unbalanced distribution of mosquito classes. This ensures precise detection and classification across all categories, addressing the competition's requirement to manage disparities in class distribution with confidence effectively. Chen et al. [5] and Mukundarajan et al. [10] thoroughly investigated mosquito species identification using acoustic data from wing beats. However, these methods encountered challenges stemming from environmental noise and variations in smartphone hardware. In the proposed work, image-based approach effectively addresses these limitations by utilizing visual data, which is more consistent and less vulnerable to external noise. This strategic shift to image data, coupled with advanced computer vision techniques, presents a highly reliable and easily scalable solution for mosquito species identification.

6   Discussion

The present discussion endeavours to explicate the nuanced implications of the obtained results and place them in the broader landscape of deep-learning mosquito surveillance applications. The findings have been contextualized to delineate their significance in the current deep learning-based mosquito surveillance scenario.

6.1   Addressing Unbalanced Class Distribution

The disproportionate distribution of mosquito classes within the dataset presents a notable challenge. The proposed model has demonstrated acceptable confidence in addressing this asymmetry and reported promising accuracies in classification across classes with dissimilar frequencies. As this feature of the model holds significant practical implications for real-world scenarios where certain mosquito species or genera may be more prevalent than others, further experiments can assist with understanding and mitigating any further class imbalances. Specifically, such a feature highlights the model's utility in the context of epidemiological studies and disease management. The model's capacity to handle asymmetry in classification is particularly noteworthy, as it provides the necessary foundations for accurate and reliable analysis of data [8,16].

6.2   Generalization to Citizen Science Data

Citizen scientists' successful integration of images underscores the model's ability to generalize to real-world, non-curated data. This inclusive approach not only enriches the diversity of the dataset but also reflects the potential for widespread public engagement in disease surveillance initiatives. The model's adaptability to citizen science data creates opportunities for scalable and collaborative approaches to mosquito monitoring. Integrating citizen science data into the model demonstrates that the model can leverage the public's collective intelligence to address public health challenges.

6.3 Future Directions

While the achieved results are promising, avenues for future research emerge. Fine-tuning strategies, ensemble methods, and integrating additional data sources could enhance the model's performance. Moreover, exploring the model's transferability to different geographic regions and incorporating temporal dynamics are promising directions for advancing the practical applications of our approach.

The further comprehension of test loss dynamics epochs presents an opportunity for refinement. It instigates the contemplation of regularisation techniques, modifications of model complexity, or fine-tuning strategies to counteract overfitting. A judicious equilibrium between learning from the training set and maintaining the model's adaptability to diverse scenarios would be advantageous in future iterations. This approach would ensure sustained accuracy across various instances of mosquito identification.

6.4 Implications for Public Health

Our deep learning model's successful development and evaluation have far-reaching implications for public health interventions. Accurately detecting and classifying mosquitoes through this model can be crucial to early intervention strategies, enabling timely responses to potential disease outbreaks. Once deployed in real-world scenarios, it has the potential to provide public health officials with a powerful tool for effective mosquito surveillance, thereby enhancing existing surveillance systems and improving the overall effectiveness of mosquito control programs. In addition to interpreting the results, the discussion highlights the broader significance of the research findings. It connects the technical details of the model and its potential impact on public health and initiatives aimed at engaging citizens.

7 Conclusion

In conclusion, our research plays a significant role in closing the loop in the cycle of disease intervention. By leveraging the power of artificial intelligence, engaging citizen scientists, and advancing our knowledge of mosquito populations, we have developed a tool that not only detects and categorizes mosquitoes but also has the potential to transform this information into practical public health interventions. This represents a crucial turning point in the ongoing fight against mosquito-borne diseases, making our work a guiding light for future initiatives at the crossroads of technology, citizen participation, and public health.

Creating datasets, developing and evaluating models, and researching mosquito detection is a collaborative effort that goes beyond traditional research methodologies. This research provides insights into mosquito detection and sets the foundation for a new, inclusive, and impactful scientific exploration era. With the fusion of deep learning and citizen science, we are at the threshold of a future where mosquito surveillance will be reshaped, contributing significantly to the field of public health.

In summary, our research contributes to closing the loop in the cycle of disease intervention. Through the power of artificial intelligence, citizen scientists, and advancing our knowledge of mosquito populations, we have created a tool that detects and classifies mosquitoes. This tool holds the promise of translating knowledge into actionable public health interventions. This marks a critical moment in the ongoing battle against mosquito-borne diseases and positions our work as a model for future endeavours at the intersection of technology, citizen engagement, and public health.

The journey from creating datasets to developing and evaluating models involves a collaborative effort that extends beyond traditional research methodologies. This research provides insights into mosquito detection's intricacies and lays the groundwork for a new, inclusive, and impactful scientific exploration era. As we evaluate our progress, we stand at the threshold of a future where the integration of deep learning and citizen science will transform the landscape of mosquito surveillance, contributing significantly to the broader field of public health.

References

1. AIcrowd. Mosquito Alert-Challenge-2023 (2023)
2. Akter, M., Hossain, M., Ahmed, T., Andersson, K.: Mosquito classification using convolutional neural network with data augmentation, pp. 865–879. NISO, February 2021
3. Alubedy, A.: Mosquito detection and classification using machine learning algorithms. Iraqi J. Intell. Comput. Inform. (IJICI) **2**, 113–129 (2023)
4. Sousa, L.B., et al.: Methodological diversity in citizen science mosquito surveillance: a scoping review. Citizen Sci. Theory Pract. **7**, 8 (2022)
5. Chen, Y., Why, A., Batista, G., Mafra-Neto, A., Keogh, E.: Flying insect detection and classification with inexpensive sensors. J. Vis. Exp. JoVE, 52111 (2014)
6. da Silva de Souza, A.L., Multini, L.C., Marrelli, M.T., Wilke, A.B.B.: Wing geometric morphometrics for identification of mosquito species (Diptera: Culicidae) of neglected epidemiological importance. Acta Tropica **211**, 105593 (2020)
7. Goodwin, A., et al.: Mosquito species identification using convolutional neural networks with a multitiered ensemble model for novel species detection. Sci. Rep. **11**, 07 (2021)
8. Isawasan, P., Abdullah, Z.I., Ong, S.-Q., Salleh, K.A.: A protocol for developing a classification system of mosquitoes using transfer learning. MethodsX **10**, 101947 (2023)

9. McFeeters, S.: Using the normalized difference water index (NDWI) within a geographic information system to detect swimming pools for mosquito abatement: a practical approach. Remote Sens. **5**(7), 3544–3561 (2013)
10. Mukundarajan, H., Hol, F., Castillo, E., Newby, C., Prakash, M.: Using mobile phones as acoustic sensors for high-throughput mosquito surveillance, September 2017
11. Murphey, Y., Guo, H., Feldkamp, L.: Neural learning from unbalanced data: Special issue: Engineering Intelligent Systems (Guest Editor: László Monostori). Appl. Intell. **21**, 09 (2004)
12. Nkya, T.E., Akhouayri, I., Kisinza, W., David, J.-P.: Impact of environment on mosquito response to pyrethroid insecticides: facts, evidences and prospects. Insect Biochem. Mol. Biol. **43**(4), 407–416 (2013)
13. Okayasu, K., Yoshida, K., Fuchida, M., Nakamura, A.: Vision-based classification of mosquito species: comparison of conventional and deep learning methods. Appl. Sci. **9**, 3935 (2019)
14. WHO. World Health Organization. World malaria report (2019). https://www.who.int/publications/i/item/9789241565721. Accessed 25 Aug 2023
15. Prechelt, L.: Early stopping - but when? Appl. Intell. (2000)
16. Abhishek, A.V.S.: ResNet18 model with sequential layer for computing accuracy on image classification dataset. Appl. Intell. **10**, 2320–2882 (2022)
17. Sáez, J.A., Krawczyk, B., Wozniak, M.: Analyzing the oversampling of different classes and types of examples in multi-class imbalanced datasets. Pattern Recogn. **57**, 164–178 (2016)
18. Wilke, A.B.B., Vasquez, C., Carvajal, A., Moreno, M., Petrie, W.D., Beier, J.C.: Mosquito surveillance in maritime entry ports in Miami-Dade County, Florida to increase preparedness and allow the early detection of invasive mosquito species. PLoS One **17**(4), e0267224 (2022)

Action Recognition for Privacy-Preserving Ambient Assisted Living

Vincent Gbouna Zakka$^{(\boxtimes)}$ ⓘ, Zhuangzhuang Dai ⓘ, and Luis J. Manso ⓘ

Aston University, Birmingham, UK
{vzakk22,z.dai1,l.manso}@aston.ac.uk

Abstract. The care challenges posed by an increasing elderly population have made ambient assisted living a significant research focus. Computer vision-based technologies can monitor older adults' daily activities in their homes, providing insights into their health and prolonging their capacity to live independently. However, despite the benefits of these technologies, their widespread adoption has been hampered due to privacy concerns. These concerns frequently stem from the need to stream user data to cloud servers for computation, posing a risk to user privacy. This study proposes a privacy-preserving method for activity recognition that enhances the accuracy of activity recognition locally, eliminating the need to stream user data to the cloud. The paper's contributions are twofold: a Temporal Decoupling Graph Depthwise Separable Convolution Network (TD-GDSCN) to address the challenges of real-time performance and a data augmentation technique to prevent accuracy degradation in real-world environmental conditions. The experimental results show that the TD-GDSCN and data augmentation techniques outperform existing methods in addressing real-time performance and degradation challenges on the NTU-RGB+D 60 and NW-UCLA datasets.

Keywords: Assisted Living · Privacy Preservation · Real-time Performance

1 Introduction

The United Nations projects that the population aged 65 and older will reach 2 billion by 2050 [16], which is expected to strain the socioeconomic stability and healthcare facilities of many nations [1]. Consequently, there is a growing interest in Ambient Assisted Living (AAL) from researchers and industry stakeholders [2,6]. AAL enhances older adults' independence, autonomy, and well-being by monitoring their behaviour, predicting anomalies, and alerting caregivers when needed [3].

In recent years, there has been a significant interest in solutions for monitoring the Activities of Daily Living (ADL) of older adults [3,8]. In the context of AAL, activity recognition involves registering the daily behaviours of individuals, which is essential for identifying patterns related to specific health conditions [3]. Compared to other computer vision-based systems for ADL recognition, skeleton-based methods have gained attention due to their robustness

X. Xie et al. (Eds.): AIiH 2024, LNCS 14976, pp. 203–217, 2024.
https://doi.org/10.1007/978-3-031-67285-9_15

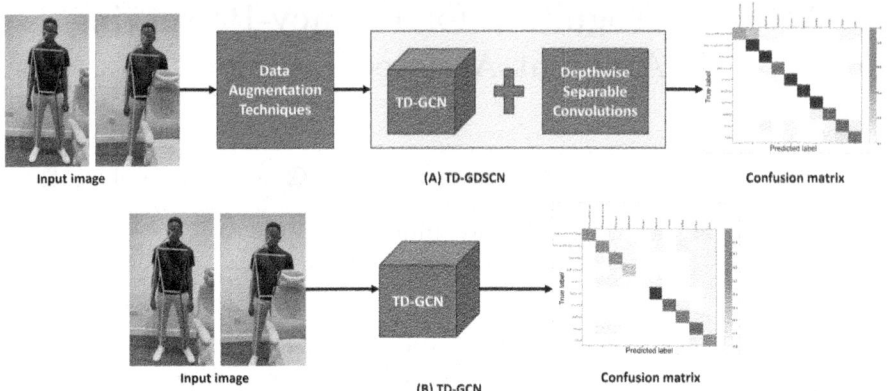

Fig. 1. Temporal Decoupling Graph Convolutional Network (TD-GCN) [12] vs. TD-GDSCN (Ours): Given input data both with and without occlusion, (A) We first apply our data augmentation techniques. The data is then trained using TD-GDSCN, and the result at test time is shown in the confusion matrix. Using the same input data, the result at test time using TD-GCN (B) is shown in the confusion matrix.

against varying backgrounds and privacy-preserving nature [4, 10]. However, privacy concerns identified as the main barrier in technology acceptance studies have significantly limited the adoption of ADL recognition for smart healthcare applications [22, 38]. Users are particularly concerned about data breaches, as most systems rely on cloud servers [26].

Recent methods have focused on developing models for real-time action recognition on edge devices to address the challenge of data streaming to the cloud [5, 17, 30, 35]. These methods improved the computational efficiency of existing methods but at the expense of accuracy. This raises the question: can we achieve higher accuracy without increasing the computational cost? In addition to the accuracy and computational cost trade-off challenge, it is key for action recognition models to be robust against real-world challenges such as noise, viewpoint variability, and differences in action execution [21, 35]. This often leads to performance degradation when these models are tested with datasets that reflect real-world environmental conditions [21, 32]. The models' performance degradation can be attributed to their limited adaptability to the disparities in data distribution between controlled and real-world environments. This is illustrated in the confusion matrix shown in Fig. 1b, where accuracy decline is observed when a SOTA model TD-GCN [12] is tested on data with occlusions. However, when data augmentation techniques were employed to manage the occlusion scenario, such performance degradation was significantly reduced, as depicted in Fig. 1a.

This paper, therefore, proposes Temporal Decoupling Graph Depthwise Separable Convolution Network (TD-GDSCN) and data augmentation techniques to reduce the computational cost and accuracy degradation in real-world conditions. The TD-GDSCN uses TD-GCN [12], which benefits from optimisation to improve its real-time performance on devices with limited computational resources. To enhance TD-GCN's computational efficiency, we incorporated depthwise separable convolution operations into TD-DCN's temporal convolution operations. For our data augmentation techniques, we considered real-world factors that impact performance and designed several strategies to enhance the adaption of TD-GDSCN to real-world environmental conditions. We conducted extensive experiments on two benchmark datasets: NTU RGB+D 60 [24] and Northwestern-UCLA [31]. TD-GDSCN outperforms existing approaches in terms of real-time performance without sacrificing accuracy, and the data augmentation techniques significantly adapted the developed model to a dataset reflecting real-world conditions. The contribution of our work can be summarised as follows: a) We propose TD-GDSCN to enhance real-time performance and privacy preservation in AAL without sacrificing accuracy. b) We propose a suite of data augmentation techniques to enhance the adaptability of TD-GDSCN in real-world conditions.

2   Related Works

2.1   Real-Time Performance of Skeleton-Based Action Recognition

The introduction of Graph Convolutional Networks (GCN) [34] in skeleton-based action recognition brought a significant breakthrough in accuracy. However, the computational cost of graph-based methods poses a challenge to meeting real-time performance requirements [21]. Recent approaches aim to address this by reducing model parameters, employing efficient feature extraction methods [5,17,30,35]. For instance, Yang et al. [35] proposed a lightweight model capable of processing 3,500 skeleton sequences per second. However, the model struggles to distinguish between actions with the same global trajectories. To overcome this challenge, Nguyen et al. [17] proposed a method to enrich the spatial information using the normalised coordinates of the joints. Furthermore, in [5,30], the model's accuracy was further improved by incorporating additional features. Although these methods improved the model's accuracy, they did so at the expense of computational cost, indicating a trade-off between accuracy and computational efficiency. The proposed TD-GDSCN aims to address this trade-off challenge.

2.2   Data Augmentation Strategies

Various data augmentation methods have been proposed to address the challenges encountered in real-world environments. One of such method is Skeleton-CutMix [11], which generates a new skeleton by exchanging some bones from the source domain skeleton with corresponding target domain skeletons to mitigate domain shift. Other methods, however, have focused on addressing a specific challenge encountered in a real-world environment. For instance, to address the

challenge of noisy skeletons, recent methods have developed techniques to simulate noisy skeletons as augmented data during training [20,28,37]. Additionally, adaptable approaches using generation-based adaptable models [27], 3D
bio-constrained skeleton model [18], and GAN [10] have been investigated to
generate data representing noisy skeletons. Addressing the challenge of diverse
viewpoints introduced by different camera angles, potential methods such as
coordinate rotation [32,33], sequence-based view-invariant transform [13], and
sequence-wise augmentation [19] has been proposed to simulate actions viewed
from different angles. In addition, to address the variability in the size of human
subjects performing an action, methods such as scaling [23,36] and phase ran-
domisation [15] have been proposed to scale the sizes of the skeleton data. While
previous approaches have individually addressed specific challenges, analysing
their relationships and contributions is essential. Moreover, it is crucial that
methods used to simulate real-world environment data reflect real-world scenarios rather than based on assumptions. Therefore, our data augmentation
techniques aim to generate augmented data that mirrors real-world environmental conditions. It also seeks to analyse the interplay between the various factors
influencing performance in the real-world environment.

3   Method

The overall framework of the proposed method is presented in Fig. 2. Given input
skeleton data, data augmentation techniques are applied to generate copies of
the input data. TD-GDSCN enhances computational efficiency by integrating
depthwise separable convolution operations.

3.1   TD-GDSCN

TD-GCN [12] applies convolutions through time and space, allowing it to capture spatio-temporal features, facilitating the understanding of temporal dynamics and spatial relationships among joints. However, the convolution operation
in TD-GCN is computationally expensive and requires a relatively high number of parameters. We decomposed the convolution operations into depthwise
and pointwise convolutions to reduce the number of parameters and enhance
TD-GCN's computational efficiency. The depthwise convolution applies a single
filter per input feature independently across all input features. This reduces the
computational cost, particularly with large input feature maps, as it operates on
individual features rather than across the entire input feature map. The subsequent pointwise convolution combines the output from the depthwise convolutions using 1×1 convolutions, enabling efficient channel-wise feature aggregation.
Our approach's reduced computational cost and improved parameter efficiency
translate into overall model efficiency, as shown below.

    In TD-GCN, the output feature map Y for each output channel C_{out} and
each input batch n is computed as a weighted sum of the input feature maps,

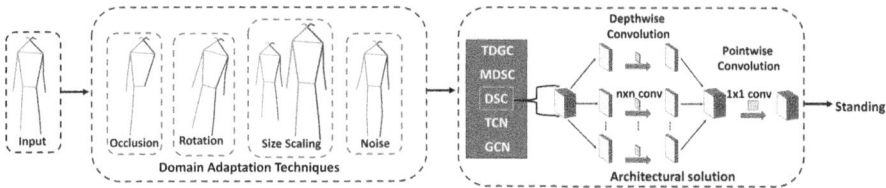

Fig. 2. Overview of the proposed method: TDGC = Temporal Decoupling Graph Convolution, MDSC = Multiscale Depthwise Separable Convolution, DSC = Depthwise Separable Convolution, TCN = Temporal Convolution Network, and GCN = Graph Convolution Network

where each output feature map is derived from all input feature maps calculated as follows:

$$Y_{n,c_{out},ij} = \sum_{c_{in}=1}^{C_{in}} \sum_{m=0}^{k-1} \sum_{n=0}^{k-1} X_{n,cin,i+m,j+n} \times F_{c_{out},c_{in},m,n}. \tag{1}$$

In Eq. 1, X is an input tensor of dimensions (C_{in}, H, W), where C_{in} is the number of input features and H, W are the height and width of the input. F is a convolutional filter of dimensions $C_{out}, C_{in}, K, K)$, where C_{out} is the number of output features, and K is the size of the kernel (assuming a square kernel for simplicity). The indices i, j refer to the height and width of the output feature map.

In our proposed approach, TD-GDSCN, the feature map computation involves convolving each input feature with its own separate filter, thus operating on each feature independently before combining them through a pointwise convolution. TD-GDSCN takes the same input tensor X as Eq. 1 but uses a set of depthwise convolutional filters D of dimensions $(C_{in}, 1, K, K)$, indicating one filter per input feature. The output feature map Y' for each input feature c_{in} and each input batch n was therefore computed as follows:

$$Y'_{n,c_{in},i,j} = \sum_{m=0}^{k-1} \sum_{n=0}^{k-1} X_{n,c_{in},i+m,j+n} \times D_{c_{in},1,m,n} \tag{2}$$

Finally, a 1×1 convolution projects the C_{in} features into C_{out} output features, employing $C_{in} \times C_{out}$ parameters. The final output Z is computed as follows:

$$Z_{n,c_{out},i,j} = \sum_{c_{in}=1}^{C_{in}} Y'_{n,c_{in},i,j} \cdot P_{c_{out},c_{in}} \tag{3}$$

The TD-GDSCN parameter efficiency is highlighted through its reduced parameter count $C_{in} \times K^2 + C_{in} \times C_{out}$ compared to the $C_{out} \times C_{in} \times K^2$ parameters of TD-GCN. For a given layer, assuming the computational cost is primarily due to multiplications, comparing the number of multiplicative operations needed for each approach highlights the efficiency of TD-GDSCN. The computational load of TD-GCN scales with $N \times C_{out} \times C_{in} \times K \times K \times H \times W$, whereas TD-GDSCN substantially lowers the computational demand to $N \times C_{in} \times K \times K \times H \times W$. The reduction is particularly significant when C_{out} is large.

3.2   Data Augmentation Techniques

In contrast to previous works, our strategies are based on real-world conditions that cause performance degradation. For instance, instead of randomly occluding frames, we recognised that an object occluding a camera view typically affects a continuous number of frames in a real-world scenario. Additionally, occlusions can occur randomly due to the unpredictable nature of real-world environments. Considering a practical scenario like this, we define the following strategies to generate augmented data to adapt TD-GDSCN to real-world environmental conditions. All the data augmentation methods use the following definition. Let $\mathbf{S}$ denote the original skeleton data, represented as a three-dimensional matrix of dimensions $N_f, N_j, 3$, where N_f is the number of frames, and N_j is the number of joints in the skeleton. Each element $\mathbf{S}_{ijk}$ of this matrix corresponds to the k-th coordinate (with $k \in \{1, 2, 3\}$ representing the 3D coordinates) of the j-th joint in the i-th frame.

Jittering: This strategy applies Gaussian noise of varying magnitude to joints within randomly selected continuous frame sequences. Two standard deviations, σ_{high} and σ_{low}, are used to control the noise magnitude. The length of each noise sequence is randomly determined from the range of $L_{\min}$ to $L_{\max}$. Let $\mathbf{J}_{\text{high}}$ denote the set of joint indices where higher magnitude noise is to be added and p the probability of frames being selected. The augmented data is obtained as follows:

For all frames, a random decision is made to determine the sequence of frames to be selected with lengths varying between $L_{\min}$ and $L_{\max}$ based on p. For the selected frame sequences, for each frame i and each joint j, the standard deviation for the noise is determined as follows:

$$\sigma = \begin{cases} \sigma_{\text{high}} & \text{if } j \in \mathbf{J}_{\text{high}} \\ \sigma_{\text{low}} & \text{otherwise} \end{cases} \tag{4}$$

Gaussian noise $\mathbf{N}_{ij}$ is then generated for each joint following a normal distribution $\mathcal{N}(0, \sigma^2)$ according to the determined standard deviation. The noise is then added to the corresponding joints in the frames as follows:

$$\mathbf{G}_{ijk} = \mathbf{S}_{ijk} + \mathbf{N}_{ijk} \tag{5}$$

where $\mathbf{G}_{ijk}$ represents the augmented value for the k-th coordinate of the j-th joint in the i-th frame. For the sequence of frames not selected, the original joint data is retained:

$$\mathbf{G}_{ijk} = \mathbf{S}_{ijk} \tag{6}$$

After processing a sequence of frames, a random skip length is computed to determine which subsequent frame to skip as follows.

$$
\text{skip\_length} = \begin{cases} \text{remaining\_frames} & \text{if remaining\_frames} < n \\ n & \text{if remaining\_frames} = n \quad (7) \\ \text{randint}(n, \text{remaining\_frames}) & \text{otherwise} \end{cases}
$$

where remaining_frames $= N_f - \text{current\_frames}$ and n is the minimum number of frames to skip. This method introduces variability in the skeleton data by applying noise of different intensities to specific joints over different temporal sequences. This reflects a likely scenario in a real-world environment.

Occlusion: This method applies erasing to random joints at random continuous frames. The following parameters control the erasing process: the erasing area se, proportion of the erased area $[s_l, s_h]$, value range for the erased area $[v_l, v_h]$, probability of erasing p, aspect ratio of the erased area $[r_1, r_2]$, and erasing sequences length range $L_{\min}$ and $L_{\max}$. The augmented data is computed as follows: Frames are considered for erasing based on probability p. Consecutive sequences of frames are then randomly selected with lengths between $L_{\min}$ and $L_{\max}$. For each selected sequence, the erasing area's dimensions (frame extent fe, keypoint extent ke, and position (xe and ye) are calculated as follows:

$$
\begin{aligned}
\text{se} &= \text{Uniform}(s_l, s_h) \times (N_f \times N_j), \\
\text{re} &= \text{Uniform}(r_1, r_2), \\
fe &= \text{int}(\sqrt{\text{se} \times \text{re}}), \\
ke &= \text{int}(\sqrt{\text{se}/\text{re}}), \\
xe &\sim \text{Uniform}(0, N_j - ke), \\
ye &\sim \text{Uniform}(\text{current\_frame}, \\
&\quad \min(\text{current\_frame} + \text{sequence\_length} - fe, N_f - fe)).
\end{aligned}
$$

If the calculated area fits within the bounds of the skeleton data ($xe + ke \leq N_j$ and $ye + fe \leq N_f$), the selected area within the sequence is then replaced with random values within the value range v_l and v_h. After each sequence, a random number of frames are skipped according to Eq. 7. The original joint data is retained for frames not selected according to Eq. 6. This method introduces variability in the skeleton data's spatial and temporal dimensions, simulating likely occlusion situations in real-world environments.

Skeleton Size Scaling: Given a set of skeleton data, each point X_i can be represented as a vector in $\mathbf{R}^3$. This approach applies a scaling transformation to uniformly adjust the size of the skeleton data in all dimensions to generate a dataset that is more adaptable to variations in the size or distance of human subjects from the camera. This is achieved by applying a scaling matrix S to each data point X_i.

$$X_i = \begin{pmatrix} x_i \\ y_i \\ z_i \end{pmatrix}, and\ S = \begin{pmatrix} s\ 0\ 0 \\ 0\ s\ 0 \\ 0\ 0\ s \end{pmatrix} \tag{8}$$

Thus, the scaled data point X_i is obtained by:

$$X_i' = S \cdot X_i = \begin{pmatrix} s\ 0\ 0 \\ 0\ s\ 0 \\ 0\ 0\ s \end{pmatrix} \begin{pmatrix} x_i \\ y_i \\ z_i \end{pmatrix} = \begin{pmatrix} s \cdot x_i \\ s \cdot y_i \\ s \cdot z_i \end{pmatrix} \tag{9}$$

Skeleton Rotation: This strategy aimed at performing a rotation transformation to simulate different viewing angles. The input data X represents the skeleton data, and agx and agy are the rotation angles around the x-axis and y-axis, respectively. The rotation matrices for the x-axis (R_x) and y-axis (R_y) are defined as follows:

$$R_x = \begin{bmatrix} 1 & 0 & 0 \\ 0 & \cos(agx) & \sin(agx) \\ 0 & -\sin(agx) & \cos(agx) \end{bmatrix} \tag{10}$$

$$R_y = \begin{bmatrix} \cos(agx) & 0 & -\sin(agy) \\ 0 & 1 & 0 \\ \sin(agx) & 0 & \cos(agx) \end{bmatrix} \tag{11}$$

where agx and agy are converted from degrees to radians. The transformed data X' is obtained by first reshaping X to a two-dimensional array. The rotation is applied as follows:

$$X' = X_{reshaped} \cdot (R_y \cdot R_y) \tag{12}$$

After the rotation, X' is reshaped back to its original dimensions to maintain the structure of the skeleton data.

4   Experiments

4.1   Datasets[1]

The **NTU RGB+D 60** [24] dataset comprises 56,880 video sequences recorded from three perspectives using Microsoft Kinect V2. It consists of 60 categories of actions performed by 40 subjects. It is organised into two benchmarks: cross-subject (CS) and cross-view (CV). The CS benchmark divides the participants into two groups, one for training and the other for evaluation. The CV benchmark uses video sequences from the second and third camera angles for training and the first camera for evaluation.

---

[1] The University Research Ethics Committee Approved the Dataset. Approval ID: EPS21036.

Table 1. Parameters and Values

Parameters	Values
p	0.5
J_{high}	elbows, wrists, hands, knees, ankles, feet
σ_{high} and σ_{low}	0.5 and 0.05
L_{min} and L_{max}	5 and 10
$[v_l, v_h]$	0,0
$[s_l, s_h]$	0.05, 0.2
$[r_1, r_2]$	0.5, 2
agx and agy	random values between -135 and 135
S	random values between 0.5 and 1.5

The Northwestern-UCLA (NW-UCLA) dataset [31] comprises 1,494 video clips spanning 10 action categories. Three Kinect cameras captured these clips from different perspectives. According to the evaluation protocol suggested by the authors, we used the videos from the first two cameras for training and the videos from the third camera for evaluation.

4.2   Implementation Details

To improve training stability for our TD-GDSCN model, we used the Stochastic Gradient Descent (SGD) with a warm-up strategy. The initial learning rate was set to 0.1, with a momentum of 0.9. The NTU RGB+D 60 was trained for 100 epochs with a batch size of 64. The learning rate decayed by a factor of 0.1 and a weight decay parameter of 0.0004 was used. The NW-UCLA dataset was trained for 200 epochs with a batch size of 16. The weight decay was set to 0.0001, and the learning rate decreased by 0.1. The model was trained on the Aston University machine learning server, funded by the EPSRC core equipment fund.

4.3   Data Augmentation Techniques

We conduct ablation experiments on the NW-UCLA dataset to evaluate the effectiveness of our data augmentation techniques. The parameter values, defined in Sect. 3.2, are given in Table 1. The results in Table 2 indicate an accuracy increase with the addition of different augmentation types. When the model was tested with data where jittering and occlusion were applied without augmentation, the accuracy was 53.02% and 29.96% for jittering and occlusion, respectively. The addition of various augmentation types led to a performance increase from 53.02% to 92.89% for jittering and from 29.96% to 92.67% for occlusion. This underscores the significance of different data augmentation techniques in adapting TD-GDSCN to real-world environmental conditions.

Table 2. Influence of Augmentation Types: N = Noise (jittering and occlusion), R = Skeleton rotation, and S = Skeleton size scaling

Noise type	Jittering (%)	Occlusion (%)
TD-GDSCN	53.02	29.96
TD-GDSCN+N	81.14	90.73
TD-GDSCN+N+R	92.03	91.38
TD-GDSCN+N+R+S	**92.89**	**92.67**

4.4   Evaluation of Computational Efficiency

We conducted ablation experiments on the NTU-RGB+D 60 and NW-UCLA datasets to evaluate the robustness of TD-GDSCN in handling the trade-off between accuracy and computational cost. TD-GDSCN, CTR-GCN [4], and TD-GCN were compared in detail using three data modalities: joint, bone, and motion. To make a fair comparison, we only replaced the convolution operation in TD-GCN with our depthwise separable convolution, keeping the training settings identical for each model. The results are presented in Tables 3, 4, and 5. For the NW-UCLA dataset (Table 3), TD-GDSCN outperforms TD-GCN and CTR-GCN in all three modalities. For the NTU-RGB+D 60 dataset (Table 4), under the CV protocol, TD-GDSCN's accuracy was higher than TD-GCN and CTR-GCN on the joint and motion modality. Conversely, TD-GCN outperformed TD-GDSCN by a small margin on bone modality. Under the CS protocol, TD-GDSCN surpassed TD-GCN and CTR-GCN in bone and motion modalities, while CTR-GCN outperformed TD-GDSCN in the joint modality. Regarding computational efficiency (Table 5), TD-GDSCN reduced the parameter count by 8.89% and 8.76% on NW-UCLA and NTU-RGB+D datasets, respectively. In addition, TD-GDSCN reduced the computational cost by 26.63%, 71.38%, and 71.52% on the NW-UCLA, NTU-RGB+D 60 CV, and CS evaluations, respectively, as indicated by the inference time. The results in Tables 3, 4 and 5 demonstrate that TD-GDSCN effectively improves both computational efficiency and accuracy, thereby addressing the trade-off challenge between accuracy and computational cost.

Table 3. Accuracy Comparison on NW-UCL dataset using Different Modalities

Modality	TD-GCN (%)	CTR-GCN (%)	TD-GDSCN (%)
Joint	94.40	93.1	**95.69**
Bone	93.75	94.39	**94.61**
Motion	89.66	89.22	**93.32**

Table 4. Accuracy Comparison on NTU-RGB+D dataset using Different Modalities

Modality	CV (%)	CS (%)
Joint (TD-GCN)	94.55	89.32
Joint (CTR-GCN)	94.56	**89.66**
Joint (TD-GDSCN)	**94.90**	89.57
Bone (TD-GCN)	**94.87**	90.13
Bone (CTR-GCN)	94.67	89.96
Bone (TD-GDSCN)	94.78	**90.15**
Motion (TD-GCN)	91.81	87.37
Motion (CTR-GCN)	91.66	87.29
Motion (TD-GDSCN)	**92.94**	**87.75**

Table 5. Comparison of Parameters and Computational Cost on NW-UCL and NTU-RGB+D dataset

Method	Parameters (%)	Inference Time (Seconds per batch)
TD-GCN (NW-UCL)	1.35M	4.13
CTR-GCN (NW-UCL)	1.43M	–
TD-GDSCN (NW-UCL)	**1.23**	**3.03**
TD-GCN (NTU-RGB+D CS)	1.37	106.45
CTR-GCN (NTU-RGB+D CS)	1.45	–
TD-GDSCN (NTU-RGB+D CS)	**1.25**	**30.47**
TD-GCN (NTU-RGB+D CV)	1.37	121.65
CTR-GCN (NTU-RGB+D CV)	1.45	–
TD-GDSCN (NTU-RGB+D CV)	**1.25**	**34.64**

4.5 Comparison to State-of-the-Art Methods

We compared our data augmentation strategy with the SOTA Denoising Autoencoder (DAE) [9] method, which uses a denoising approach to adapt the model to real-world conditions on the NTU-RGB+D 60 dataset. To ensure a fair comparison, we used the same settings as DAE for the jittering and occlusion noise as follows: we applied random jittering and occlusion to all frames and joints, occlusion and jittering probabilities were set as shown in Table 6 and 7, σ was set to 0.1, and the CS protocol was used. The results, presented in Table 6 and 7, show that TD-GDSCN outperforms DAE across all the jittering and occlusion probabilities. This demonstrates the robustness of TD-GDSCN under various degrees of noise present in data, regardless of the temporal effect as determined by the probability values.

Table 6. Recognition accuracy towards random jittering noise on NTU-RGB+D 60 CS: The suffice "w" denotes the use of DAE denoising method

Method	Jittering Probability				
	0	0.05	0.1	0.2	0.3
EfficientGCN [29]w [9]	87.62	87.57	87.59	87.60	87.58
ST-GCN++ [7]w [9]	87.89	87.80	87.75	87.58	87.31
CTR-GCN [4]w [9]	89.07	89.11	89.03	89.09	88.76
AAGCN [25]w [9]	88.57	88.59	88.65	88.65	88.45
MS-G3D [14]w [9]	88.60	88.64	88.62	88.61	88.34
TD-GDSCN (Ours)	**89.69**	**89.30**	**89.43**	**89.28**	**89.10**

Table 7. Recognition accuracy towards random occlusion noise on NTU-RGB+D 60 CS: The suffice "w" denotes the use of DAE denoising method

Method	Occlusion Probability				
	0	0.08	0.1	0.12	0.15
EfficientGCN [29]w [9]	87.74	87.66	87.66	87.57	87.51
ST-GCN++ [7]w [9]	87.80	87.47	87.37	87.38	87.23
CTR-GCN [4]w [9]	89.20	89.19	89.19	89.12	88.12
AAGCN [25]w [9]	88.71	88.42	88.42	88.37	88.42
MS-G3D [14]w [9]	88.75	88.71	88.68	88.67	88.57
TD-GDSCN (Ours)	**89.51**	**89.53**	**89.37**	**89.97**	**89.59**

5   Conclusion

This paper proposes TD-GDSCN and data augmentation techniques to address the trade-off challenge between accuracy and computational cost and enhance performance in real-world conditions. To improve the performance of the existing method, we introduced depthwise separable convolution and detailed data augmentation techniques. The effectiveness of our method is demonstrated on NW-UCLA and NTU-RGB+D datasets. TD-GDSCN and our data augmentation techniques outperform SOTA methods on datasets reflecting real-world conditions and computational efficiency.

Disclosure of Interests. The authors have no competing interests to declare that are relevant to the content of this article.

References

1. Ahmed, S., Irfan, S., Kiran, N., Masood, N., Anjum, N., Ramzan, N.: Remote health monitoring systems for elderly people: a survey. Sensors **23**(16) (2023). https://doi.org/10.3390/s23167095, https://www.mdpi.com/1424-8220/23/16/7095

2. van den Broek, G., Cavallo, F., Wehrmann, C.: AALIANCE ambient assisted living roadmap, vol. 6. IOS press (2010)

3. Buzzelli, M., Albé, A., Ciocca, G.: A vision-based system for monitoring elderly people at home. Appl. Sci. **10**(1) (2020). https://doi.org/10.3390/app10010374, https://www.mdpi.com/2076-3417/10/1/374

4. Chen, Y., Zhang, Z., Yuan, C., Li, B., Deng, Y., Hu, W.: Channel-wise topology refinement graph convolution for skeleton-based action recognition (2021)

5. Deng, Z., Gao, Q., Ju, Z., Yu, X.: Skeleton-based multifeatures and multistream network for real-time action recognition. IEEE Sens. J. **23**(7), 7397–7409 (2023). https://doi.org/10.1109/JSEN.2023.3246133

6. Dohr, A., Modre-Opsrian, R., Drobics, M., Hayn, D., Schreier, G.: The internet of things for ambient assisted living. In: 2010 Seventh International Conference on Information Technology: New Generations, pp. 804–809. IEEE (2010)

7. Duan, H., Wang, J., Chen, K., Lin, D.: Pyskl: towards good practices for skeleton action recognition (2022)

8. Guerra, B.M.V., et al.: Ambient assisted living for frail people through human activity recognition: state-of-the-art, challenges and future directions. Front. Neurosci. **17** (2023). https://api.semanticscholar.org/CorpusID:263632991

9. Guo, J., Ji, Q., Shan, G.: Overcomplete graph convolutional denoising autoencoder for noisy skeleton action recognition. IET Image Processing pp. n/a–n/a (10 2023). https://doi.org/10.1049/ipr2.12944

10. Huang, X., et al.: Graph contrastive learning for skeleton-based action recognition (2023)

11. Liu, H., Liu, Y., Mu, T.J., Huang, X., Hu, S.M.: Skeleton-cutmix: mixing up skeleton with probabilistic bone exchange for supervised domain adaptation. IEEE Trans. Image Process. **32**, 4046–4058 (2023). https://doi.org/10.1109/TIP.2023.3293766

12. Liu, J., Wang, X., Wang, C., Gao, Y., Liu, M.: Temporal decoupling graph convolutional network for skeleton-based gesture recognition. IEEE Trans. Multimed. **PP**, 1–13 (2023). https://doi.org/10.1109/TMM.2023.3271811

13. Liu, M., Liu, H., Chen, C.: Enhanced skeleton visualization for view invariant human action recognition. Pattern Recogn. **68**, 346–362 (2017). https://doi.org/10.1016/j.patcog.2017.02.030, https://www.sciencedirect.com/science/article/pii/S0031320317300936

14. Liu, Z., Zhang, H., Chen, Z., Wang, Z., Ouyang, W.: Disentangling and unifying graph convolutions for skeleton-based action recognition. In: 2020 IEEE/CVF Conference on Computer Vision and Pattern Recognition (CVPR), pp. 140–149 (2020). https://doi.org/10.1109/CVPR42600.2020.00022

15. Mitsuzumi, Y., Irie, G., Kimura, A., Nakazawa, A.: Phase randomization: A data augmentation for domain adaptation in human action recognition. Pattern Recogn. **146**, 110051 (2024). https://doi.org/10.1016/j.patcog.2023.110051, https://www.sciencedirect.com/science/article/pii/S0031320323007483

16. Nations, U.: World population ageing 2019. Department of Economic and Social Affairs PD (2019)

17. Nguyen, T.T., Pham, D.T., Vu, H., Le, T.L.: A robust and efficient method for skeleton-based human action recognition and its application for cross-dataset evaluation. IET Comput. Vis. **16**(8), 709–726 (2022). https://doi.org/10.1049/cvi2.12119, https://ietresearch.onlinelibrary.wiley.com/doi/abs/10.1049/cvi2.12119

18. Nie, Q., Wang, J., Wang, X., Liu, Y.: View-invariant human action recognition based on a 3d bio-constrained skeleton model. IEEE Trans. Image Process. **28**(8), 3959–3972 (2019). https://doi.org/10.1109/TIP.2019.2907048

19. Park, J., Kim, C., Kim, S.C.: Enhancing robustness of viewpoint changes in 3d skeleton-based human action recognition. Mathematics **11**(15) (2023). https://doi.org/10.3390/math11153280, https://www.mdpi.com/2227-7390/11/15/3280

20. Rao, H., Xu, S., Hu, X., Cheng, J., Hu, B.: Augmented skeleton based contrastive action learning with momentum lstm for unsupervised action recognition (2021)

21. Sanchez, J., Neff, C., Tabkhi, H.: Real-world graph convolution networks (rw-gcns) for action recognition in smart video surveillance. In: 2021 IEEE/ACM Symposium on Edge Computing (SEC), pp. 121–134 (2021). https://doi.org/10.1145/3453142.3491293

22. Schomakers, E.M., Ziefle, M.: Privacy perceptions in ambient assisted living. In: International Conference on Information and Communication Technologies for Ageing Well and e-Health (2019). https://api.semanticscholar.org/CorpusID:174804297

23. Shahid, A.R., Nawaz, M., Fan, X., Yan, H.: View-adaptive graph neural network for action recognition. IEEE Trans. Cognitive Dev. Syst. **15**(2), 969–978 (2023). https://doi.org/10.1109/TCDS.2022.3204905

24. Shahroudy, A., Liu, J., Ng, T., Wang, G.: NTU RGB+D: a large scale dataset for 3D human activity analysis. In: 2016 IEEE Conference on Computer Vision and Pattern Recognition (CVPR), pp. 1010–1019. IEEE Computer Society, Los Alamitos, CA, USA, June 2016. https://doi.org/10.1109/CVPR.2016.115, https://doi.ieeecomputersociety.org/10.1109/CVPR.2016.115

25. Shi, L., Zhang, Y., Cheng, J., Lu, H.: Skeleton-based action recognition with multistream adaptive graph convolutional networks. IEEE Trans. Image Process. **29**, 9532–9545 (2020). https://doi.org/10.1109/TIP.2020.3028207

26. Singh, D., Kropf, J., Hanke, S., Holzinger, A.: Ambient assisted living technologies from the perspectives of older people and professionals. In: Holzinger, A., Kieseberg, P., Tjoa, A.M., Weippl, E. (eds.) CD-MAKE 2017. LNCS, vol. 10410, pp. 255–266. Springer, Cham (2017). https://doi.org/10.1007/978-3-319-66808-6_17

27. Song, S., Liu, J., Lin, L., Guo, Z.: Learning to recognize human actions from noisy skeleton data via noise adaptation. IEEE Trans. Multimed. **24**, 1152–1163 (2022). https://doi.org/10.1109/TMM.2021.3120631

28. Song, Y.F., Zhang, Z., Shan, C., Wang, L.: Richly activated graph convolutional network for robust skeleton-based action recognition. IEEE Trans. Circuits Syst. Video Technol. **31**(5), 1915–1925, May 2021. https://doi.org/10.1109/tcsvt.2020.3015051, http://dx.doi.org/10.1109/TCSVT.2020.3015051

29. Song, Y.F., Zhang, Z., Shan, C., Wang, L.: Constructing stronger and faster baselines for skeleton-based action recognition. IEEE Trans. Pattern Anal. Mach. Intell. **45**(2), 1474–1488 (2023). https://doi.org/10.1109/TPAMI.2022.3157033

30. Ul Hassan Asif Mattoo, F., Khan, U.S., Nawaz, T., Rashid, N.: Deep learning-based feature fusion for action recognition using skeleton information. In: 2023 International Conference on Robotics and Automation in Industry (ICRAI), pp. 1–6 (2023). https://doi.org/10.1109/ICRAI57502.2023.10089577

31. wang, J., Nie, X., Xia, Y., Wu, Y., Zhu, S.C.: Cross-view action modeling, learning and recognition (2014)

32. Xin, C., Kim, S., Park, K.S.: A comparison of machine learning models with data augmentation techniques for skeleton-based human action recognition. In: Proceedings of the 14th ACM International Conference on Bioinformatics, Computational Biology, and Health Informatics. BCB '23. Association for Computing Machinery, New York (2023). https://doi.org/10.1145/3584371.3612999, https://doi.org/10.1145/3584371.3612999

33. Xu, B., Shu, X., Song, Y.: X-invariant contrastive augmentation and representation learning for semi-supervised skeleton-based action recognition. IEEE Trans. Image Process. **31**, 3852–3867 (2022). https://doi.org/10.1109/TIP.2022.3175605

34. Yan, S., Xiong, Y., Lin, D.: Spatial temporal graph convolutional networks for skeleton-based action recognition (2018)

35. Yang, F., Sakti, S., Wu, Y., Nakamura, S.: Make skeleton-based action recognition model smaller, faster and better (2020)

36. Yao, L., Yang, W., Huang, W.: A data augmentation method for human action recognition using dense joint motion images. Appl. Soft Comput. **97**, 106713 (2020). https://doi.org/10.1016/j.asoc.2020.106713

37. Zeng, Q., Liu, C., Liu, M., Chen, Q.: Contrastive 3d human skeleton action representation learning via crossmoco with spatiotemporal occlusion mask data augmentation. IEEE Trans. Multimed. **25**, 1564–1574 (2023). https://doi.org/10.1109/TMM.2023.3253048

38. Ziefle, M., Rocker, C., Holzinger, A.: Medical technology in smart homes: Exploring the user's perspective on privacy, intimacy and trust. In: Proceedings of the 2011 IEEE 35th Annual Computer Software and Applications Conference Workshops, COMPSACW 2011, pp. 410–415. IEEE Computer Society, USA (2011). https://doi.org/10.1109/COMPSACW.2011.75

Digital Twinning, Virtual Pathology and Oncology

Weight Perturbations for Simulating Virtual Lesions in a Convolutional Neural Network

W. Joseph MacInnes[1]([⊠]), Natalia Zhozhikashvili[2], and Matteo Feurra[2]

[1] Department of Computer Science, Swansea University, Swansea, Wales
william.macinnes@swansea.ac.uk

[2] Centre for Cognition and Decision Making, HSE University, Moscow, Russia

Abstract. Convolutional Neural Networks (CNNs) match human performance in many visual tasks like the classification of images, however they may not simulate the underlying biological processes. We implemented a CNN to try replicate results from an object inversion experiment with Transcranial Magnetic Stimulation (TMS). After training on upright faces, the CNN model went through three stages of testing: checking (1) for overall accuracy, (2) for the presence of the Face Inversion Effect (FIE) and (3) for an FIE reduction after weight perturbations. Results of the model were compared with human performance in an analogous experiment, where disruption of the extrastriate cortex (the Occipital Face Area (OFA) and the control Occipital Place Area (OPA)) was performed using TMS. The resulting model (1) showed a level of accuracy similar to humans, but (2) did not show the FIE, but rather showed a general object inverted effect. Disruption with TMS (3) led to a reduction in the FIE, however disruption of model layers only led to reduction of the general object inverted effect. Thus, CNNs were observed to successfully simulate some results of objects recognition in general, but are unable to simulate the specific mechanisms of modularity and face processing. CNNs are certainly a useful metaphor for human visual processing, but it's important to understand the limits of that metaphor if they are to be used as models in medicine and neuroscience.

Keywords: Deep learning · TMS · virtual lesions

1 Introduction

1.1 Human Visual Recognition

One of the most enduring questions in cognitive science is how we derive meaning from low-level visual information. After light has reached the retina, our visual cortex computes a series of operations that include edge detection, orientation, curvature, luminance, depth, color, movement and eventually recognition of particular objects. Humans can discriminate between thousands of object categories and learn new categories from just a single example. Visual object recognition reflects our ability to assign a label or meaning to an image of an object regardless of the precise size, position, illumination or context [1]. Humans demonstrate incredible results in object recognition - effortlessly

© The Author(s), under exclusive license to Springer Nature Switzerland AG 2024
X. Xie et al. (Eds.): AIiH 2024, LNCS 14976, pp. 221–234, 2024.
https://doi.org/10.1007/978-3-031-67285-9_16

and instantaneously discriminating between thousands of image categories, despite huge variations that images of the same object produce on the retina [2]. Feature-matching theories suggest that viewpoint invariance is achieved by discrete analysis of object features such as color, shape and direction of motion, and then by integrating these features together at a later stage [3]. The earliest theory of hierarchical object recognition was the pandemonium architecture, and it used a metaphor of screaming demons in four layers to represent weights and features [4].

A similar mechanism has been assumed by most hierarchical models of face recognition, where detection of discrete features was followed by global analysis. The visual cortex shows signs of category selectivity fairly early, with a classic example highlighting regions for place-scenes versus faces. Information is transmitted from early visual cortex to more specialized areas that include the Occipital Face Area (OFA), where basic features of a face are analyzed and is followed by integration of information into a more global representation in areas like the Fusiform Face Area (FFA). Scene recognition follows similar logic: from early visual areas information is passed to the Occipital Place Area (OPA) for the local analysis of scene elements and is further transmitted to the Parahippocampal Place Area (PPA) [5]. TMS studies have shown early dissociation in selectivity for these areas with TMS over right OPA disrupting performance on scene categorization but not faces and vice versa for right OFA [6].

1.2 Computational Models

Computational models of human vision share many techniques with computer vision, but there is often a difference in purpose. Where computer vision tasks typically try to solve a visual processing task in the most effective way, computer models of human vision have the goal of simulating and understanding human visual processing. These models simulate a hypothetical mechanism of processing visual information by the brain. Such models test the validity of proposed mechanisms by comparing simulated results to human data (Lewandowsky & Farrell, 2010). If a model performs a task like a human (with a human accuracy level and typical human errors), we have more confidence that the mechanism of the model may accurately describe the mechanism of the studied human cognitive process. Models simulating operation of the visual cortex are usually organized hierarchically. For example, contemporary hierarchical models of object recognition - the Neocognitron (Fukushima, 1980) and HMAX (Riesenhuber & Poggio, 1999) were inspired from the Hubel & Wiesel pioneering research on the visual cortex (Hubel & Wiesel, 1962, 1968) and attempted to imitate the work of the cortex in accordance with wide a range of parameters, including receptive field sizes and number of layers.

1.3 CNNs as Computational Models

Convolutional Neural Networks (CNNs) revolutionized machine learning by, for the first time, approaching human-level performance in object recognition [7]. Just like its predecessors, the Neocognitron and HMAX, CNNs were inspired from the research on visual cortex and by-design share with it such features as hierarchical organization and local connectivity. Similarly to these earlier models, rich invariant representations are acquired through the sequence of increasingly complex layers [8]. CNNs do not mimic biology as precisely as the Neocognitron and HMAX - for instance, current state-of-art solutions [9, 10] are stacks of over 50 layers versus only seven layers in HMAX. Instead, CNNs were designed for engineering goals and solving real world problems including character recognition, speech processing, security and navigation [11]. Nevertheless, initial studies comparing representational dissimilarity matrices (RDMs) from primate neural responses and internal representations of the model indicated remarkable correspondence between hidden layers of a CNN and hierarchical processing stages of primate visual cortex [12]. Layers of a CNN predict neural responses across ventral stream better than any other models [13]. Initial convolutional layers better describe early stages of visual processing [14], while inferotemporal (IT) cortex responses best correspond to ultimate fully-connected layer of the network [15]. Finally, Eickenberg [16] used linear predictive models to generate synthetic maps of brain activation from a CNN. Attempts to quantify the similarity between CNNs and cortical processing have resulted in metrics like the 'Brainscore' [17] that tries to capture given CNNs similarity to ventral processing and rates models on a multitude of behavioral and neural benchmarks.

To consider these networks as models of cognitive processing, however, we need to understand their limitations as well as their strengths [18]. For example, CNNs are time invariant and as such neglect the complex dynamic properties of biological neurons. Secondly, CNNs take images as an input in a 'spatiotopic' rectangular grid, which has fixed spatial resolution. Alternatively, humans tend to actively search through the scene with saccades and fixate on the target with the fovea, where spatial resolution is highest. Combined, this places CNNs as spatiotopic models even though the human cortex is primarily retinotopic. In addition to organizational differences, it is unlikely that humans and CNNs use similar strategies for recognizing objects. Deep Learning algorithms conventionally require thousands of examples to learn a classification problem, while for a child or even a monkey it is possible to generalize from single example [19]. Some degree of viewpoint invariance can often be achieved by deep learning solutions using a large number of training images of the same object under multiple conditions but they only learn the invariance of the input. However, it is unlikely that a similar approach of scanning an image across different positions is implemented in the brain. Thus, some researchers argue that the large amount of training data that CNNs need to accurately perform classification task is not biologically realistic [20]. Popular theories of human face representation like that of the 'face space' have recently been modelled [20] and may provide a better framework for determining the overlap between human and machine face presentation.

1.4 Aim and Hypothesis of the Study

In some ways, trained neural networks are remarkably similar to the visual cortex, while on the other hand, the structure of computational neurons and their learning mechanism is clearly different from humans. In this study, we tested the applicability of CNNs to simulate specific aspects of facial recognition. The extent that CNNs can be used as a metaphor and model of human visual processing has been well discussed [22], so we chose to test the limits of that metaphor on a few key aspects namely, modularity, category specificity and the face inversion effect. As with other models, we compare the accuracy of the CNN model to human accuracy, but we also propose a novel comparison of task specific errors.

We tested the trained model for specific human visual effects reflecting the peculiarity of visual information processing by the brain [23]. For face recognition, one such classic effect is the Face Inversion Effect (FIE). Although recognition with any inverted object is difficult in contrast to upright, inversion of a face impairs recognition performance more dramatically than the inversion of non-face objects [24]. This is likely due to the way that humans process faces more holistically than other object types. We decided to test whether a trained neural network could show a similar FIE after being trained on upright images. Its presence would suggest additional similarity of operational mechanisms for the model and of the visual cortex in facial recognition and the possibility of explaining the occurrence of this effect in terms of neural networks.

Lesion studies have been instrumental in psychology and neuroscience to uncover how and where key functions are implemented in the brain. Transcranial Magnetic Stimulation (TMS) is a non-invasive tool that enables neuroscientists to causally link brain areas to specific functions. By directing a magnetic field to the cortical regions of interests it is possible to induce various effects that depend on the choice of stimulation parameters, such as frequency and intensity [25]. Previous studies indicated that repetitive TMS (rTMS) delivered at 10 Hz over the right Occipital Face Area (rOFA) impairs recognition of both upright and inverted faces, but has no effect on recognition of objects [25], whereas rTMS delivered at 10 Hz over the right Occipital Place Area (rOPA) impairs recognition of scenes, but has no effect on recognition of either faces or objects [6].

Simulating TMS Lesions with Weight Perturbations. We tried to simulate this TMS effect in a CNN by disrupting specific layers that might potentially reflect activity in the extrastriate cortex. For simulating TMS, we adapted the neural network lesioning method coined by Cheney as weight perturbations [27]. We proposed that if the CNN structure is useful as a model visual cortex, then it should also share modular characteristics of visual processing beyond simple accuracy of classification.

1.5 Five Incremental Goals

In particular, we wanted to test the limits of CNNs as a metaphor for human visual processing to answer a number of questions. These are arranged in what we expect to be an order of increasing difficulty for a CNN to achieve:

1. Can a CNN match human performance on simultaneous presentation, identity matching task?
2. Will a CNN trained on upright faces/objects show a cost when tested on inverted images?
3. Will that cost be greater for faces than for other objects (the FIE)?
4. Can we 'lesion' a CNN to disrupt processing in a way similar to the effect of TMS on humans?
5. Can we find CNN lesion locations that show modular specialization (OFA, OPA)?

We chose a CNN that rated high on the Brainscore [17] and trained it to classify pairs of upright faces and houses as same or different and compared the results to human data in a side-by-side matching task. First, response accuracy and the presence of FIE were compared between human and CNN responses. We then tried to disrupt the FIE in humans using TMS inhibition of the Occipital Face Area (OFA), and in the trained CNN using disruption of layers imitating this area (weight perturbations method). We first present human data from the TMS study, then the results of the CNN model and compare their response accuracy levels, the FIEs and disruption effects.

2 Experiment Materials and Methods

2.1 Matching Task

We used an adapted version of the face matching task (Burton, White & McNeill, 2010), where two samples are displayed on the screen at the same time. Participants were shown two images and were instructed to decide if the left and the right half of the screen depict different views of the same identity (e.g. same person, same house), or different identities (e.g. different persons, different houses).

Stimuli. Stimuli were greyscale photographs of faces and houses pairs. Faces were a set from Glasgow Face Matching Task (GFMT) [28] and houses were from an unpublished set generated for use with the face dataset.

Both faces and houses contained multiple views of the same item and were combined to create equal numbers of same and different pairs using MATLAB. For 'same' pairs, images were never completely identical, but they differed from one another in brightness, proportion and/or camera angle, with face stimuli additionally differing in expression and hairstyle. Thereby, the task required matching of object identity, not sets of visual features.

Procedure. On each trial, a fixation cross appeared at the centre of the screen for a random duration of 300–500 ms. This was followed by a paired image (faces or houses, upright or inverted), also presented at the center of the screen, with a duration of one second. After the image disappeared, participants were shown a blank screen for up to one more second to submit their decision. The next trial began either immediately after a participant's response, or after a two-second decision limit had been reached. Participants responded with their right or left button on a Microsoft Xbox controller, whether they believed the pair were the same or different identity (buttons were counterbalanced across participants).

Each participant completed a total of 12 blocks of 40 trials with each block being part of the three (TMS Site: OFA, OPA, Sham) x two (Stimuli type: face, house) x two (Stimuli orientation: upright, inverted) design. The order of blocks was counterbalanced across participants.

Statistical Analysis. We used the 'lme4', 'CAR' and 'emmeans' packages in R to perform linear mixed effect analysis (LME). Four models in total were built: Separately for each of the stimuli types (Faces and Houses) - one model with accuracy as dependent variable, the other with reaction time (RT) as dependent variable. The Face Inversion effect was determined primarily using the Accuracy scores, though RT scores were tested to look for speed accuracy trade-offs.

All models included fixed effects for TMS Site (Sham, OFA, OPA) and Stimuli Orientation (Upright, Inverted) and their interactions. The base level of fixed effects used for model intercepts was the "Sham, Upright" condition. All models included both random slopes and intercepts with Subject as a random effect. For accuracy analysis, binomial linear mixed effect model was used ('glmer' function), while for RT analysis, simple linear mixed effect model was used ('lmer' function), since RT was observed to be closer to normal distribution.

3   Experiment Results

3.1   Accuracy

Accuracy for the Sham Condition (Face Inversion Effect). The baseline test for the FIE was conducted for accuracy on the sham condition separately to ensure the typical interaction was observed. The resulting model showed a main effect of Orientation (Chisq (1) = 27.8, p < 0.001), Stimulus Type (Chisq (1) = 5.2, p = 0.023) and an interaction between the Stimulus Orientation and Stimulus Type predictors (Chisq (1) = 8.1, p = 0.005).

According to the post-hoc tests, subjects were significantly more accurate at matching upright stimuli in contrast to inverted stimuli ($z = 5.5$, p < 0.001), as well as at matching faces stimuli in contrast to houses stimuli ($z = 2.6$, p = 0.009). Also, there was a significant difference in accuracy for faces upright compared to houses upright stimuli ($z = 3.6$, p < 0.001), while no such difference was observed in inverted stimuli data ($z = 0.2$, p > 0.05). Thus, the experiment replicated the Face Inversion Effect.

Accuracy for the Face Stimuli. The resulting model showed a main effect of Stimulus Orientation (Chisq (1) = 20.6, p < 0.001) and an interaction between the Stimulus Orientation and TMS Site (Chisq (2) = 6.1, p = 0.046).

According to the post-hoc analysis, subjects were significantly more accurate at matching upright faces in contrast to inverted faces ($z = 4.6$, p < 0.001). The post-hoc analysis also showed that stimulation of both OFA and OPA areas decreases accuracy of upright face recognition ($z = 2.4$, p = 0.038 and $z = 2.5$, p = 0.045, respectively). The post-hoc analysis did not reveal the effect of the stimulation on recognition of inverted faces ($z = -0.6$, p = 0.83 for OFA; $z = 0.09$, p = 0.99 for OPA). For both upright and inverted faces, there was no difference between OFA and OPA stimulation conditions ($z = 0.2$, p = 0.97; $z = 0.6$, p = 0.84, respectively.

Accuracy for the Houses Stimuli. The resulting model showed only a main effect of Stimulus Orientation (Chisq (1) = 4.7, p = 0.029) but no other effects nor interactions were significant. According to the post-hoc analysis, subjects were significantly more accurate at matching upright houses in contrast to inverted houses ($z = 2.2$, p = 0.028).

3.2   Reaction Times

Reaction times (RT) for the Face Stimuli. The resulting model showed no significant main effects but only a significant interaction between Stimulus Orientation and TMS

Site (Chisq (2) $=$ 6.3, p $=$ 0.043). However, the post-hoc comparisons with Tukey adjustment did not reveal any significant paired differences, although inspection did suggest a nonsignificant trend where subjects were faster at matching inverted faces during OPA inhibition in contrast to the Sham condition (t $=$ 2.5, p $=$ 0.052; p $>$ 0.5 for all other comparisons).

RT for House Stimuli. The resulting model again showed no significant main effects but did show an interaction between the Stimulus Orientation and TMS Site (Chisq (2) $=$ 29.9, p $<$ 0.001). Post-hoc comparisons with Tukey adjustment did not reveal significant pairwise comparisons, although a non-significant trend suggested that subjects were slower at matching upright faces in contrast to inverted faces during OPA inhibition (t $=$ 2.3, p $=$ 0.078) and OFA inhibition (t $=$ 2.4, p $=$ 0.063) compared to the Sham condition (p $>$ 0.5 for all other comparisons)

3.3 TMS Experiment Discussion

We replicated the Face Inversion Effect, which confirmed the correctness of the experiment and the stimulus material and allowed us to carry out further analysis. However, we did not reproduce Pitcher and Dilks double dissociation studies results, since our TMS effect was not site-specific. Nevertheless, TMS reduced the Face Inversion Effect by impairing discrimination accuracy of upright faces pairs. TMS of the same areas did not affect house matching, which means that we managed to reveal the Face Inversion Effect using the single dissociation method.

We did not obtain significant effects in the reaction time analysis. Thus, participants did not demonstrate a speed-accuracy trade-off, which allowed us to further explore accuracy as our sole task performance indicator. We decided to continue our attempt at simulating this pattern with a CNN by perturbing proportions of weights in the convolutional layers.

4 Modeling

4.1 Modeling Approach

In the modeling part of our study, we investigated a CNN as a candidate model of the human visual cortex. Paramount CNN layers are "Convolutional" - which multiply local areas of the image (patch) with a small filter to see how well the patch corresponds to the feature represented by the filter; and pooling layers, which perform down sampling and either the maximum or average filter response in the patch is selected over other filter results.

For the CNN architecture we chose the DenseNet [10] implementation in Keras with 200 CNN layers and initialized weights. DenseNet was chosen, in part, due to its relatively high rating on Brainscore (rated in the top 5 of convolutional neural nets at the time of training). We used the Google Colab environment to train the network exclusively on upright images of face and house pairs. The training set consisted of an equal number of same and different pairs of faces and houses that were not used in the TMS experiment (in total, 1256 image pairs). The testing data consisted of an equal number of same and different pairs of faces and houses that were used in the TMS experiment (in total, 480 image pairs). Image augmentation was implemented offline before training by randomly changing illumination in a range of 10%, rotating in the range of 5% or zooming in/out an image in the range of 5% using.

The model was trained using the Adam optimizer, with binary cross entropy as the loss function and accuracy as the metric, and trained for 30 epochs, with a batch size of 16. The checkpoint with maximum validation accuracy was saved for testing. The learning rate of 0.001 was reduced by a factor of 0.5 after 2 epochs without improvement in the accuracy.

Weight Perturbations. Recently, Cheney and colleagues introduced a technique for lesioning artificial networks, which they coined as weight perturbations [27]. The authors pointed out that in the case of a disturbance to an embedded circuit via application of noise or damage, weights can be altered in a way that causes temporary detriment in the network performance.

This procedure is implemented by modifying each individual weight value within a layer according to a random amount drawn from Gaussian distribution centered at zero and standard deviation of the original standard deviation of this layer.

Here we propose to test if this approach might be used to simulate biological TMS procedure for artificial neural networks. We have consequentially applied weight perturbations to convolutional layers choosing those layers, disruption of which maximally accurately repeated the TMS effect obtained in humans. Thus, we tried to replicate the effect of the drop in accuracy for upright faces only (not for inverted faces, nor for normal and inverted houses). Previous studies indicated that lower convolutional layers better correspond to V1 features, while the inferior temporal cortex (IT) responses are best described by the last fully connected layer [14]. Considering that occipitotemporal areas, OPA and OFA to which stimulation was applied in the TMS experiment lie between IT and V1 in the visual cortex hierarchy, we assumed that we would find such effects in the middle layers of the model.

We disrupted 1 layer as well as 6 layers at time (i.e. 3 blocks of the DenseNet model). We did also try smaller regions of the CNN, but they had no significant effect on network accuracy. Layer selection for perturbation was handled sequentially through the network, and each experiment (each disruption) was carried out 20 times to account for variation of results.

4.2 Modeling Results

The purpose of this analysis was to answer 5 key questions that tested the degree to which a CNN might match specific quirks of human visual processing. To do this we trained our CNN on upright pairs of houses and faces and tested the trained network on inverted faces and also disrupted the work of certain layers of the model to replicate the TMS effect we obtained on humans (Fig. 1).

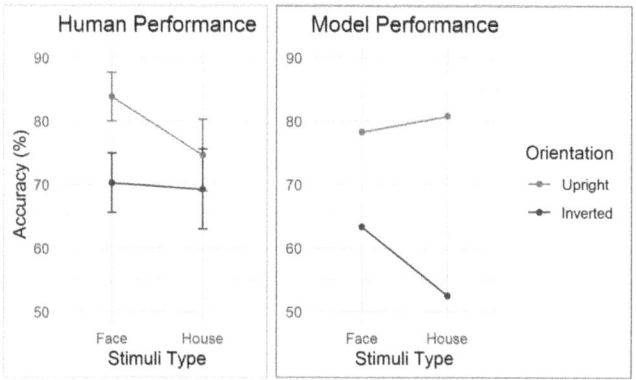

Fig. 1. Interaction between Stimuli Type and Orientation. Face Inversion Effect. Only the results of the Sham condition are shown. For each plotted condition, the estimated marginal mean accuracy and confidence interval are indicated.

The overall accuracy of the best performing CNN was 69% and it was much better at discriminating normal faces than inverted (78% vs 63%) and much better at discriminating normal houses than inverted (81% vs 53%).

In line with Cheney's findings, higher convolutional layers in DenseNet demonstrated more robustness to perturbations than earlier layers. According to this feature of the model, but not in accordance with our assumptions, the most veridical fit to the human TMS data was observed when we perturbed the first 3 blocks of convolutional layers in the initial convolutional section of DenseNet.

We did not manage to obtain an exact match of the TMS 3-way interaction in which TMS impacted accuracy for upright faces, but not inverted faces, upright houses nor inverted houses. The model did not have such a layer or 3 blocks of layers, for which perturbations led to a drop in accuracy only for normal faces. It was, however, possible to replicate an effect only for faces: the first 3 blocks of convolutional layers in the first convolutional section of DenseNet perturbations led to a drop in accuracy only for normal faces, but not for inverted ones, which is consistent with the results obtained in humans. At the same time, such a disruption led to a drop in accuracy for upright houses and an increase in accuracy for inverted houses, which is inconsistent with the results obtained in humans (Fig. 2).

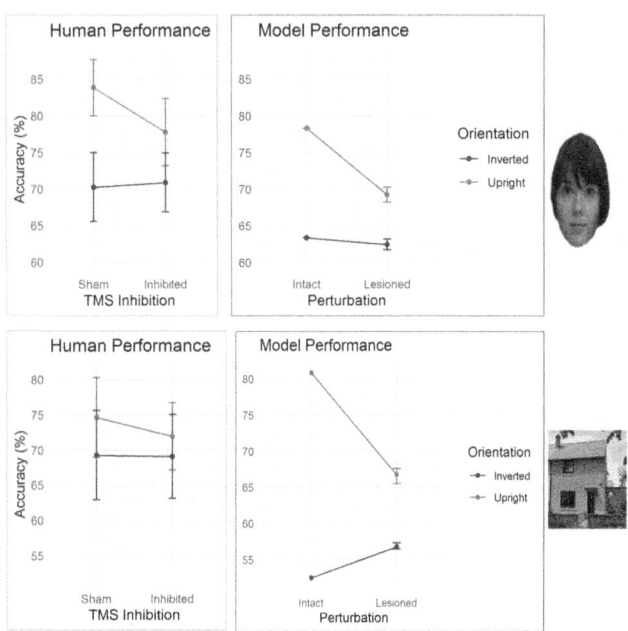

Fig. 2. (Top) The TMS effect on the accuracy for the Face condition. Interaction between Stimuli Orientation and TMS Site. For each plotted condition, the estimated marginal mean accuracy and confidence interval are indicated. (Bottom) The TMS effect on the accuracy for the House condition. The Interaction between Stimuli Orientation and TMS Site was not significant. For each plotted condition, the estimated marginal mean accuracy and confidence interval are indicated.

5 Discussion

We implemented a Convolution Neural network to test whether this style of deep learning algorithm could replicate key results from an object inversion experiment with TMS. Namely we trained the network on upright houses and faces, and then tested to see if the network was able to match: human performance on baseline accuracy for a side-by-side matching task; The classic Face Inversion Effect result; and results from TMS intervention using a new artificial network lesioning technique.

5.1 Hypothesis Questions

Can a CNN Match Human Performance on Simultaneous Presentation, Identity Matching Task? (YES). The Best performing CNN, DenseNet-201 came close to reproduce overall human-level accuracy for normal image pairs discrimination (80% vs 78% for the CNN and human respectively in "Sham" condition). As expected, matching this level of human performance was trivial for the CNN.

Will a CNN Trained on Upright Faces/Objects Show a Cost for Inverted? (YES). If we look solely at the pattern for face discrimination, it was reproduced very well for both for upright faces pairs discrimination (80% vs 78% for the CNN and human respectively in "Sham" condition) and for inverted faces pairs discrimination (63% vs 69%). House accuracy was less well represented by the model with upright house performing better than human, and inverted houses performing worse. Thus, model results replicated human impaired perception of inverted objects. Again, this level of performance was expected, and since both human and computer classifiers will typically show a performance hit as the stimuli deviate more from their usual presentation.

Will that Cost be Greater for Faces Than for Other Objects (the FIE)? (NO*). While the trained CNN did show a cost of inversion, it did not replicate the Face Inversion Effect. Overall, our CNN did not show the pattern of the expected Face Inversion Effect, but instead showed a "General Inversion Effect". This suggests that features that the CNN learned for matching house pairs were not viewpoint invariant, but were more tuned for upright orientation than faces. We suspect that the CNN exploited background information available in the houses images which was specific for scenes, and this information became irrelevant for matching inverted house pairs. Humans process faces more globally than other types of objects, and are therefore more impacted when the typical upright representation is inverted. Our CNN did not show this pattern, suggesting that human and computer classifiers do not process faces in the same way despite similar accuracies for upright faces. The fact that we did observe a non-FIE interaction, does suggest an interesting path for future research.

Can we 'Lesion' a CNN to Disrupt Processing Similar to TMS? (NO*). We were able to disrupt CNN performance with our perturbation technique, though the best results came from perturbations to the first 3 network layers. Perturbations to single layers or less had little effect on classification accuracy. We were able to find layers that impacted face classification more than house, those results were not able to match the three-way interaction we observed in the human data.

Can we Find CNN Lesions that Show Modular Specialization (OFA, OPA)? (NO*). The human results from our TMS experiment did not demonstrate region specific effects for OFA and OPA stimulation shown in previous dissociation studies [6, 26, 29]. We used a side-by-side matching task rather the sequential task from previous research in order to remove complications from a recurrent or memory based deep learning model. The aforementioned studies also used prestimulation fMRI localizer for the localization of individual co-ordinates for subsequent application of TMS, whereas our experiment used mean co-ordinates from previous studies in combination with participants' struc-tural MRI. Indeed, having an fMRI localizer would have been the optimal way to ensure a more robust and precise effect. On the other hand, there is a plenty of evidence about the use of rTMS on face processing by using the average location of the cortical targets by extracting coordinates form similar fMRI studies (e.g. [30]). It is possible that our TMS manipulation managed to temporarily impair generic visual processing composite of OFA and OPA. However, despite the lack of regional TMS results, we did success-fully reduce the Face Inversion Effect using single dissociation method: TMS impaired accuracy of upright faces discrimination and did not affect neither inverted faces, nor houses discrimination.

The results of the TMS experiment were replicated in the CNN model only for faces pairs stimuli. Perturbing weights in its first 3 blocks of convolutional layers resulted in the impairment of network performance at matching upright faces, but not inverted faces. Thus, subjects and the model showed the same results on the face discrimination task. However, perturbing weights of the model also resulted in the impairment of network performance at matching upright houses, while TMS did not affect houses discrimination in humans. Such results could mean similar processing of houses and faces in the model, which does not correspond with perception in humans.

5.2 Summary

In summary, our results show that there are some similarities in the underlying mechanisms of human and CNN strategies in performing a side-by-side matching task. Both humans and the model were worse at recognizing inverted objects, while disruption of information processing reduced this effect for faces stimuli. However, the results revealed rather different strategies in side-by-side matching task performance for humans and the CNN model. CNN models don't seem to process faces in a configural way as evidenced by the lack of an FIE, though we did observe other differences in face vs house processing. For our perturbation vs TMS comparison, we did observe an effect of lower layer perturbation on the CNN, though the results were not able to match the same pattern observed in the human TMS data.

DLNNS certainly share hierarchical processing with human vision, but they do not appear to be as modular. Another key difference is that 'Mid' layers of human lesioning seem best matched 'early' layers of CNN lesioning. Despite that currently CNNs are considered to model visual cortex on the state-of-the-art level of biological fidelity, our results cue at their limitations and suggest that the quest for the ultimate algorithm capable of delineating computational mechanisms of visual processing in the human brain is not over yet. To complete the quest, future research is needed and more techniques have to be developed for the comparison between human participants and computational models at cognitive tasks, and more experimental data should be acquired to identify how damage to artificial neural networks corresponds to either real or virtual lesions to visual cortex.

To conclude, these results may not be surprising to researchers in these fields, but it is always useful to test the limits of the metaphors we employ. For researchers building better algorithms for computer vision, these metaphors may not even be that important, but for those wishing to build computational models of human vision, we should certainly consider whether models match the quirks of human vision as well as the accuracy.

Acknowledgments. The TMS data collected for this article was an output of a research project implemented as part of the Basic Research Program at the National Research University Higher School of Economics (HSE University) and was carried out using HSE Automated system of non-invasive brain stimulation.

References

1. DiCarlo, J.J., Yoccolan, D., Rust, N.C.: How does the brain solve visual object recognition? Neuron **73**(3), 415–434 (2012). https://doi.org/10.1016/j.neuron.2012.01.010

2. Hung, C.P., Kreiman, G., Poggio, T., DiCarlo, J.J.: Fast readout of object identity from macaque inferior temporal cortex. Science **310**(5749), 863–866 (2005). https://doi.org/10.1126/science.1117593
3. Sternberg, R.J., Sternberg, K.: Cognitive Psychology, 6th edn., Wadswort, USA (2012)
4. Selfridge, O.G.: Pandemonium: a paradigm for learning in mechanisation of thought processes. In: Mechanisation of Thought Processes in Proceedings of a Symposium Held at the National Physical Laboratory, pp. 513–526 (1958)
5. Kamps, F.S., Julian, J.B., Kubilius, J., Kanwisher, N., Dilks, D.D.: The occipital place area represents the local elements of scenes. Neuroimage **132**, 417–424 (2016). https://doi.org/10.1016/j.neuroimage.2016.02.062
6. Dilks, D.D., Julian, J.B., Paunov, A.M., Kanwisher, N.: The occipital place area is causally and selectively involved in scene perception. J. Neurosci. **33**(4), 1331–1336 (2013)
7. Krizhevsky, A., Sutskever, I., Hinton, G.E.: ImageNet classification with deep convolutional neural networks. In: Advances in Neural Information Processing Systems, pp. 1–9 (2012). https://doi.org/10.1016/j.protcy.2014.09.007
8. Kriegeskorte, N.: Deep neural networks: a new framework for modeling biological vision and brain information processing. Annu. Rev. Vis. Sci. **1**(1), 417–446 (2015). https://doi.org/10.1146/annurev-vision-082114035447
9. He, K., Zhang, X., Ren, S., Sun, J.: Delving deep into rectifiers: surpassing human-level performance on ImageNet classification. CoRR, abs/1502.0. https://doi.org/10.1109/ICCV.2015.123(2015)
10. Huang, G., Liu, Z., Van Der Maaten, L., Weinberger, K.Q.: Densely connected convolutional networks. In: Proceedings - 30th IEEE Conference on Computer Vision and Pattern Recognition, CVPR 2017, January 2017, pp. 2261–2269 (2017). https://doi.org/10.1109/CVPR.2017.243
11. LeCun, Y., Bengio, Y.: Convolutional networks for images, speech, and time series. In: The Handbook of Brain Theory and Neural Networks, vol. 3361, pp. 255–258 (1995). https://doi.org/10.1109/IJCNN.2004.1381049
12. Khaligh-Razavi, S.M., Kriegeskorte, N.: Deep supervised, but not unsupervised, models may explain IT cortical representation. PLoS Comput. Biol. **10**(11) (2014). https://doi.org/10.1371/journal.pcbi.1003915
13. Cadieu, C.F., et al.: Deep neural networks rival the representation of primate IT cortex for core visual object recognition. PLoS Comput. Biol. **10**(12) (2014). https://doi.org/10.1371/journal.pcbi.1003963
14. Güçlü, U., van Gerven, M.A.J.: Deep neural networks reveal a gradient in the complexity of neural representations across the brain's ventral visual pathway **35**(27), 10005–10014 (2014). https://doi.org/10.1523/JNEUROSCI.5023-14.2015
15. Yamins, D.L.K., Hong, H., Cadieu, C.: Hierarchical modular optimization of convolutional networks achieves representations similar to Macaque IT and human ventral stream. Adv. Neural Inf. Process. Syst., 1–9 (2013)
16. Eickenberg, M., Gramfort, A., Varoquaux, G., Thirion, B.: Seeing it all: convolutional network layers map the function of the human visual system. NeuroImage **152**, 184–194 (2017). https://doi.org/10.1016/j.neuroimage.2016.10.001
17. Schrimpf, M., et al.: Brain-score: which artificial neural network for object recognition is most brain-like? BioRxiv, 407007 (2018)
18. Cichy, R.M., Kaiser, D.: Deep neural networks as scientific models. Trends Cogn. Sci. **23**(4), 305–317 (2019). https://doi.org/10.1016/j.tics.2019.01.009
19. Anselmi, F., Leibo, J.Z., Rosasco, L., Mutch, J., Tacchetti, A., Poggio, T.: Unsupervised learning of invariant representations. Theoret. Comput. Sci. **633**, 112–121 (2016). https://doi.org/10.1016/j.tcs.2015.06.048

20. Medathati, N.V.K., Neumann, H., Masson, G.S., Kornprobst, P.: Bioinspired computer vision: towards a synergistic approach of artificial and biological vision. Comput. Vis. Image Underst. **150**, 1–30 (2015). https://doi.org/10.1016/j.cviu.2016.04.009

21. Jozwik, K.M., O'Keeffe, J., Storrs, K.R., Guo, W., Golan, T., Kriegeskorte, N.: Face dissimilarity judgments are predicted by representational distance in morphable and image-computable models. Proc. Natl. Acad. Sci. **119**(27), e2115047119 (2022)

22. Hill, M.Q., et al.: Deep convolutional neural networks in the face of caricature. Nat. Mach. Intell. **1**(11), 522–529 (2019)

23. Sinha, P., Balas, B., Ostrovsky, Y., Russell, R.: Face recognition by humans: nineteen results all computer vision researchers should know about. Proc. IEEE **94**(11), 1948–1962 (2006)

24. Epstein, R.A., Higgins, J.S., Parker, W., Aguirre, G.K., Cooperman, S.: Cortical correlates of face and scene inversion: a comparison. Neuropsychologia **44**(7), 1145–1158 (2006)

25. O'Shea, J., Walsh, V.: Transcranial magnetic stimulation. Curr. Biol. **17**(6), 81 (2006). https://doi.org/10.1097/PRA.0000000000000221

26. Pitcher, D., Duchaine, B., Walsh, V., Yovel, G., Kanwisher, N.: The role of lateral occipital face and object areas in the face inversion effect. Neuropsychologia **49**(12), 3448–3453 (2011). https://doi.org/10.1016/j.neuropsychologia.2011.08.020

27. Cheney, N., Schrimpf, M., Kreiman, G.: On the robustness of convolutional neural networks to internal architecture and weight perturbations (2017). http://arxiv.org/abs/1703.08245

28. Megreya, A.M., Burton, A.M.: Unfamiliar faces are not faces: evidence from a matching task. Mem. Cognit. **34**(4), 865–876 (2006). https://doi.org/10.3758/BF03193433

29. Pitcher, D., Charles, L., Devlin, J.T., Walsh, V., Duchaine, B.: Triple dissociation of faces, bodies, and objects in extrastriate cortex. Curr. Biol. **19**(4), 319–324 (2009). https://doi.org/10.1016/j.cub.2009.01.007

30. Candidi, M., Stienen, B.M., Aglioti, S.M., de Gelder, B.: Virtual lesion of right posterior superior temporal sulcus modulates conscious visual perception of fearful expressions in faces and bodies. Cortex **65**, 184–194 (2015)

Using GANs to Visualise Class-Specific Features in Digital Histopathology Images

Catherine Little, Richard Gault$^{(\boxtimes)}$ ⓘ, Stephanie Craig ⓘ, and Jacqueline James

Queen's University, Belfast, UK
{clittle12,richard.gault,stephanie.criag,j.james}@qub.ac.uk

Abstract. Oropharyngeal squamous cell carcinoma (OPSCC) patients have an increased likelihood of testing positive for human papillomavirus (HPV). Additionally, people with OPSCC and HPV have a better prognosis than those without HPV. Improving our understanding of the relationship between HPV and OPSCC may improve diagnosis and treatment for OPSCC patients. There are known molecular and clinical entities that differentiate the two cohorts. Whilst it is beneficial to be able to computationally classify the HPV status of patients from histological images, it is important to understand which features a computational model is utilising to make such a prediction. Generative Adversarial Networks (GANs) can be trained to generate hematoxylin and eosin (H&E) stained biopsy samples of cancerous tissues with a specified HPV status, it may be possible to use its understanding of the image domain to gain insight into the connection between OPSCC and HPV. This paper proposes a novel model, PathologyAC-GAN, which combines the class labeling aspect of Auxiliary Classier GANs with the high image fidelity achieved by PathologyGAN to generate images of a specified HPV status. Through qualitative and quantitative assessment, this paper finds that PathologyAC-GAN can learn distinguishing morphological characteristics that distinguish the HPV status of OPSCC patients creating biological insights.

Keywords: GAN · Digital Pathology · AC-GAN · PathologyAC-GAN · Pathology-GAN · HPV

1 Introduction

Approximately 34% of patients diagnosed with oropharyngeal squamous cell carcinoma (OPSCC) in Northern Ireland also test positive for human papillomavirus (HPV) [4]. People with OPSCC who are HPV positive have an improved prognosis compared with those without HPV [1]. Whilst HPV status is usually determined by molecular testing, recent studies have used deep learning to accurately predict HPV status from Haematoxylin and Eosin (H&E) stained biopsy and resection specimens [5]. Such classification studies explore **if** HPV status can be differentiated from specimen images, but it is important to ask "**how** does HPV impact these specimens?". Whilst explainable AI methods could be used to extract features at a sample level, this study will explore the challenge across many samples.

Generative adversarial networks (GANs) are an example of a deep learning system that could potentially provide us with insight into the learnt features of a deep neural network. Although diffusion models have gained much publicity for the fidelity of the synthetic images they generate, they also come with computationally expensive, and poor denoising can lead to unrealistic image generation. Due to these constraints, in this work we explore GANs as a methodology to explore what features indicate the HPV status of a patient; either HPV+ or HPV-. This paper proposes a novel GAN architecture to generate synthetic images of H& E stained OPSCC tissue that reflects a specified HPV status.

2   Literature Review

PathologyGAN [13] seeks a deep understanding of the morphological characteristics of cancerous tissue. The model uses the same structure as BigGAN [3], but with the addition of the mapping layer and style mixing regularisation from the StyleGAN [7] model, and the use of a relativistic discriminator [6] as a loss function. It is trained on a custom dataset of 249K H&E breast cancer tissue images. The result is a model that can more accurately depict biological structures found in tissue specimens. To demonstrate this, linear interpolation is used between the structured latent space of two images, one that resembles a benign tissue sample and one that resembles a malignant tissue sample. With the mapping layer and the style mixing regularisation, the transition from benign to malignant tissue is represented by an increase in the number of cancerous cells which, according to Quiros et al., is representative of real-life cancer cell population growth. This illustrates how GANs can be used to gain insight in morphological features that distinguish subgroups within histopathology datasets. While PathologyGAN produced interpretable synthetic images, the images generated are class agnostic.

Some GANs have been adapted to utilise class information to allow for images of a specified class to be generated and identified. Examples of existing class-aware GANs include Conditional GAN (C-GAN) [9] and Auxiliary Classifier GAN (AC-GAN) [12]. C-GAN is an early example of class labels being used to condition both the generator and the discriminator. It demonstrates how the generator can be developed to produce an image of a specified class. It also explores the potential for the C-GAN to produce 'tags' that explain the contents of the input image using a set of labels. In the context of digital pathology, this method could be used to identify biological features of a sample, for example a biopsy scan could be tagged with 'stroma tissue, TIL, tumour, necrotic tissue". However, this particular style of 'word tagging' may not be suitable for HPV diagnosis, where a probability distribution between 'positive' and 'negative' is more appropriate. An expert looking into HPV status identification is only interested in whether the sample is positive or negative, and so the use of multiple tags adds no additional value.

AC-GAN is a type of C-GAN that arguably fits a diagnosis problem better as the discriminator gives both a prediction for the image source and the class label. The class label is passed into the generator alongside the latent space. The discriminator will attempt to classify the images produced by the generator, and this prediction, alongside the authenticity prediction, is used to calculate the generator loss. A major shortcoming of AC-GAN typically achieves a lower Inception Score and higher Fréchet inception distance (FID) than models such as BigGAN and SA-GAN [15] when trained on the ImageNet1000 dataset. This suggests the images produced are less varied, less classifiable, and less representative of the ImageNet1000 image set. In the context of exploring HPV and OPSCC through generative methods, the generated images must be of high enough quality so the images are interpretable in the pathology sector whilst maintaining class-specific details.

There is a need to benefit from the high fidelity of the synthetic images generated through the capabilities of models like PathologyGAN and StyleGan while leveraging class-specific structuring of the latent space as captured by models like AC-GAN. Combining the advantages of PathologyGAN and AC-GAN into a new computational model may enable high image fidelity and the generation of class-specific image features. Section 3 outlines a novel GAN, PathologyAC-GAN, that aims to generate synthetic images with high quality and accuracy, while the class aspects could allow further analysis into the biological structures that differentiate between HPV+ and HPV- samples. We hypothesise that this will enable experts to use the model's understanding of class-specific biological features to explore the relationship between HPV and OPSCC.

3   Methodology

The proposed model, PathologyAC-GAN, consists of 3 main sections, the mapping network, the generator, and the discriminator. The overall architecture of the proposed model is shown in Fig. 1c alongside the architectures of PathologyGAN and AC-GAN in Figs. 1a and b. Note that the class label, c, is fed into the mapping network, rather than through the generator. This is so that the mapping layer learns to shape the structured latent spaces based on the target class. The rational behind this step is that the structured latent space is generally responsible for dictating what high-level features are present in the final image [7]. If the mapping layer can learn to create structured latent spaces based on a given class, the high-level features in the final image should be more representative of that class. This in turn may produce more coherent results when these structured latent spaces are used in the Linear Interpolation step.

In the mapping network, two unstructured latent spaces, each with a similar class label, are used to produce the structured latent space. Figure 2c shows how a latent space and class label are concatenated together, transformed into a (n, z_{dim}) tensor using a dense layer, where n is the number of images in the batch, and z_{dim} (=128) is the size of the latent space. It is then fed into 4 consecutive ResNet layers, and passed to the final dense layer. This whole process

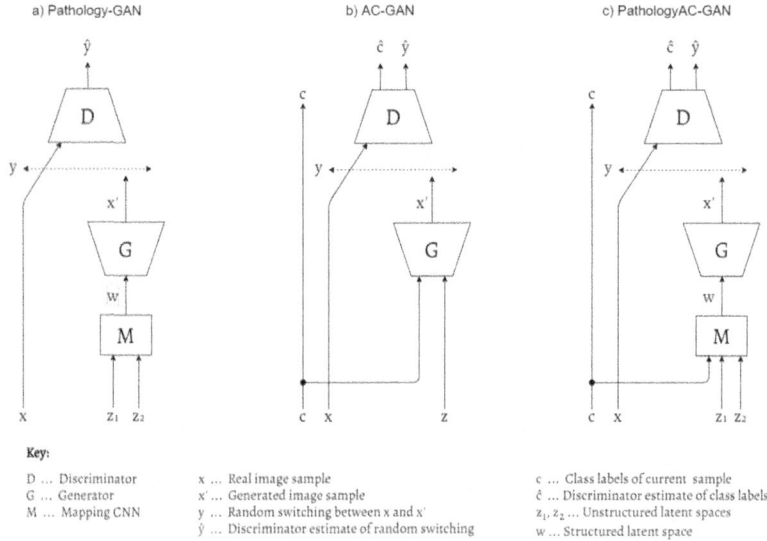

Fig. 1. Architectures of the PathologyGAN [13], AC-GAN [12] and the proposed model PathologyAC-GAN

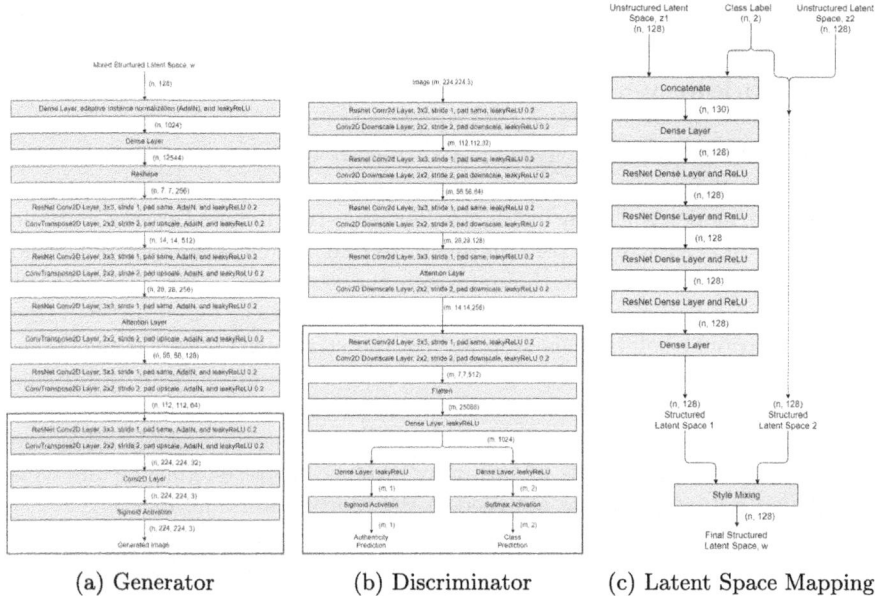

(a) Generator   (b) Discriminator   (c) Latent Space Mapping

Fig. 2. The structures of the generator, discriminator, and the latent space mapping components

is conducted twice to produce 2 structured latent spaces, and then style mixing is used to produce the final structured latent space. Once the structured latent space is created, it is passed to the generator, which is a mirror of the generator found in PathologyGAN.

Figure 2a shows how the generator is predominantly comprised of a series of 'ResBlocks'. These blocks consist of a ResNet layer and a convolution layer. The use of ResBlocks is based on the structure of PathologyGAN, which in turn was based on BigGAN. An attention layer, first developed by Bahdanau et al. [2] for use in language translation, is used in the middle block to help the model focus on relevant information and therefore enhance performance.

The discriminator is fed images from both the dataset, as well as from the generator. It will predict both the authenticity and the class of the image. Like the generator, the discriminator is built using mostly ResBlocks, with an attention layer. As shown in Fig. 2b, the last two layers are split so that 2 predictions are made. One prediction is for class, and the other is for authenticity. The class prediction uses a dense layer to achieve a tensor of size $(n, 2)$, for one-hot conditioning of 2 classes; namely HPV+ and HPV-. It is then fed to a softmax activation layer so that the 2 values represent the probability of each class. The authenticity prediction also has a dense layer but uses sigmoid activation to give a likelihood of authenticity. Softmax is not used for the authenticity prediction in order to preserve the use of the Relativistic Average Discriminator [6] from PathologyGAN, which requires sigmoid activation.

3.1 Dataset

The dataset used in these experiments consists of a combination of 2 existing datasets referred to as OPC and TCGA. Ethical approval and access to the OPC image dataset was granted through the Northern Ireland Biobank (NIB19-0312). Additional images were also obtained from the National Cancer Institute Genomic Data Commons Data Portal and form the TCGA dataset. Both these datasets have been identified, annotated for HPV status, and pre-processed to extra patches of size 224×224 from whole slide images of H&E stained tumour tissue. This combined dataset, herein called OPC-TCGA, is used to compensate for the small size of each individual set, and therefore provide a meaningful sample size for the model to learn from during training. Utilising data from two sources also improves the chances of the model being more generalisable to the problem of HPV status detection and less susceptible to inter-laboratory variability [10, 11]. Additionally, data augmentation was applied to every image in the dataset to boost model performance. The augmentations applied are a horizontal flip, 180-degree rotation, and a combination of the flip and rotation. There are 82936 images in total with 80% of those images isolated to form the training set, and the remaining 20% used to form the test set.

3.2   Training

In training of the PathologyGAN model, the loss is calculated in terms of image authenticity predictions defined L_{auth}^{D} and L_{auth}^{G} outlined in Eqs. 1 and 2 respectively. The expectation of image x_r in the distribution of real data $\mathbb{P}$, is represented by $\mathbb{E}_{x_r \sim \mathbb{P}}$. The expectation of image x_f in the distribution of fake data $\mathbb{Q}$, is represented by $\mathbb{E}_{x_f \sim \mathbb{Q}}$. The raw discriminator authenticity output is represented by $C(x)$ where the input x can be a real image x_r or a fake image x_f.

$$L_{auth}^{D} = -\mathbb{E}_{x_r \sim \mathbb{P}}[log(\tilde{D}_{auth}(x_r))]$$
$$- \mathbb{E}_{x_f \sim \mathbb{Q}}[log(1 - \tilde{D}_{auth}(x_f))] \tag{1}$$

$$L_{auth}^{G} = -\mathbb{E}_{x_f \sim \mathbb{Q}}[log(\tilde{D}_{auth}(x_f))$$
$$- \mathbb{E}_{x_r \sim \mathbb{P}}[1 - log(\tilde{D}_{auth}(x_r))] \tag{2}$$

where $\tilde{D}_{auth}(x_r)$ and $\tilde{D}_{auth}(x_r)$ are calculated using Eqs. 3 and 4 respectively.

$$\tilde{D}_{auth}(x_r) = sigmoid(C(x_r) - \mathbb{E}_{x_f \sim \mathbb{Q}}C(x_f)) \tag{3}$$

$$\tilde{D}_{auth}(x_f) = sigmoid(C(x_f) - \mathbb{E}_{x_r \sim \mathbb{P}}C(x_r)) \tag{4}$$

The loss from the discriminator class predictions, L_{class}, will be the same for both the discriminator and the generator. Class loss can be calculated using Eq. 5 where n is the number of predictions made, $\mathbb{C}$ is the set of possible classes, $t_{ic} = 1$ when i belongs to class c, and y_{ic} is the probability that i belongs to class c.

$$L_{class} = \frac{1}{n} \sum_{i=1}^{n} \sum_{c \sim \mathbb{C}} t_{ic} log(y_{ic}) \tag{5}$$

In PathologyAC-GAN the optimisation goal is that the discriminator is trying to minimise its loss in regards to authenticity predictions, as well as for class predictions. The generator is trying to maximise loss for the authenticity prediction, however, it is also trying to minimise loss for class predictions. Like PathologyGAN, PathologyAC-GAN will make use of the Relativistic Average Discriminator [6] when calculating authenticity loss. The class loss will be calculated using softmax cross entropy as this is appropriate for classification tasks where the classes are mutually exclusive. This is important because there is only one correct answer for this classifier; a sample cannot be both HPV+ and HPV-.

Given the architectural similarities of PathologyGAN and PathologyAC-GAN, it is appropriate to use transfer learning to improve domain representation and variability between images by transferring the weights from the original PathologyGAN model to PathologyAC-GAN. This would allow PathologyAC-GAN to benefit from high-level features that would be relevant for both models.

Only fine-tuning will occur with the layers highlighted in red in Fig. 2a and b permitted to be trainable, while the layers above will be frozen. All layers of the Mapping network are trainable (denoted M in Fig. 1c). This decision was informed by an early preliminary experiment with different transfer learning configurations.

4 Experimentation

This section outlines three experiments to evaluate PathologyAC-GAN for domain representation and class-specific sample generation compared with PathologyGAN and AC-GAN from which it is developed. All models were developed using Python 3.6 and utilising Tensorflow and PyTorch. All models were trained for 45 epochs at a batch size of 20 using a GeForce GTX 1080. Further consistent hyperparameter values across all models can be found in Table 1.

Table 1. Hyperparameters of experiment A

Parameter	PathologyGAN	PathologyAC-GAN	AC-GAN
Latent space dimension	128	128	128
Gradient penalty coefficient	0.65	0.65	–
Adam optimiser beta 1	0.5	0.5	0.5
Adam optimiser beta 2	0.9	0.9	0.9
Image shape	$224 \times 224 \times 3$	$224 \times 224 \times 3$	$224 \times 224 \times 3$
Alpha for LeakyReLU	0.2	0.2	0.2
Regulariser Scale	0.2	0.2	–
Generator Learning Rate	1e-5	1e-4	1e-5
Discriminator Learning Rate	1e-5	1e-5	1e-5
Style mixing probability threshold	0.5	0.5	–

4.1 Domain Representation - Comparison Between Models

This experiment aims to evaluate the performance of the novel PathologyAC-GAN in its ability to represent a given domain. This will give insight into how well PathologyAC-GAN can generate domain-accurate images compared with the models from which it has been derived. From the review of current literature conducted in Sect. 2, it is anticipated that PathologyGAN (and by construction PathologyAC-GAN) should be better at domain representation than AC-GAN.

4.2 Domain Representation - Class-Specific Representation of HPV Status

The goal of this experiment is to better understand the model's capability to generate samples of a specific class. A FID score will be calculated using the generated samples of each class and a test dataset for each class comprised of images from the test dataset. The OPC-TCGA training set consists of 46% HPV- samples and 54% HPV+ samples. Similarly, the test set contains 47% HPV- samples and 53% HPV+. This experiment will also establish if the model is better at generating one particular class more than the other.

4.3 Linear Interpolation

The style mixing and mapping layers (M in Fig. 1a and 1c) of PathologyGAN and PathologyAC-GAN are able to use a structured latent space as input to the generator. The values in this structured latent space are responsible for the high level features of the final generated image. In the context of the OPC-TCGA dataset, the rational is that a structured latent space generated using a given class label will contain values that represent biological features specific to the given class. Linear Interpolation can then be used to produce a series of intermediary points between the HPV- latent space and the HPV+ latent space. It is possible that the high-level feature changes necessary to change a sample's class may be documented via these mid-way latent spaces. The images generated using these latent spaces may give us insight into how the biological structures differ as HPV status differs. Experts in digital pathology will review the generated images providing insight into the model's understanding of the image domain according to experts.

5 Results

5.1 Domain Representation - Comparison Between Models

PathologyGAN had the best performance (FID=55.2), whilst PathologyAC-GAN (FID=82.9) significantly outperformed AC-GAN (FID=392.3). This is unexpected with one possible explanation that the addition of the class loss value has interfered with the model's ability to learn how to generate the images. However, another potential cause is that for the OPC-TCGA dataset, HPV status was determined at a patient level by pathologists rather than at an individual image level. It is likely that some of the HPV+ images do not display any HPV+ characteristics, therefore resembling a HPV- sample, despite the overall rating for a patient in the dataset being HPV+. This may have a negative effect on the GANs ability to learn efficiently.

Example output from PathologyGAN, AC-GAN and PathologyAC-GAN can be found in Figs. 3 and 4 respectively. A subjective view of the results correlates with the objective FID scores. AC-GAN produces images (Fig. 3) that can only be interpreted as noise with minor appreciation of the colour spectra of H&E

images, while PathologyGAN and PathologyAC-GAN (Fig. 4a and 4b respectively) produce images with characteristics and features relating to biological structures. This interpretation has been verified by pathologists.

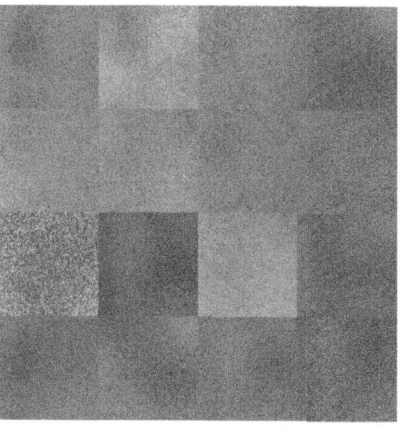

Fig. 3. Example of 16 generated images from the AC-GAN Model following training with the OPC-TCGA dataset.

5.2 Domain Representation - Class Specific Representation of HPV Status

This experiment aimed to see how well PathologyAC-GAN represented samples of a particular class. The HPV+ samples had an FID score of 119.1 whilst HPV- samples had a score of 86.1. Additionally, HPV+ generated images are represented more poorly than HPV- generated images, suggesting that the models understanding of the OPC-TCGA dataset is bias towards HPV- samples. It is possible that the imbalance of HPV- and HPV+ images in the training set may have impacted the class-specific FID scores. Another potential factor is the integrity of the class labels mentioned in Sect. 5.1. Classifying samples at a patient level may have caused the model to learn a less accurate representation for HPV+ samples specifically as some extracted tiles may not reflect the patient's HPV status.

5.3 Linear Interpolation - Transition from HPV- to HPV+

Figure 5 shows 2 arbitrarily selected examples of linear interpolation. They demonstrate the transformation from generated HPV- images (leftmost) to generated HPV+ images (rightmost). The mapping layer was given the same unstructured latent space for each image, but with different class labels, and so

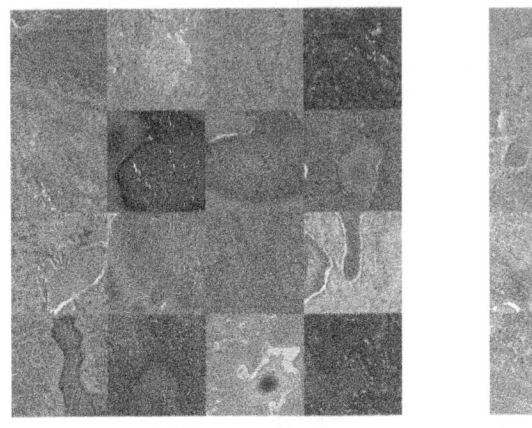

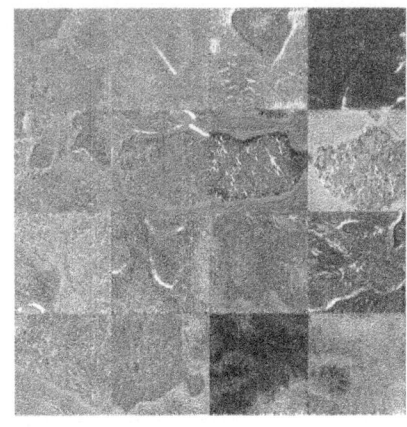

(a) PathologyGAN   (b) PathologyAC-GAN

Fig. 4. Example of 16 generated images from the PathologyGAN and PathologyAC-GAN models.

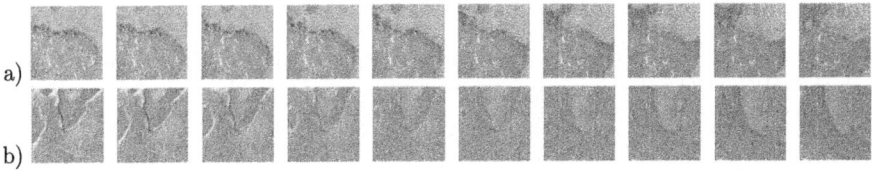

Fig. 5. Two examples of Liner Interpolation on images generated by PathologyAC-GAN. Each row shows the steps taken to transform a HPV- sample to a HPV+ sample

any changes displayed are as a direct result of the different class label. Consolation with digital pathology researchers has provided possible biological explanations for some features present in the generated images. The area high-lighted in blue in Fig. 6 (from Fig. 5 row a)) is indicative of stroma tissue. In HPV-generated images this stroma tissue is less uniform, with a wavy texture. As the generated images become more like the HPV+ class, this area becomes denser with cells and more uniform, and also shows an increase in small dark structures.

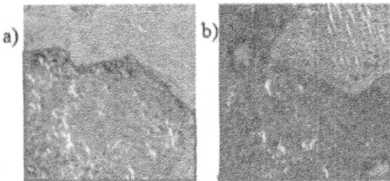

Fig. 6. Examples taken from row b) of Fig. 5. Areas highlighted in blue are indicative of stroma tissue.

These small dark structures may be indicative of an increase in Tumour infiltrating lymphocytes (TILs). Denser TIL population is a recognised biological feature of tissue sampled from OPSCC patients with HPV [14], suggesting that the model has learnt some class specific high-level features that correlate with real-life understanding of the domain. Additionally, the area in Fig. 7a) (from Fig. 5 row b)) circled in blue presents characteristics of necrotic tissue. Necrotic tissue is a common characteristic of HPV- OPSCC [8] and, as shown in Fig. 7b), this area disappears as the image class changes from HPV- to HPV+. Overall, while PathologyAC-GAN may not generate images that are as representative of the data as PathologyGAN, the model still has potentially learnt some high-level biological features that are consistent with existing biological theory regarding HPV and OPSCC.

6   Discussion

PathologyAC-GAN was created with the goal of providing insight into the relationship between HPV and OPSCC. This required the development of a novel computational GAN that extends the methodology of the current state-of-the-art GANs in this area to include class-specific information whilst providing synthetic images with high fidelity. By examining the generated images, insight into the key biological structures that determine HPV status may have been gained.

The qualitative analysis of the linear interpolation results outlined in Sect. 5.3, suggests that the model was able to learn biologically relevant features that correlated with current knowledge on the relationship between HPV and OPSCC. Digital pathology researchers were able to find areas in the generated images that may be indicative of an increase in TIL population in Fig. 6 and the presence of necrotic tissue in Fig. 7. This gives us insight into how the generator is making decisions and provides some level of interpretation as to the computational decision making that is being used to differentiate HPV status.

However, overall the PathologyAC-GAN did not perform as well as expected with respect to generating realistic histopathology images. The FID score calculated shows that while it was significantly better at creating accurate images than the simplified AC-GAN, it performed slightly worse than PathologyGAN (Sect. 5.1). While the reasons for the less than desirable FID scores are not fully

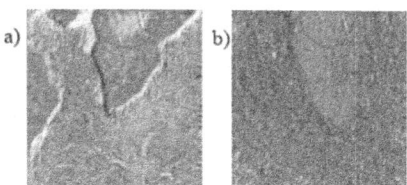

Fig. 7. Examples taken from row d) of Fig. 5. Areas highlighted in blue are indicative of necrotic tissue in (a) with the same characteristic absent in (b) (Color figure online).

clear, it is possible that the fact that images in the OPC-TCGA dataset are classified at a patient level rather than a individual image level has had a significant negative impact on the models ability to learn advanced class specific features. This means some samples labelled HPV+ may not contain features indicative of an HPV+ sample, despite being labelled as such as other patches for that patient do contain HPV+ related features. This may lead to the model mistaking HPV- features for HPV+ features.

Future development of the PathologyAC-GAN may benefit from a review of how the class loss is integrated into the overall loss function. Throughout the training of PathologyAC-GAN, the loss calculated for class prediction was consistently much lower than the loss calculated for authenticity prediction. By adding the two values together, it is possible that the lower value was being overshadowed. A loss function that was more sensitive to the class prediction may yield better results, although it is possible that placing less value on the authenticity prediction could also harm the overall image quality. Further investigation would be required to confirm this statement.

7   Conclusion

Understanding of the morphological distinctions between OPSCC patients who are HPV+ and those who are HPV- is important to help us understand the role HPV status has on the underlying biology associated with OPSCC. This work explored how computational approaches, in particular GANs, can be used to learn the distinguishing features of HPV status in a data-driven way. The computationally extracted features may overlap with existing expert knowledge or even highlight features that were previously not considered. This could subsequently support the investigation into

Overall, PathologyAC-GAN in its current state has some ability to generate images that represent biological features that are relevant to a given class. Using linear interpolation of the structured latent space allowed the visual transformation from a HPV- sample to a HPV+ sample. This enables the learnt features of a model to be visually inspected by pathologists, which would in turn support interpretability within the model. However, improvement in image quality and class representation would likely be necessary before valuable or clinically relevant insight can be gained from the model.

References

1. Albers, A.E., Qian, X., Kaufmann, A.M., Coordes, A.: Meta analysis: Hpv and p16 pattern determines survival in patients with HNSCC and identifies potential new biologic subtype. Sci. Rep. **7**(1), 1–14 (2017)
2. Bahdanau, D., Cho, K., Bengio, Y.: Neural machine translation by jointly learning to align and translate. In: Bengio, Y., LeCun, Y. (eds.) 3rd International Conference on Learning Representations, ICLR 2015, San Diego, CA, USA, May 7-9, 2015, Conference Track Proceedings (2015). arXiv:1409.0473

3. Brock, A., Donahue, J., Simonyan, K.: Large scale GAN training for high fidelity natural image synthesis. CoRR **abs/1809.11096** (2018). arXiv:1809.11096

4. Craig, S.G., et al.: Recommendations for determining HPV status in patients with oropharyngeal cancers under tnm8 guidelines: a two-tier approach. Br. J. Cancer **120**(8), 827–833 (2019). https://doi.org/10.1038/s41416-019-0414-9

5. Craig, S.G., et al.: A deep learning alternative to regional molecular testing for hpv status (2023). https://www.aacr.org/professionals/meetings/previous-aacr-meetings/previous-aacr-meetings-2023/. aACR-AHNS Head and Neck Cancer Conference: Innovating through Basic, Clinical, and Translational Research

6. Jolicoeur-Martineau, A.: The relativistic discriminator: a key element missing from standard GAN. CoRR **abs/1807.00734** (2018), arXiv:1807.00734

7. Karras, T., Laine, S., Aila, T.: A style-based generator architecture for generative adversarial networks. In: Proceedings of the IEEE/CVF Conference on Computer Vision and Pattern Recognition (CVPR) (June 2019)

8. Lewis, J.S.: Morphologic diversity in human papillomavirus-related oropharyngeal squamous cell carcinoma: catch me if you can! Mod. Pathol. **30**(1), S44–S53 (2017)

9. Mirza, M., Osindero, S.: Conditional generative adversarial nets. CoRR **abs/1411.1784** (2014), arXiv:1411.1784

10. Moyes, A., Gault, R., Zhang, K., Ming, J., Crookes, D., Wang, J.: Multi-channel auto-encoders for learning domain invariant representations enabling superior classification of histopathology images. Med. Image Anal. **83**, 102640 (2023)

11. Moyes, A., Zhang, K., Wang, L., Ji, M., Crookes, D., Zhou, H.: A novel method for unsupervised scanner-invariance with dcae model. In: British Machine Vision Conference (BMVC 2018), p. 1. BMVC (Sep 2018)

12. Odena, A., Olah, C., Shlens, J.: Conditional image synthesis with auxiliary classifier GANs. In: Precup, D., Teh, Y.W. (eds.) Proceedings of the 34th International Conference on Machine Learning. Proceedings of Machine Learning Research, vol. 70, pp. 2642–2651. PMLR, International Convention Centre, Sydney, Australia (06–11 Aug 2017). http://proceedings.mlr.press/v70/odena17a.html

13. Quiros, A.C., Murray-Smith, R., Yuan, K.: Pathologygan: Learning deep representations of cancer tissue. In: Arbel, T., Ayed, I.B., de Bruijne, M., Descoteaux, M., Lombaert, H., Pal, C. (eds.) Proceedings of the Third Conference on Medical Imaging with Deep Learning. Proceedings of Machine Learning Research, vol. 121, pp. 669–695. PMLR, Montreal, QC, Canada (06–08 Jul 2020). http://proceedings.mlr.press/v121/quiros20a.html

14. Wood, O., et al.: Gene expression analysis of TIL rich HPV-driven head and neck tumors reveals a distinct b-cell signature when compared to hpv independent tumors. Oncotarget **7**(35), 56781 (2016)

15. Zhang, H., Goodfellow, I., Metaxas, D., Odena, A.: Self-attention generative adversarial networks. In: Chaudhuri, K., Salakhutdinov, R. (eds.) Proceedings of the 36th International Conference on Machine Learning. Proceedings of Machine Learning Research, vol. 97, pp. 7354–7363. PMLR, Long Beach, California, USA (09–15 Jun 2019). http://proceedings.mlr.press/v97/zhang19d.html

Artificial Intelligence for Predicting Responses to Thyroid Cancer Treatment

Alaa Abd-Alrazaq[1]([⊠]) [iD], Rawan AlSaad[1] [iD], Arfan Ahmed[1] [iD], Hania Aslam[1] [iD], Babul Salam[2] [iD], Sarah Aziz[1] [iD], and Javaid Sheikh[1] [iD]

[1] Weill Cornell Medicine-Qatar, Doha, Qatar
{aaa4027,rta4003,ara4013,haa4018,saa4038,
jsheikh}@qatar-med.cornell.edu
[2] Gulf University for Science and Technology, Hawally, Kuwait
babul.s@gust.edu.kw

Abstract. Thyroid cancer, one of the most prevalent endocrine malignancies, presents diverse treatment responses among patients, underscoring the necessity for personalized treatment strategies. This study aims to develop and evaluate AI models that can accurately predict the initial treatment response among patients with well-differentiated thyroid cancer. We trained and validated various machine learning and deep learning models using a dataset that comprises demographic and clinicopathological features. This dataset was collected from a retrospective cohort of 383 patients diagnosed with thyroid cancer at a single medical center. Models in all experiments achieved an average accuracy of 72.2%, average precision of 76.2%, average recall of 68%, average F1 score of 70.6%, and average AUC of 80.5%. Multi-layer Perceptron achieved the highest accuracy (85.7%), recall (75%), and F1 score (81.7%) in this study when it was used for predicting binary treatment response using all features, excluding those weakly correlated with the treatment response. However, Naive Bayes attained the highest precision (95.1%) and AUC (88.7%) in this study when it was used for predicting binary treatment response using all features. Models used for predicting binary treatment responses outperformed those used for predicting multi-class treatment responses. AI demonstrates satisfactory performance in predicting the response to thyroid cancer treatment, yet there is room for optimization. Healthcare providers should not solely rely on our models; combining them with other tools is advised until further studies validate their optimal performance. Future research should enhance predictive capabilities by including additional features, exploring alternative models, and utilizing larger and balanced datasets.

Keywords: Artificial Intelligence · Thyroid Cancer · Treatment Response

1 Introduction

Thyroid cancer is one of the most common endocrine malignancies that results from abnormal growth and division of cells in the thyroid, a gland located beneath the voice box at the front of the throat [1]. Worldwide, it is estimated that over 586,202 new cases

© The Author(s), under exclusive license to Springer Nature Switzerland AG 2024
X. Xie et al. (Eds.): AIiH 2024, LNCS 14976, pp. 248–260, 2024.
https://doi.org/10.1007/978-3-031-67285-9_18

of thyroid cancer emerged in 2020 [2]. The typical approach to treating thyroid cancer usually starts with surgery, followed by radioactive iodine therapy, thyroid hormone therapy, and external beam radiation therapy if needed. For more aggressive or advanced cases, targeted therapies and chemotherapy may also be employed [3].

Response to thyroid cancer treatment is categorized into "Excellent", "Indeterminate", "Biochemical incomplete", and "Structural incomplete" [3]. An "Excellent Response" indicates that physical examinations, imaging tests, and blood tests show no signs of the disease. The "Indeterminate Response" category is applied when the results are unclear or uncertain, such as ambiguous imaging findings that cannot definitively be identified as cancer. A "Biochemical Incomplete Response" suggests that, despite the absence of cancer on imaging, elevated thyroglobulin levels in the blood imply the likely presence of unseen cancer cells. Lastly, a "Structural Incomplete Response" is characterized by visible evidence of remaining cancer on imaging tests, regardless of thyroglobulin levels, indicating that structural remnants of the disease persist despite the treatment. Because thyroid cancer varies in type, stage, and how it affects each person, treatment responses can differ significantly. In other words, the effectiveness of thyroid cancer treatment is highly individualized.

Numerous studies showed promising results in using Artificial Intelligence (AI) in several applications related to thyroid cancer such as detecting and differentiating between different types of thyroid tumors [4–6], predicting its recurrence [7–9], and stratifying its risk [10]. However, very few studies assessed the effectiveness of AI in predicting the response of thyroid cancer treatment [11–13]. These studies also have some limitations. Firstly, they did not consider important features in their models such as current smoking status, past smoking history, presence of goiter, and presence of adenopathy [11–13]. Secondly, they did not compare the performance of AI in predicting a 4-class treatment response versus a 2-class treatment response [11–13]. Thirdly, the follow-up period after the treatment was short (<10 years) [11–13]. Lastly, they did not compare the performance of different AI models [11, 12]. Therefore, the aim of the study is to examine the performance of AI in predicting the treatment response among patients with well-differentiated thyroid cancer.

2   Methods

2.1   Dataset Information

This study used a dataset published by Shiva Borzooei in the UC Irvine Machine Learning Repository [14]. The dataset consists of 383 participants, comprising 312 females and 71 males. On average, the participants were 40.7 years old (standard deviation 15.1). The dataset encompasses 17 features, including age, gender, smoking status, history of smoking, history of radiation therapy, thyroid function, presence of goiter, presence of adenopathy, pathological type of thyroid cancer, focality, risk assessment according to American Thyroid Association (ATA) guidelines, extent and severity of cancer based on (1) primary tumor size and extent (T), (2) involvement of nearby lymph nodes (N), and (3) presence of distant metastasis (M), overall cancer stage based on T, N, and M, recurrence of cancer, and treatment response.

2.2 Data Preprocessing

There are no missing values in all variables. The feature "recurrence of cancer" was used as the target variable in the original study [7] where the data was collected and hence was not considered in the present study. The dataset predominantly consists of categorical variables, except for 'age,' which is continuous. Accordingly, we applied label encoding to the categorical variables to prepare them for modeling. We also performed a correlation analysis between the target variable and the predictors to determine the most relevant features for model development.

2.3 Experiments

The correlation heatmap revealed that certain features exhibit a weak correlation (<0.1) with the target variable, whereas others demonstrate moderate to high correlations (≥ 0.30) with it (Figs. 1 and 2). For this reason, this study used 3 different sets of features: (1) all features, (2) all features without weakly correlated features, and (3) only moderately to strongly correlated features. There was an imbalance in the number of participants across classes within the target variable (i.e., treatment response): 208 in the Excellent class, 91 in the Structural incomplete class, 61 in the Indeterminate class, and 23 in the Biochemical incomplete class. Therefore, the target variable in this study was both multi-class (i.e., Excellent, Structural incomplete, Indeterminate, and Biochemical incomplete) and binary (i.e., Excellent and Non-Excellent (others)). In total, 6 experiments were carried out, varying the combinations of features and the number of classes utilized (Table 1).

Table 1. Experiments' details

Experiment #	Features	Number of classes
Experiment 1	All features	4
Experiment 2	All features without thyroid function and pathology	4
Experiment 3	Only smoking status, presence of adenopathy, focality, risk assessment, cancer stage based on T, cancer stage based on N, and overall cancer stage	4
Experiment 4	All features	2
Experiment 5	All features without thyroid function, pathology, and smoking history	2
Experiment 6	Only smoking status, presence of adenopathy, focality, risk assessment, cancer stage based on T, cancer stage based on N, and overall cancer stage	2

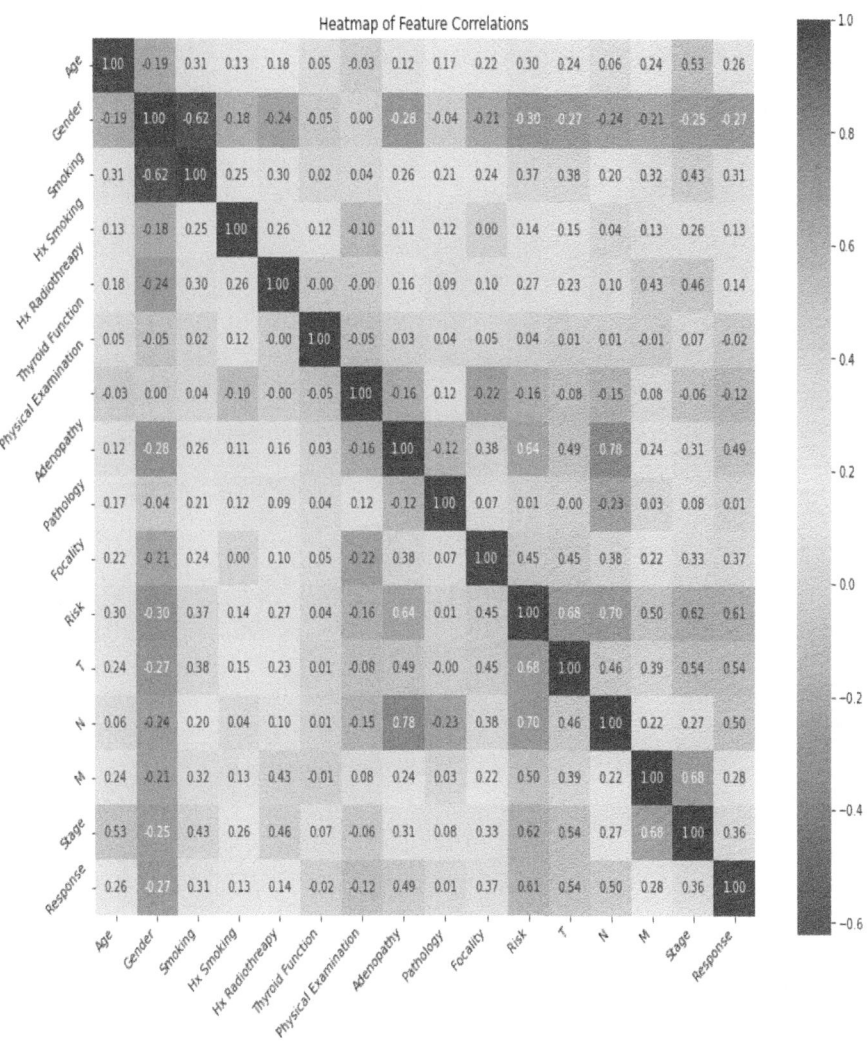

Fig. 1. Heatmap of correlations between all features when using multi-class target variable

2.4 Model Development and Evaluation

In this study, we developed and evaluated different AI models including Logistic Regression (LogR), Decision Trees (DT), Random Forests (RF), Support Vector Machines (SVM), Naïve Bayes (NB), and K-Nearest Neighbor (KNN) and Multi-layer Perceptron (MLP). These models underwent training utilizing 80% of the dataset and were subsequently evaluated using the remaining 20% of the dataset. The following performance metrics were used to evaluate the effectiveness of these models:

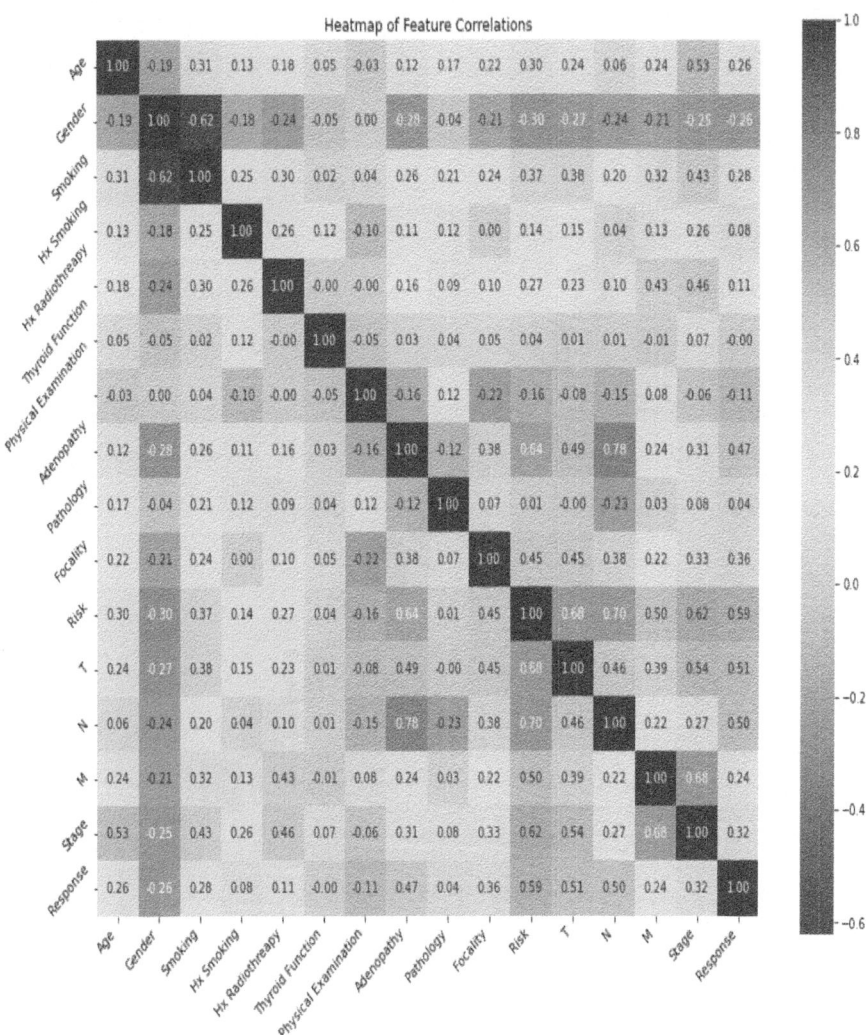

Fig. 2. Heatmap of correlations between all features when using binary target variable

1. Accuracy: It represents the proportion of correct predictions made by the model across the entire dataset. It is calculated as the ratio of true positives (TP) and true negatives (TN) to the total number of samples.
2. Recall: It assesses how well the model catches all the positive cases. It is calculated as proportion of TP predictions among all the actual positive samples in the dataset.
3. Precision: It is the measure of the accuracy of the positive predictions. It is calculated as the proportion of true positive predictions among all the positive predictions made by the model.
4. F1 score: It is the harmonic mean of precision and recall. It is calculated as follows:
   F1 = 2 TP/(2 TP + FP + FN)

5. Area under the Curve (AUC): It measures the overall performance of a model by calculating the area underneath the Receiver Operating Characteristic (ROC) curve. The ROC curve is a plot of the true positive rate (recall) against the false positive rate (1 - specificity).

T-tests and one-way ANOVA were conducted to determine the statistical significance of differences in model performance while predicting varying numbers of classes in the target variable using distinct feature sets, respectively. Differences in performance were considered to be statistically significant if the p-value was below 0.05.

3   Results

3.1   Overall Performance

The highest accuracy, recall, and F1 score across all experiments were 85.7%, 79.5%, and 85.0%, respectively, as bolded in Table 2. These results were achieved by Multi-layer Perceptron when it was used for predicting binary treatment response using all features, excluding those weakly correlated with the treatment response. However, the highest precision and AUC across all experiments were 96.3% and 91.6%, respectively. These results were attained when using Naive Bayes for predicting binary treatment response using all features. As shown in Table 3, models in all experiments achieved an average accuracy of 72.2%, average precision of 76.2%, average recall of 68%, average F1 score of 70.6%, and average AUC of 80.5%. It is worth mentioning that the following sampling techniques were used in Experiments 1, 2, and 3 to overcome the imbalance issue in the target variable: Synthetic Minority Over-sampling Technique (SMOTE), RandomOverSampler, and RandomUnderSampler. However, the models exhibited superior performance in most results when no sampling strategies were used (Fig. 1, 2 and 3 in Appendix).

Table 2. Results of each experiment

Models	Accuracy	Precision	Recall	F1 Score	AUC
Experiment 1					
Decision Tree	0.610	0.646	0.610	0.626	0.687
Naive Bayes	0.519	0.728	0.519	0.578	0.788
K-Nearest Neighbor	0.727	0.650	0.727	0.676	0.752
Random Forest	0.701	0.694	0.701	0.694	0.792
Support Vector Machine	0.688	0.595	0.688	0.597	0.859
Logistic Regression	0.714	0.644	0.714	0.675	0.753
Multi-layer Perceptron	0.675	0.635	0.675	0.654	0.759

(*continued*)

Table 2. (*continued*)

Models	Accuracy	Precision	Recall	F1 Score	AUC
Experiment 2					
Decision Tree	0.610	0.622	0.610	0.616	0.670
Naive Bayes	0.390	0.707	0.390	0.465	0.799
K-Nearest Neighbor	0.649	0.616	0.649	0.622	0.759
Random Forest	0.714	0.697	0.714	0.705	0.787
Support Vector Machine	0.688	0.595	0.688	0.597	0.858
Logistic Regression	0.753	0.633	0.753	0.685	0.757
Multi-layer Perceptron	0.727	0.619	0.727	0.665	0.724
Experiment 3					
Decision Tree	0.701	0.672	0.701	0.685	0.734
Naive Bayes	0.740	0.683	0.740	0.707	0.796
K-Nearest Neighbor	0.701	0.641	0.701	0.666	0.745
Random Forest	0.701	0.672	0.701	0.685	0.728
Support Vector Machine	0.753	0.642	0.753	0.693	0.875
Logistic Regression	0.740	0.630	0.740	0.680	0.767
Multi-layer Perceptron	0.701	0.659	0.701	0.678	0.734
Experiment 4					
Decision Tree	0.727	0.780	0.727	0.753	0.731
Naive Bayes	0.753	0.963	0.591	0.732	0.916
K-Nearest Neighbor	0.688	0.857	0.545	0.667	0.849
Random Forest	0.753	0.791	0.773	0.782	0.842
Support Vector Machine	0.662	0.846	0.500	0.629	0.800
Logistic Regression	0.805	0.914	0.727	0.810	0.911
Multi-layer Perceptron	0.805	0.914	0.727	0.810	0.886
Experiment 5					
Decision Tree	0.727	0.765	0.667	0.712	0.719
Naive Bayes	0.779	0.958	0.590	0.730	0.887
K-Nearest Neighbor	0.740	0.828	0.615	0.706	0.801
Random Forest	0.792	0.829	0.744	0.784	0.848
Support Vector Machine	0.727	0.950	0.487	0.644	0.878

(*continued*)

Table 2. (*continued*)

Models	Accuracy	Precision	Recall	F1 Score	AUC
Logistic Regression	0.818	0.903	0.718	0.800	0.869
Multi-layer Perceptron	0.857	0.912	0.795	0.850	0.854
Experiment 6					
Decision Tree	0.727	0.811	0.682	0.741	0.815
Naive Bayes	0.844	0.944	0.773	0.850	0.886
K-Nearest Neighbor	0.779	0.829	0.773	0.800	0.808
Random Forest	0.766	0.825	0.750	0.786	0.832
Support Vector Machine	0.805	0.914	0.727	0.810	0.852
Logistic Regression	0.805	0.914	0.727	0.810	0.874
Multi-layer Perceptron	0.779	0.886	0.705	0.785	0.837

Table 3. Summary of overall performance of all models in all experiments

	Accuracy	Precision	Recall	F1 Score	AUC
Mean	0.722	0.762	0.680	0.706	0.805
SD	0.083	0.123	0.088	0.082	0.064
Max	0.857	0.963	0.795	0.850	0.916
Min	0.390	0.595	0.390	0.465	0.670

3.2 Performance Based on the Number of Classes

As outlined in Table 4, our AI models generally exhibited superior performance in predicting a binary treatment response (Excellent and Non-excellent) compared to predicting multi-class treatment responses (Excellent, biochemical incomplete, structurally incomplete, indeterminate classes) in terms of all metrics: accuracy (76.8% vs. 67.6%), precision (87.3% vs. 65.1%), recall (68.3% vs. 67.6%), F1 score (76.1% vs. 65%), and AUC (84.3% vs. 76.8%). However, the difference in the performance was statistically significant ($p < 0.05$) in terms of all metrics except for recall ($p = 0.8081$).

3.3 Performance Based on Features Used

As presented in Table 5, in general, the performance of our AI models in predicting a multi-class treatment response using moderately-to-strongly correlated features was higher than using all features without weakly correlated features or all features in terms of accuracy (72% vs. 64.7% vs. 66.2%), recall (72% vs. 64.7% vs. 66.2%), and F1 score (68.5% vs. 62.2% vs. 64.3%). On the other hand, their performance was comparable in terms of precision (65.7% vs. 64.1% vs. 65.6%) and AUC (76.8% vs. 76.5% vs. 77%).

Table 4. Summary of overall performance of all models based on number of classes in the target variable.

Metrics	Multi-class prediction				Binary prediction				p-value
	Mean	SD	Max	Min	Mean	SD	Max	Min	
Accuracy	0.676	0.086	0.753	0.390	0.768	0.049	0.857	0.662	0.0001
Precision	0.651	0.036	0.728	0.595	0.873	0.062	0.963	0.765	0.0001
Recall	0.676	0.086	0.753	0.390	0.683	0.092	0.795	0.487	0.8081
F1 Score	0.650	0.057	0.707	0.465	0.761	0.062	0.850	0.629	0.0001
AUC	0.768	0.052	0.875	0.670	0.843	0.051	0.916	0.719	0.0001

However, there was no statistically significant difference in models' performance in terms of all metrics.

Table 5. Summary of the overall performance of all models in predicting multi-class treatment response based on different sets of features.

	All features				Without weakly correlated				With moderately-to-strongly correlated				p-value
	Mean	SD	Max	Min	Mean	SD	Max	Min	Mean	SD	Max	Min	
Accuracy	0.662	0.074	0.727	0.519	0.647	0.123	0.753	0.390	0.720	0.024	0.753	0.701	0.261
Precision	0.656	0.043	0.728	0.595	0.641	0.043	0.707	0.595	0.657	0.020	0.683	0.630	0.678
Recall	0.662	0.074	0.727	0.519	0.647	0.123	0.753	0.390	0.720	0.024	0.753	0.701	0.261
F1 Score	0.643	0.044	0.694	0.578	0.622	0.080	0.705	0.465	0.685	0.013	0.707	0.666	0.106
AUC	0.770	0.052	0.859	0.687	0.765	0.059	0.858	0.670	0.768	0.053	0.875	0.728	0.984

As exhibited in Table 6, our AI models generally showed superior performance in predicting a binary treatment response when utilizing moderately-to-strongly correlated features compared to scenarios involving all features, either with or without weakly correlated features. This superiority was evident in terms of accuracy (78.6% compared to 77.7% and 74.2%), recall (73.4% compared to 65.9% and 65.6%), and F1 score (79.7% compared to 74.6% and 74%). On the other hand, their performance showed similarity in precision (87.5% compared to 87.8% and 86.6%) and AUC (84.3% compared to 83.7% and 84.8%). However, there was no statistically significant difference in models' performance in terms of all metrics.

Table 6. Summary of the overall performance of all models in predicting binary treatment response based on different sets of features.

	All features				Without weakly correlated				With moderately-to-strongly correlated				p-value
	Mean	SD	Max	Min	Mean	SD	Max	Min	Mean	SD	Max	Min	
Accuracy	0.742	0.054	0.805	0.662	0.777	0.049	0.857	0.727	0.786	0.037	0.844	0.727	0.207
Precision	0.866	0.068	0.963	0.780	0.878	0.072	0.958	0.765	0.875	0.053	0.944	0.811	0.943
Recall	0.656	0.108	0.773	0.500	0.659	0.105	0.795	0.487	0.734	0.034	0.773	0.682	0.207
F1 Score	0.740	0.070	0.810	0.629	0.746	0.069	0.849	0.644	0.797	0.033	0.850	0.741	0.175
AUC	0.848	0.066	0.916	0.731	0.837	0.059	0.887	0.719	0.843	0.029	0.886	0.808	0.925

4 Discussion

4.1 Principal Findings

This study aimed to examine the performance of AI in predicting the treatment response among patients with well-differentiated thyroid cancer. Our experiments showed that AI has an acceptable performance in predicting the response of thyroid cancer treatment, but it is not optimal. Notably, the Multi-layer Perceptron exhibited superior performance in accuracy, recall, and F1 score whereas Naive Bayes emerged as the top-performing model in terms of precision and AUC. Further, this study showed that our AI models had superior performance in predicting a binary treatment response compared to predicting multi-class treatment responses. In this study, the performance of our AI models in predicting a binary or multi-class treatment response using moderately-to-strongly correlated features was higher than using all features without weakly correlated features or all features, however, this difference in performance was not statistically significant in terms of all metrics.

Our findings align closely with the findings reported in Sa et al.'s study [13]. To elaborate, Sa et al. investigated the performance of six algorithms (Logistic Regression, Support Vector Machine, Random Forest, Neural Networks, Adaptive Boosting, and Gradient Boost) in predicting responses (effective response vs. non-effective response) to radioiodine therapy and thyrotropin (TSH) suppression therapy in patients with differentiated thyroid cancer but without structural disease, based on pre-treatment information [13]. The study showed that Random Forest outperformed other models in predicting responses to radioiodine therapy (accuracy of 81.3%, sensitivity of 79.5%, and AUC of 0.896) and thyrotropin (TSH) suppression therapy (accuracy of 78.7%, sensitivity of 79.7%, and AUC of 0.857).

However, the AI models in our research demonstrated superior predictive capabilities in predicting treatment response compared to the findings presented in Grani et al.'s study [11]. Specifically, Grani et al.'s [11] study assessed the effectiveness of 2 decision tree models to predict treatment response among patients with differentiated thyroid cancer. The highest sensitivity achieved by the decision tree models was 49%. This inconsistency in results may be attributed to several factors: (1) this study used decision trees as the sole AI model, (2) the follow-up period was shorter (< 7 years) than the follow-up period in the data used in our study, (3) several features were not used in their models such as smoking status, history of radiation therapy, presence of goiter, presence of adenopathy, and risk assessment according to ATA guidelines.

4.2 Practical and Research Implications

Considering that our models did not achieve optimal performance in predicting the response to thyroid cancer treatment, healthcare providers should not rely exclusively on our models for treatment response predictions. Instead, they should utilize our models in combination with other tools and approaches until further studies show optimal performance of the AI models. Our research indicates that there is still potential for enhancing AI's ability to predict treatment responses. As a result, future investigations should focus on refining this predictive capability by incorporating additional features not considered in our study, such as body mass index, tumor size, Thyroglobulin level, family history of thyroid cancer, radioiodine uptake (RAIU%), surgical approach, surgical margins, presurgical cytology, and number of removed lymph nodes. Moreover, exploring alternative models like Adaptive Boosting, Gradient Boost, and Deep Neural Networks, as well as employing larger and more balanced datasets, could contribute to improved predictions. Additionally, it is imperative for future studies to use other validation techniques (e.g., k-fold cross-validation and leave-one-out cross-validation) when splitting a dataset, especially when the dataset size is small. Furthermore, researchers should assess the performance of AI models in predicting responses to various types of thyroid cancer treatments, including total thyroidectomy, partial thyroidectomy (thyroid lobectomy), and thyroidectomy plus Radioactive Iodine Therapy. Prioritizing the prediction of multi-class treatment responses is also essential, given its greater clinical significance compared to predicting binary responses.

4.3 Limitations

Despite the significance of this study, several noteworthy limitations should be acknowledged. Firstly, the generalizability of our models to datasets beyond our specific dataset is uncertain because external validation was impossible due to the absence of comparable data from other institutions. Secondly, the internal validation dataset closely mirrors the training dataset, raising the possibility of potential model overfitting. Thirdly, the study used only a training-test split method for dividing the dataset, instead of employing alternative techniques like K-fold cross-validation. Fourthly, the limited size of the dataset constrained the development of more advanced deep learning techniques. Lastly, this paper cannot provide insights into the performance of AI in predicting the response of specific thyroid cancer treatments, as the dataset lacked information on the types of treatments administered.

5 Conclusion

While AI demonstrates satisfactory performance in predicting the response to thyroid cancer treatment, there remains room for optimization. Notably, our AI models used for predicting binary treatment responses outperformed AI models used for predicting multi-class treatment responses. The highest accuracy, recall, and F1 score in all experiments were achieved by Multi-layer Perceptron when it was used for predicting binary treatment response using all features, excluding those weakly correlated with the treatment response. However, the highest precision and AUC across all experiments were attained when using Naive Bayes for predicting binary treatment response using all features.

While our models fell short of optimal performance in predicting thyroid cancer treatment response, it is crucial for healthcare providers to consider these tools as part of a broader diagnostic and decision-making framework rather than as standalone solutions. The integration of model insights with clinical expertise ensures a more comprehensive approach to patient care and treatment. Combining our models with other tools is recommended until further studies establish their optimal performance. Future research should enhance predictive capabilities by including additional features, exploring alternative models, and utilizing larger and balanced datasets. Validation techniques like k-fold and leave-one-out cross-validation are crucial, especially with small datasets. Evaluating AI models across various thyroid cancer treatments and prioritizing multi-class responses remains imperative for comprehensive clinical insights.

Disclosure of Interests. The authors have no competing interests to declare that are relevant to the content of this article.

Appendix. The appendix can be accessed through the following link: https://github.com/DrA laaalzoubi/Artificial-Intelligence-for-Predicting-Responses-to-Thyroid-Cancer-Treatment/tree/main.

References

1. Nguyen, Q.T., Lee, E.J., Huang, M.G., Park, Y.I., Khullar, A., Plodkowski, R.A.: Diagnosis and treatment of patients with thyroid cancer. Am. Health Drug Benefits **8**(1), 30–40 (2015). PMID: 25964831
2. Pizzato, M., Li, M., Vignat, J., Laversanne, M., Singh, D., La Vecchia, C., et al.: The epidemiological landscape of thyroid cancer worldwide: GLOBOCAN estimates for incidence and mortality rates in 2020. The Lancet Diabetes & Endocrinology. 2022 2022/04/01/, 10(4), 264–72. https://doi.org/10.1016/S2213-8587(22)00035-3
3. Haugen, B.R., Alexander, E.K., Bible, K.C., Doherty, G.M., Mandel, S.J., Nikiforov, Y.E., et al.: 2015 American Thyroid Association Management Guidelines for Adult Patients with Thyroid Nodules and Differentiated Thyroid Cancer: The American Thyroid Association Guidelines Task Force on Thyroid Nodules and Differentiated Thyroid Cancer. Thyroid : official journal of the American Thyroid Association. 2016 Jan, 26(1):1–133. PMID: 26462967. https://doi.org/10.1089/thy.2015.0020
4. Ma, X., Xi, B., Zhang, Y., Zhu, L., Sui, X., Tian, G., et al.: A machine learning-based diagnosis of thyroid cancer using thyroid nodules ultrasound images. Current Bioinform. **15**(4), 349–58 (2020). https://doi.org/10.2174/1574893614666191017091959
5. Bellantuono, L., Tommasi, R., Pantaleo, E., Verri, M., Amoroso, N., Crucitti, P., et al.: An eXplainable Artificial Intelligence analysis of Raman spectra for thyroid cancer diagnosis. Sci. Rep. **13**(1), 16590 (2023). https://doi.org/10.1038/s41598-023-43856-7
6. Zhu, Y.-C., Du, H., Jiang, Q., Zhang, T., Huang, X.-J., Zhang, Y., et al.: Machine Learning Assisted Doppler Features for Enhancing Thyroid Cancer Diagnosis. **41**(8), 1961–1974 (2022). https://doi.org/10.1002/jum.15873

7. Borzooei, S., Briganti, G., Golparian, M., Lechien, J.R., Tarokhian, A.: Machine learning for risk stratification of thyroid cancer patients: a 15-year cohort study. European archives of oto-rhino-laryngology : official journal of the European Federation of Oto-Rhino-Laryngological Societies (EUFOS): affiliated with the German Society for Oto-Rhino-Laryngology - Head and Neck Surgery. 2023 Oct 30. PMID: 37902840. https://doi.org/10.1007/s00405-023-082 99-w

8. Park, Y.M., Lee, B.-J.: Machine learning-based prediction model using clinico-pathologic factors for papillary thyroid carcinoma recurrence. Sci. Rep. **11**(1), 4948 (2021). https://doi.org/10.1038/s41598-021-84504-2

9. Kil, J., Kim, K.G., Kim, Y.J., Koo, H.R., Park, J.S.: Deep learning in thyroid ultrasonography to predict tumor recurrence in thyroid cancers. Taehan Yongsang Uihakhoe chi. **81**(5):1164–74. PMID, 36238043 (2020). https://doi.org/10.3348/jksr.2019.0147

10. Li, Y., Wu, F., Ge, W., Zhang, Y., Hu, Y., Zhao, L., et al.: Risk stratification of papillary thyroid cancers using multidimensional machine learning. Int. J. Surg. **110**(1) (2024)

11. Grani, G., Gentili, M., Siciliano, F., Albano, D., Zilioli, V., Morelli, S., et al.: A data-driven approach to refine predictions of differentiated thyroid cancer outcomes: a prospective multicenter study. J. Clin. Endocrinol. Metabolism **108**(8), 1921–8 (2023). PMID: 36795619. https://doi.org/10.1210/clinem/dgad075

12. Lubin, D.J., Tsetse, C., Khorasani, M.S., Allahyari, M., McGrath, M.: Clinical predictors of I-131 therapy failure in differentiated thyroid cancer by machine learning: a single-center experience. World J. Nuclear Med. **20**(3), 253–9 (2021). PMID: 34703393. https://doi.org/10.4103/wjnm.WJNM_104_20

13. Sa, R., Yang, T., Zhang, Z., Guan, F.: Random Forest for Predicting Treatment Response to Radioiodine and Thyrotropin Suppression Therapy in Patients With Differentiated Thyroid Cancer But Without Structural Disease. The Oncologist **29**(1), e68-e80. PMID: 37669005 (2024). https://doi.org/10.1093/oncolo/oyad252

14. Borzooei, S., Tarokhian, A.: Differentiated Thyroid Cancer Recurrence. 2023, 09 Mar 2023. https://archive.ics.uci.edu/dataset/915/differentiated+thyroid+cancer+recurrence

Patient Data, Privacy and Ethics

ZMAM: A ZKP-Based Mutual Authentication Scheme for the IoMT

Chaoyue Lv[1], Di Lu[1](✉), Yuanyuan Zhang[2](✉), Xindi Ma[3],
Yulong Shen[1], Liping Wang[2], and Jianfeng Ma[3]

[1] School of Computer Science and Technology, Xidian University, Shaanxi, China
tsunaley@stu.xidian.edu.cn, dlu@xidian.edu.cn
[2] Honghui Hospital, Xi'an Jiaotong University, Shaanxi, China
zhangyuanyuan_8811@126.com
[3] School of Cyber Engineering, Xidian University, Shaanxi, China

Abstract. In the era of smart healthcare, the Internet of Medical Things (IoMT) ubiquitously collects, evaluates, monitors, and prescribes treatments for patients. Despite its significant benefits, IoMT faces substantial risks related to unauthorized access to confidential medical information, largely due to the vulnerability of wireless communication channels. Furthermore, IoMT devices are constrained by limitations in computation, energy, and storage, which hinder the implementation of complex authentication protocols. To address these challenges, we propose a novel IoMT authentication scheme called ZMAM, which is based on zero-knowledge proof for mutual authentication between IoMT sensors and gateway servers. ZMAM ensures device integrity, confidentiality, and protection from cyber threats while minimizing computational and communication resource consumption.

Keywords: Internet of Medical Things · Mutual Authentication · Zero Knowledge Proof

1 Introduction

The Internet of Medical Things (IoMT) merges medical devices with the Internet of Things (IoT), which allows doctors, care providers, and patients to collect and exchange health data electronically and perform remote treatment, such as insulin pumps and smartwatches. The current IoMT architecture, as depicted in Fig. 1, consists of four layers [7], the sensor layer, gateway layer, cloud layer, and visualization layer.

However, open wireless networks, complex functions, and lack of suitable authentication schemes have increased cyberattack vulnerabilities. In 2019, the U.S. FDA warned patients and healthcare providers that certain Medtronic MiniMed insulin pumps were being recalled due to cybersecurity risks, allowing unauthorized users to potentially connect wirelessly and change settings [18]. Since treatment plans depend on patients' physiological data measured by IoMT, ensuring device authenticity is crucial. However, traditional authentication schemes are unsuitable for communicating between the sensor and gateway

X. Xie et al. (Eds.): AIiH 2024, LNCS 14976, pp. 263–278, 2024.
https://doi.org/10.1007/978-3-031-67285-9_19

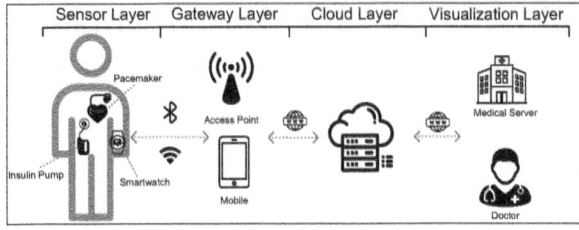

Fig. 1. IoMT architecture.

layers due to the limited energy, computational, and storage resources of sensor-layer devices.

We assume that the device's integrity is the premise of ensuring device authenticity. Thus, the data generated or processed by the device can be trusted only when the device is free of being tampered with.

However, achieving integrity protection for IoMT devices still faces some challenges: 1)Due to the resource limitations of IoMT devices, a lightweight authentication scheme is required to meet real-time requirements. 2)For specific medical devices like pacemakers and insulin pumps, it is vital to provide an emergency and secure access method to the devices when patients are in emergencies or in an unfamiliar environment. 3)Since IoMT devices typically operate in an open network environment, they are at risk of tampering from inevitable cyberattacks and need robust integrity assurance.

To meet the growing secure demands of IoMT while ensuring authenticity and real-time requirements, we have proposed ZMAM (**Z**ero-knowledge proof-based **M**utual **A**uthentication scheme for the Io**MT**), a scheme based on the zero-knowledge proof and device measurement values to ensure the device's integrity and authentication of IoMT devices between the sensor layer and gateway layer. The contributions of the paper are summarized as follows:

- Firstly, we have designed a mutual authentication scheme for IoMT based on zero-knowledge proof (ZKP) and elliptic curve cryptography (ECC) named ZMAM, including "registration protocol (RP)," "Normal Communication Protocol (NCP)," and "Communication in Emergency Protocol (CEP)". Both communication protocols mutually authenticate the device's identity. Moreover, they ensure that attackers cannot infer any information related to the device's identity during the whole mutual authentication process.
- Secondly, NCP mutually verifies device integrity and authenticates its identity. Considering people's mobility, it contains a reconnect phase based on the last session key, significantly reducing the reconnect delay. In CEP, the trusted third party verifies the gateway device identity and distributes a temporary shared key for a fast connection in an emergency.
- Finally, we have implemented ZMAM on ultra-low-power microcontrollers (STM32L475) and Raspberry Pi, evaluated and investigated ZMAM's robustness against cyberattacks through formal and informal analysis. Additionally, we compared ZMAM's performance with typical security protocols.

The remainder of this article is structured as follows: Sect. 2 reviews the related work, while Sect. 3 covers the background, threat model and assumptions. Section 4 demonstrates the proposed scheme, followed by the security analysis in Sect. 5. Performance and comparative analysis are discussed in Sect. 6. Finally, we conclude this article in Sect. 7.

2   Related Work

Several authentication schemes have been proposed to safeguard IoMT privacy, including non-cryptographic, cryptographic, blockchain-based, and physical unclonable function (PUF) methods. However, many suffer from limitations.

Non-cryptographic authentication methods typically rely on physiological features [3,10] and channel characteristics [24]. In the first scheme, devices share a symmetric key using simultaneously measured physiological features like electrocardiogram (ECG) values [3]. However, these methods often have a high rate of false alarms because it is difficult for two devices to generate physiological features with the same accuracy, and some devices cannot collect physiological data [13]. In [24], Zhang et al. utilize a channel characteristics similarity estimation mechanism to authenticate legitimate sensors, but these schemes often require advanced hardware or an extensive feature learning phase [17].

Cryptographic-based schemes use pre-shared keys, encryption, and decryption algorithms to prevent unauthorized access. Wazid et al. [21] introduced a three-factor remote user authentication protocol using ECC for implantable medical devices. Vijayakumar et al. [19] proposed an anonymous authentication framework that allows mutual authentication between doctors and patients. However, these schemes cannot mutually verify device integrity and prevent physical attacks. In the event of device compromise, remote devices remain unaware if the device they are communicating with has been compromised.

Blockchains, which are distributed ledgers with securely linked records, have also been explored for IoMT authentication. Miao et al. [15] proposed a privacy-protection authentication management protocol for communication between users and medical sensor nodes based on blockchains. In [6], Garg et al. proposed a blockchain-based authentication and key management scheme for the IoMT environment, which also considered the private blockchain in the design. However, these schemes still cannot determine if the device has been tampered with.

Physical unclonable function (PUF) relies on the uniqueness of unpredictable physical factors introduced during manufacturing. These integrated circuit (IC) features ensure that any system alteration will change the PUF output. PUF-based authentication schemes can ensure the physical security and integrity of the devices [23]. However, PUF-based protocols are vulnerable to modeling attacks, such as approximation attacks [14].

3   Background, Threat Model and Assumptions

3.1   Background: Zero-Knowledge Proof, Trusted Boot

Zero-knowledge proof [8] is an agreement involving two parties. One party (the prover) can prove to another party (the verifier) that a given statement is true while avoiding conveying any information beyond the mere fact of the statement's truth to the verifier. The zero-knowledge proof protocol is considered secure if it follows three characteristics.

- Completeness: if the prover's statement is true, the verifier will be convinced of this fact by the prover.
- Soundness: if the prover's statement is false, it is nearly impossible for a cheating prover to convince the verifier that it is true.
- Zero-knowledge: if the statement is true, no verifier learns anything other than the fact that the statement is true. In other words, the verifier can learn nothing from the proof except the statement is true.

Trusted Boot verifies each stage of the boot process to ensure that only trusted software is loaded. It relies on digital signatures as measurement values to verify the integrity and authenticity of the boot components. Trusted boot security is ensured by trusted components such as the trusted platform module (TPM) and trusted execution environment (TEE). For resource-constrained devices, the memory protection unit (MPU) provides memory protection, which can implement lightweight access control by dividing physical memory into regions and setting permissions on these regions. In [2] and [9], they achieved the MPU-based security architecture for tiny embedded devices, which can provide lightweight trusted boot.

3.2   Threat Model and Assumption

In this paper, we consider the DY-adversary model [4] as our threat model, in which communication between entities is conducted over insecure channels. The attacker has complete control over the public channel, enabling them to intercept, tamper with, forge, or inject malicious code into messages to launch attacks and gain unauthorized access to the system. Additionally, the attacker can also gain permission to access memory to steal critical data or interfere with code execution.

We assume that cryptographic primitives are well-secured and cannot be corrupted by the adversary's computational power. Additionally, we assume that the trusted third party is trusted and tamper-proof. The integrity of the entities in the scheme is guaranteed by the trusted computing base (TCB), such as the MPU. We also assume that communication with the trusted third party during entity registration is secure.

4   ZMAM Scheme Design

ZMAM scheme is composed of three primary protocols, "Registration Protocol (RP)," "Normal Communication Protocol (NCP)," and "Communication in Emergency Protocol (CEP)," which handle communication between the sensor and gateway layers under different situations. In the following sections, the design of the three protocols will be elaborated in detail. Table 1 lists the notations used in scheme descriptions.

Table 1. Notations used in scheme descriptions.

Notations	Descriptions	Notations	Descriptions
MV	The measurement values	H	Hash function
p_i, h, ω	Hash values	P_i, X, G, N	Point on eliptic curve
ID_i	Nodes identity	σ	Sent message
r, n	Random number	$\|$	Concatenation
sk, pk	Private key, public key	z, m, c	Computation result
s	Signature	K	key
Enc, Dec	Asymmetric encrypt, decrypt	$Sign$	Public key signature

4.1   System Components

The typical IoMT application scenario in our research work can be abstracted as Fig. 2, which includes a Trusted Authority (TA), Gateway Server (GS), and Medical Sensor Node (MSN).

- TA: TA performs as a trusted third party that initializes and registers the communication entities. It is responsible for generating and managing cryptographic parameters, and performing certification and pre-calculations.
- MSN: MSN continuously monitors physiological data and provides necessary treatments.
- GS: GS sends the collected data to the cloud for further analysis by doctors and other professionals. Additionally, it controls MSNs based on doctors' advice to conduct treatments.

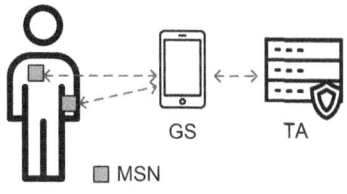

Fig. 2. Typical IoMT application scenario.

4.2   Security Goals

To eliminate the threats during the authentication in IoMT, we design an authentication scheme to satisfy the following security goals (**SG**):

- Mutual authentication (**SG$_1$**): The participants should verify the authenticity and integrity of each other's identities.
- Defense against various attacks: The scheme can resist various typical attacks, such as man-in-the-middle attacks (**SG$_2$**), replay attacks (**SG$_3$**), modification and impersonation (**SG$_4$**). Additionally, the IoMT should quickly identify DoS attacks targeting energy consumption (**SG$_5$**) and resistant to physical attacks (**SG$_6$**).
- Forward security (**SG$_7$**): Attackers cannot obtain any useful information about the previous session from the information about the current session.
- Unlinkability(**SG$_8$**): The attacker cannot identify or link the MSN even if the GS is compromised or the wireless channel is controlled.
- Anonymity (**SG$_9$**) and traceability (**SG$_{10}$**): The real identity is kept secret during the entire authentication procedure. Attackers cannot infer any relevant information about IoMT's real identity. If the MSN has been compromised, the TA can trace its identity.

4.3   Registration Protocol (RP)

The registration protocol (RP) is the premise of NCP and CEP, which initializes and sends the parameters for zero-knowledge proof and the keys used in the subsequent protocols. It includes two phases, the GS registration phase and the MSN registration phase, which are discussed below:

1. The GS initially registers the device at the TA, as depicted in Fig. 3(a). Using its measurement value MV_{GS} and a random number r, the GS computes $p_{GS} = H(MV_{GS}||r)$, then calculates $P_{GS} = p_{GS}G$ for ZKP and sends its ID and P_{GS} to the TA. The TA stores this data and sends back its public key.
2. Figure 3(b) shows the registration of the MSN. Like the GS's registration, the MSN uses its measurement value and a random number to compute p_{MSN} and P_{MSN}, then sends its ID and P_{MSN} to the TA. The TA stores the data and generates K_{MSN}, which will be sent back to the MSN as a shared key.

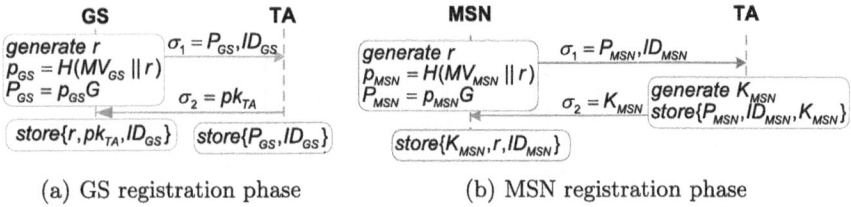

(a) GS registration phase   (b) MSN registration phase

Fig. 3. Registration protocol.

4.4 Normal Communication Protocol

The Normal Communication Protocol (NCP) is designed for routine situations. This protocol is initiated when the MSN needs to exchange information with the GS, which the MSN and the GS mutually verify their identity and establish a shared key. Firstly, the TA verifies the GS's integrity through ZKP and generates a certification for the MSN to authenticate the GS. Then, the MSN authenticates the GS using the certification, and the GS verifies the MSN's integrity through ZKP. Figure 4 shows the complete validation process, which is discussed below:

1. The MSN generates a random number, n_1, and sends it along with its ID to the GS. The GS sends its ID and the MSN's ID to the TA. The TA generates a random number, r, and sends it back to the GS.
2. The GS generates two random values, n_2 and x, and computes $N_2 = n_2 G$ and $X = xG$. It uses the hash function to compute $h_1 = H(r||N_2||P_{GS}||X)$ and $z_1 = n_2 - h_1 p_{GS}$, forming the message $\{h_1, z_1, X, n_1\}$ and transports to the TA.
3. Upon receiving the message from the GS, the TA evaluates the authenticity of the GS by computing:

$$N_2' = z_1 G + h_1 P_{GS} = (n_2 - h_1 p_{GS})G + h_1(p_{GS}G) = n_2 G = N_2$$

Then, the TA computes the same hash value h_2, and compares it with h_1. This process proves that the GS possesses the secret value p_{GS} and will not disclose it to the TA.
4. After validating the authenticity of the GS, the TA computes:

$$\omega = H(K_{MSN}||n_1||ID_{MSN}||ID_{GS}||X)$$

for the MSN to check the GS's authenticity. Then it computes:

$$h_3 = H(\omega||X||ID_{MSN}||ID_{GS}||P_{MSN})$$

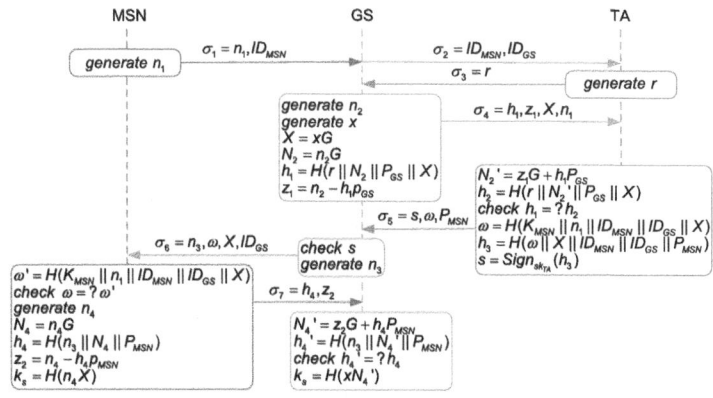

Fig. 4. Normal Communication Protocol (NCP).

$$s = Sign_{sk_{TA}}(h_3)$$

The TA sends $\{s, \omega, P_{MSN}\}$ to the GS.

5. The GS checks the sign and generates a random value n_3. Finally, the GS sends $\{n_3, \omega, X, ID_{GS}\}$ to the MSN.

6. The MSN checks ω to verify the GS's authenticity. Then, it generates a random value n_4 and computes $N_4 = n_4 G$, $h_4 = H(n_3||N_4||P_{MSN})$ and $z_2 = n_4 - h_4 p_{MSN}$. Then, it computes the symmetric key $K_s = H(n_4 X)$. The MSN sends $\{h_4, z_2\}$ back to the GS.

7. The GS computes and checks the h_4, and then computes the symmetric key $k_s = H(x N_4)$ for symmetric encrypt.

ZKP has enabled the GS and the MSN to prove they have correct measurement values without revealing any secret information over the vulnerable wireless channel, thus assuring privacy and resistance to cyber-attacks.

The Fast Reconnect Phase, which complements NCP, is designed for rapid reconnection and symmetric key update in case of disconnection between the MSN and the GS due to people's mobility. This phase enables the reuse of the last session key k_s, facilitating a quick restart without needing another complete authentication procedure. The steps of the fast reconnect procedure are shown in Fig. 5.

1. The MSN generates a random number n, and sends n to the GS. The new session key is $k'_s = H(k_s||n||ID_{MSN}||ID_{GS})$.

2. The GS computes the new session key k'_s using the same method.

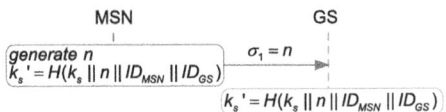

Fig. 5. Fast reconnect phase.

4.5 Communication in Emergency Protocol

As mentioned above, some IoMT devices used for remote treatments, interventional therapy, and vital signs monitoring require emergency access to deal with extraordinary cases. For example, a pacemaker suddenly malfunctions in an unfamiliar environment and requires immediate checking and repair, or a medical staff member urgently needs to access the IoMT device within an unconscious patient [25]. In such cases, the IoMT devices immediately switch to emergency mode by analyzing patient physiological data or by being manually triggered by healthcare professionals close to the patient in order to support secure and fast access via the communication in emergency protocol (CEP), whose process is given in Fig. 6.

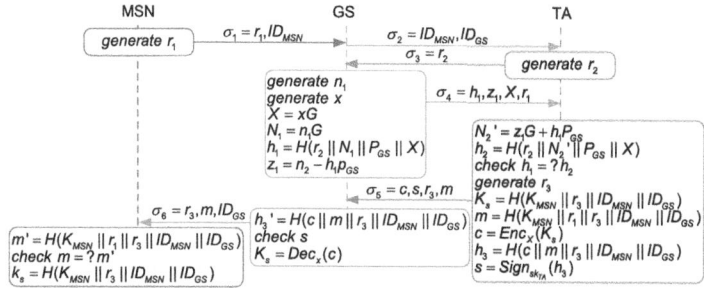

Fig. 6. Communication in Emergency Protocol (CEP).

In the CEP, for rapid connections, the TA generates the symmetric key after it verifies the GS's identity, which may increase the burden on the TA. However, this situation is expected to occur infrequently. The GS forgoes integrity verification for faster emergency access because patients are typically in hospitals with medical personnel during emergencies, and it becomes challenging for attackers to tamper with the devices. The steps of CEP are as follows:

1. Similar to the NCP, the MSN generates a random number for the GS, and then the GS proves its authenticity to the TA.
2. After validating the GS, the TA generates a random value r_3 and computes the symmetric key: $k_s = H(K_{MSN}||r_3||ID_{MSN}||ID_{GS})$ for the GS and the MSN. The TA computes $m = H(K_{MSN}||r_1||r_3||ID_{MSN}||ID_{GS})$ for the MSN to check the GS's authenticity, then encrypts k_s with X. And it computes $h_3 = H(c||m||r_3||ID_{MSN}||ID_{GS})$, signs h_3 and sends c, s, r_3, m to the GS.
3. The GS computes h_3' and checks s, then decrypts the k_s.
4. The MSN checks m and computes $k_s = H(K_{MSN}||r_3||ID_{MSN}||ID_{GS})$ for symmetric encrypt.

In this protocol, the GS and the TA perform the most computationally intensive tasks, while the MSN only calculates the hash function, which is faster.

5 Security Analysis

5.1 Formal Analysis

This section demonstrates the robustness of the presented scheme against various attacks such as replay, MITM, modification, etc. Verification was conducted using the automated tool ProVerif [1], which supports major cryptographic primitives. If an attack is identified, Proverif lists the steps for the attacker to violate the desired security feature. ProVerif has been widely used in recent literature to formally verify the security of cryptographic protocols [11,16,22].

A ProVerif model of a protocol, written in the typed pi-calculus, typically consists of three main parts: declarations, process macros, and the main process. Declarations formalize the behavior of cryptographic primitives, such as hash functions, zero-knowledge proof, public key signatures, etc. Process macros define sub-processes, specifying the behavior of entities like the MSN, the GS, and the TA. The main process utilizes these process macros to encode the entire protocol.

To verify the protocol's security property, we define four events:

- *begin_A_event*: Both the MSN and the GS have their own begin event, written in B's process macros, which signifies that entity B is started by entity A.
- *end_A_event*: The MSN and the GS both have their own end event, written in A's process macros, which signifies that entity A has completed its role in the protocol.

We conducted the tests to validate the security features offered by the ZMAM scheme. The output is shown in Fig. 7. Assume that the private key of GS (*secret_skGS*), the measurement value of nodes (*secret_mv_MSN* and *secret_mv_GS*) and all the symmetric key (*secret_KMNS* and *secret_Ks*) are securely stored locally on the devices. The output of the ProVerif provides as follows:

1. *not attacker(elem)*: Which means that the attacker cannot know the value *elem*.
2. *inj-event(end_A_event)* ==>*inj-event(begin_A_event)*: This expression checks whether the execution of event *begin_A_event* has occurred before the execution of event *end_A_event*. If *begin_A_event* has been executed prior to *end_A_event*, the expression evaluates to true; otherwise, it evaluates to false. This expression ensures the mutual authentication property, preventing an attacker from impersonating entities. Suppose the attacker impersonates B to communicate with A. The actual entity B fails to execute *begin_A_event*. Consequently, if entity A attempts to end with *end_A_event*, the expression evaluates to false, indicating a breach in mutual authentication.

As shown in Fig. 7, we observe the following: 1)The MSN and the GS can mutually verify each other, and the scheme demonstrates resilience against typical attacks such as MITM, replay, modification, and impersonation attacks. 2)The attacker cannot access all the secret values. The positive output verifies that the two devices, GS and MSN, are mutually authenticated, and the protocol is against typical attacks according to the DY-adversary model.

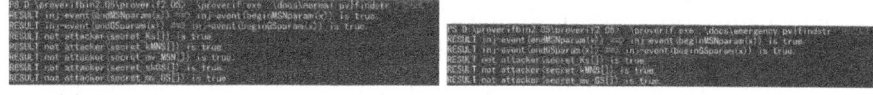

(a) Security verification of NCP.   (b) Security verification of CEP.

Fig. 7. Screenshots of the output provided by the ProVerif automatic tool.

5.2   Informal Analysis

This section uses the security fundamentals and logical reasoning to evaluate the strength of the ZMAM against malicious threats.

Prevention from MITM, Modification and Impersonation Attacks: In ZMAM, intercepted messages do not reveal any identity details or secret information. Moreover, each step of the scheme verifies the authenticity of the involved entities and checks the signatures. Consequently, the scheme eliminates opportunities for adversaries to carry out these attacks successfully.

Resistant to Replay Attacks: If the attacker captures and replays a message, such as σ_4 in NCP, it cannot pass the verification of $h_2 = h_1$ with the old nonce r. This inability to verify the old nonce prevents the attacker from successfully replaying messages. Similarly, other messages are also not susceptible to replay attacks.

Resilient to Physical Attacks: If the adversary physically captures the MSN or the GS for tampering or cloning purposes, their attempts would be thwarted. This is because the MSN and the GS mutually verify their measurement values. If the entity has been tampered with, it will fail to produce the correct measurement value, rendering it unable to prove its legitimacy.

Forward Security and Unlinkability: In ZMAM, the attacker cannot compute previous keys using the current session key due to the properties of the hash function employed. Additionally, the adversary cannot obtain any information about the entities even if another entity is compromised because of ZKP. Thus, ZMAM ensures forward security and unlinkability.

Anonymity and Traceable: Each entity's ID serves as a temporary identity, and the values of P_{MSN} and P_{GS} can be altered by selecting another random number r, thereby ensuring the anonymity of the entities' identities. The TA can utilize K_{MNS} to trace the MSN if it has been tampered with.

Considerations on Energy-depletion Attacks: In ZMAM, the MSN can detect the presence of attacks by computing just one hash function, which does not consume excessive time or computational resources. Subsequently, devices sending malicious requests can be blacklisted to prevent DoS attacks.

6   Experiments and Evaluation

In this section, we evaluate the ZMAM scheme on various parameters, including security attributes and communication expenses, comparing it with those of Gaba's [5], Wan's [20], and Li's [12].

Table 2. Comparison of ZMAM vs. conventional schemes. SG: Security goals, SG_1: Mutul authentication, SG_2: MITM, SG_3: Replay, SG_4: Modification and impersonation, SG_5: DoS, SG_6: Physical attack SG_7: Forward security, SG_8: Unlinkability, SG_9: Anonymity, SG_{10}: Traceability.

SG	SG_1	SG_2	SG_3	SG_4	SG_5	SG_6	SG_7	SG_8	SG_9	SG_{10}
ZMAM	✔	✔	✔	✔	✔	✔	✔	✔	✔	✔
Gaba's [5]	✓	✓	✓	✓	✓	✓	✓	✓	✓	✗
Wan's [20]	✓	✓	✓	✓	✗	✓	✓	✓	✓	✗
Li's [12]	✓	✓	✓	✓	✗	✗	✓	✓	✓	✗

6.1   Security Attributes

Table 2 shows that the proposed scheme is more robust than existing schemes. While Gaba's [5], Wan's [20], Li's [12], and ZMAM can provide anonymity for sensor nodes, but they fail to provide traceability for TA. Furthermore, Wan's [20] and Li's [12] do not protect against Dos attacks, and Li's [12] is vulnerable to physical attack.

6.2   Performance Comparisons

Table 3 lists the computation notions used throughout this section, and Table. 4 illustrates the computation cost spent by different entities in the ZMAM scheme.

We employed the STM32L475 microcontroller, manufactured by STMicroelectronics, as the MSN. This microcontroller is characterized by its low-power design and utilizes the ARM Cortex-M4 core. It has 512 KB of Flash memory for program storage and 128 KB of SRAM for variable and temporary data storage. Additionally, we utilized the Raspberry Pi 4 Model B, equipped with a Broadcom BCM2711 SoC featuring a quad-core ARMv8-A 64-bit processor clocked at 1.5 GHz and 4 GB of RAM, as both the GS and the TA. The test results show in Table 5 that the primary time consumption is scalar-point multiplication in the MSN, requiring 353.98 ms.

Table 3. Computations and descriptions

Notions	Descriptions	Notions	Descriptions
C_M	Scalar-point multiplication	C_H	Hash
C_{AE}	Asymmetric encrypt or decrypt	C_S	Sign
C_{SE}	Symmetric encrypt or decrypt	C_{SC}	Scalar computation
C_R	Generate random number	C_A	Scalar-point addition
cre C_{PUF}	Physical unclonable function		

Table 4. Computation cost of ZMAM. P: Protocol, P1: RP, P2: NCP, P3: NCP reconnection phase, P4: CEP.

P	MSN	GS	TA
P1	$C_H + C_M + C_R$	$C_H + C_M + C_R$	C_R
P2	$3C_H + 2C_M + C_R + C_{SC}$	$2C_H + C_A + 5C_M + 3C_R + C_S + C_{SC}$	$3C_H + C_A + 2C_M + C_R + C_S$
P3	$C_H + C_R$	C_H	
P4	$2C_H + C_R$	$2C_H + 2C_M + 2C_R + C_{AE} + C_S + C_{SC}$	$4C_H + C_A + 2C_M + 2C_R + C_{AE} + C_S$

Table 5. Time consumption of ZMAM. P: Protocol, P1: RP, P2: NCP, P3: NCP reconnection phase, P4: CEP.

P	MSN	GS	TA
P1 (ms)	355.87	1.35	0.0011
P2 (ms)	713.88	9.44	5.39
P3 (ms)	1.88	0.0007	
P4 (ms)	3.78	6.76	8.09

For the convenience of analysis, We primarily focus on the computation of relatively complex: C_M, C_H, C_S, C_{SE}, C_{AE}, and C_{PUF}. To evaluate the communication costs of different schemes, we assume that the entities' ID, hash function outputs, and random numbers are all 160 bits. The subgroup G of ECC is 160 bits, and the element size in G is 320 bits. Additionally, the block size of symmetric cryptography is 128 bits, and timestamps are 32 bits.

Table 6 lists the performance comparisons between the NCP of ZMAM and the schemes proposed in [5,12,20]. ZMAS's efficiency on the MSN node is the same as Li's [12], which involves twice scalar-point multiplication. Gaba's [5] has only one scalar-point multiplication but has extra symmetric encryption and physical unclonable function computations. ZAMA's complex calculations mainly occur in the GS. The GS is rich in computing resources, and these computations are not burdensome.

Table 6. Performance comparisons.

	ZMAM	Gaba's [5]	Wan's [20]	Li's [12]
MSN	$3C_H + 2C_M$	$C_H + C_M + C_{SE} + C_{PUF}$	$14C_H + 3C_M$	$4C_H + 2C_M$
GS	$2C_H + 5C_M + C_S$	$C_H + 2C_M + C_{SE} + C_{PUF}$	$11C_H + 3C_M$	$8C_H + 3C_M$
TA	$3C_H + 2C_M + C_S$	$4C_M + 2C_{SE}$		$7C_H + C_M$

Table 7 compares communication and storage costs. The NCP of ZMAM communication cost is higher than Wan's [20] and Li's [12]. However, in ZMAM, more than half of the communication occurs between the GS and the TA, making the burden on the MSN acceptable. Additionally, the storage overhead of MSN in ZMAM is also lower.

Table 7. Communication and storage cost comparisons.

	ZMAM	Gaba's [5]	Wan's [20]	Li's [12]
Communication cost (bits)	3360	3520	1536	2720
Storage cost (bits)	480	640	960	320

7   Conclusion

This paper proposes a novel mutual authentication and key agreement scheme based on ZKP to secure the IoMT. The scheme achieves essential security features through ZKP, integrity validation, etc. We consider various situations that may arise in IoMT during the scheme design. Security analysis and evaluations demonstrate that the scheme preserves security against typical attacks and provides anonymity and unlinkability. In the future, we aim to further improve the scheme's efficiency and reduce its dependence on trusted third parties.

Acknowledgement. This work was supported by Natural Science Basic Research Program of Shaanxi (Program No. 2024JC-YBMS-745), Key Research and Development Program of Shaanxi (Grant No. 2023-YBSF-206, 2023-ZDLGY-52), the National Natural Science Foundation of China (Grant No. 62372350), Key R&D Program of Shandong Province(Grant No.2023CXPT056), Shenzhen Science and Technology Program(CJGJZD20220517142005013).

References

1. Blanchet, B.: Automatic verification of correspondences for security protocols (2008)
2. Brasser, F., El Mahjoub, B., Sadeghi, A.R., Wachsmann, C., Koeberl, P.: Tytan: tiny trust anchor for tiny devices. In: 2015 52nd ACM/EDAC/IEEE Design Automation Conference (DAC), pp. 1–6 (2015). https://doi.org/10.1145/2744769. 2744922

3. Dodangeh, P., Jahangir, A.H.: A biometric security scheme for wireless body area networks. J. Inform. Secur. Appl. **41**, 62–74 (2018). https://doi.org/10.1016/j.jisa.2018.06.001, https://www.sciencedirect.com/science/article/pii/S2214212617306251X

4. Dolev, D., Yao, A.: On the security of public key protocols. IEEE Trans. Inf. Theory **29**(2), 198–208 (1983)

5. Gaba, G.S., Hedabou, M., Kumar, P., Braeken, A., Liyanage, M., Alazab, M.: Zero knowledge proofs based authenticated key agreement protocol for sustainable healthcare. Sustain. Cities Society **80**, 103766 (2022). https://doi.org/10.1016/j.scs.2022.103766, https://www.sciencedirect.com/science/article/pii/S2210670722000956

6. Garg, N., Wazid, M., Das, A.K., Singh, D.P., Rodrigues, J.J.P.C., Park, Y.: Bakmp-Iomt: design of blockchain enabled authenticated key management protocol for internet of medical things deployment. IEEE Access **8**, 95956–95977 (2020). https://doi.org/10.1109/ACCESS.2020.2995917

7. Ghubaish, A., Salman, T., Zolanvari, M., Unal, D., Al-Ali, A., Jain, R.: Recent advances in the internet-of-medical-things (Iomt) systems security. IEEE Internet Things J. **8**(11), 8707–8718 (2021). https://doi.org/10.1109/JIOT.2020.3045653

8. Goldwasser, S., Micali, S., Rackoff, C.: The knowledge complexity of interactive proof-systems, pp. 203–225. Association for Computing Machinery (Oct 2019). https://doi.org/10.1145/3335741.3335750

9. Koeberl, P., Schulz, S., Sadeghi, A.R., Varadharajan, V.: Trustlite: a security architecture for tiny embedded devices. In: Proceedings of the Ninth European Conference on Computer Systems. EuroSys '14, Association for Computing Machinery, New York, NY, USA (2014). https://doi.org/10.1145/2592798.2592824

10. Koya, A.M., P. P., D.: Anonymous hybrid mutual authentication and key agreement scheme for wireless body area network. Comput. Netw. **140**, 138–151 (2018). https://doi.org/10.1016/j.comnet.2018.05.006, https://www.sciencedirect.com/science/article/pii/S1389128618302044

11. Kumar, D., Grover, H.S.: Adarsh: a secure authentication protocol for wearable devices environment using ECC. J. Inform. Security Appl. **47**, 8–15 (2019). https://doi.org/10.1016/j.jisa.2019.03.008, https://www.sciencedirect.com/science/article/pii/S2214212618303727

12. Li, X., Niu, J., Bhuiyan, M.Z.A., Wu, F., Karuppiah, M., Kumari, S.: A robust ECC-based provable secure authentication protocol with privacy preserving for industrial internet of things. IEEE Trans. Industr. Inf. **14**(8), 3599–3609 (2018). https://doi.org/10.1109/TII.2017.2773666

13. Liu, B., Luo, H., Chen, C.W.: A novel authentication scheme based on acceleration data in wban. In: 2017 IEEE/ACM International Conference on Connected Health: Applications, Systems and Engineering Technologies (CHASE), pp. 120–126 (2017). https://doi.org/10.1109/CHASE.2017.70

14. Mall, P., Amin, R., Das, A.K., Leung, M.T., Choo, K.K.R.: Puf-based authentication and key agreement protocols for Iot, WSNS, and smart grids: a comprehensive survey. IEEE Internet Things J. **9**(11), 8205–8228 (2022). https://doi.org/10.1109/JIOT.2022.3142084

15. Miao, J., Wang, Z., Wu, Z., Ning, X., Tiwari, P.: A blockchain-enabled privacy-preserving authentication management protocol for internet of medical things. Expert Syst. Appl. **237**, 121329 (2024). https://doi.org/10.1016/j.eswa.2023.121329, https://www.sciencedirect.com/science/article/pii/S0957417423018316

16. Tedeschi, P., Sciancalepore, S., Eliyan, A., Di Pietro, R.: Like: lightweight certificateless key agreement for secure Iot communications. IEEE Internet Things J. **7**(1), 621–638 (2020). https://doi.org/10.1109/JIOT.2019.2953549

17. Umar, M., Wu, Z., Liao, X.: Channel characteristics aware zero knowledge proof based authentication scheme in body area networks. Ad Hoc Netw. **112**, 102374 (2021). https://doi.org/10.1016/j.adhoc.2020.102374, https://www.sciencedirect.com/science/article/pii/S1570870520307149

18. U.S. Food and Drug Administration: Fda warns patients and health care providers about potential cybersecurity concerns with certain medtronic insulin pumps (2019).   https://www.fda.gov/news-events/press-announcements/fda-warns-patients-and-health-care-providers-about-potential-cybersecurity-concerns-certain, june 27, 2019

19. Vijayakumar, P., Obaidat, M.S., Azees, M., Islam, S.H., Kumar, N.: Efficient and secure anonymous authentication with location privacy for Iot-based WBANs. IEEE Trans. Industr. Inf. **16**(4), 2603–2611 (2020). https://doi.org/10.1109/TII.2019.2925071

20. Wan, T., Wang, L., Liao, W., Yue, S.: A lightweight continuous authentication scheme for medical wireless body area networks. Peer-to-Peer Network. Appl. **14**(6), 3473–3487 (2021). https://doi.org/10.1007/s12083-021-01190-7

21. Wazid, M., Das, A.K., Kumar, N., Conti, M., Vasilakos, A.V.: A novel authentication and key agreement scheme for implantable medical devices deployment. IEEE J. Biomed. Health Inform. **22**(4), 1299–1309 (2018). https://doi.org/10.1109/JBHI.2017.2721545

22. Xu, Z., Liang, W., Li, K.C., Xu, J., Zomaya, A.Y., Zhang, J.: A time-sensitive token-based anonymous authentication and dynamic group key agreement scheme for industry 5.0. IEEE Trans. Indust. Inform. **18**(10), 7118–7127 (2022). https://doi.org/10.1109/TII.2021.3129631

23. Yanambaka, V.P., Mohanty, S.P., Kougianos, E., Puthal, D.: Pmsec: physical unclonable function-based robust and lightweight authentication in the internet of medical things. IEEE Trans. Consum. Electron. **65**(3), 388–397 (2019). https://doi.org/10.1109/TCE.2019.2926192

24. Zhang, P., Ma, J.: Channel characteristic aware privacy protection mechanism in WBAN. Sensors **18**(8), 2403 (2018). https://doi.org/10.3390/s18082403

25. Zheng, G., Shankaran, R., Orgun, M.A., Qiao, L., Saleem, K.: Ideas and challenges for securing wireless implantable medical devices: a review. IEEE Sens. J. **17**(3), 562–576 (2017). https://doi.org/10.1109/JSEN.2016.2633973

Demystifying the Ethical Framework for Generative AI in Healthcare: A Data Science Perspective

R. Vani Lakshmi[1]([✉]) [iD], Rahul Sheshan Clare[2] [iD], and Asha Kamath[1] [iD]

[1] Department of Data Science, Prasanna School of Public Health, Manipal Academy of Higher Education, Manipal 576 104, India
vani.lakshmi@manipal.edu
[2] Centre for Digital Health, Applied Research and Technology, Manipal Academy of Higher Education, Manipal 576 104, India
rahul.clare@manipal.edu

Abstract. Generative Artificial Intelligence, also known as Generative AI has enhanced the capabilities of what is known to be AI to the world by its capability to generate text, image, or other forms of media through the extensive use of Large Language Models (LLMs). While the roots of LLM can be traced back to the Markovian theories proposed in 1906, Generative AI is the outcome of advancements in transformer-based deep neural networks which extend the machine learning paradigm. Fundamentally, there is a definitive need to store, manage, and use data to generate data that matches consumer needs. Generative AI-based tools today free users from the need to master programming language. This has paved the way for easy access to data generation, analytics, and subsequent dissemination of findings as per the consumer's needs, often with or without a subscription fee. The ethical frameworks of AI are built on the four key principles, namely, beneficence, non-maleficence, autonomy, and justice. In recent years, explicability, which incorporates intelligibility and accountability, was added as the fifth crucial principle in the framework. The use of AI by organizations have also led to reputational, regulatory, and legal risks, resulting in widespread discussions on Ethical AI or the ethical use of AI.

In India, the Indian Council of Medical Research (ICMR, India) has released guidelines for the Ethical Use of AI in Healthcare. Protecting data privacy at the individual (or citizen) level has been one of the crucial challenges in the healthcare sector. With the advent of Generative AI, these challenges have also experienced a multiplicative effect. In addition, the post-COVID-19 era has led to increased use of digital health technologies, fueling data privacy and security risks apart from misinformation (leading to infodemics) and bias. Such concerns often affect developing countries, especially in the healthcare sector.

The present research provides a state-of-the-art review of the ethical frameworks for Generative AI in healthcare. The study also provides an overview of privacy-preserving Generative AI paradigms, enabling the policy-makers (government, private, and other not-for-profit entities) to plan, propose, and disseminate policies that preserve the privacy of the data shared at an individual level. The study will benefit researchers by developing methodologies that align with the

X. Xie et al. (Eds.): AIiH 2024, LNCS 14976, pp. 279–289, 2024.
https://doi.org/10.1007/978-3-031-67285-9_20

ethical framework for Generative AI, thus aligning with the principles of using AI for Good.

Keywords: Generative AI · healthcare · privacy · ethics · policy · regulations · framework

1 Introduction

Generative Artificial Intelligence (AI), also known as Gen AI [1], is a unique form of artificial intelligence capable of generating text, images, videos, or other data using generative models. One of the earliest deliberations of a precursor to generative AI that is familiar to us today was its illustrious start at a research workshop held at Dartmouth College in 1956. The first historical example of generative AI was ELIZA, a talking computer program created in 1961 by Joseph Weizenbaum [1]. It was one of the first examples of Natural Language Processing (NLP). It was designed to simulate conversations with a human user by generating responses based on the text it received [2–5].

Generative AI has a long history with notable milestones from the 1940s to the present. From a data science perspective, here are some key milestones in the Gen AI journey.

- 1948: Claude Shannon publishes his paper "A Mathematical Theory of Communications", which references the idea of n-grams, which was An essential element of Google until 2018.
- 1950: Alan Turing published his seminal paper "Computing Machinery and Intelligence", which introduces the Turing Test.
- 1952: The first machine learning algorithm was developed by Arthur Samuel for playing checkers.
- 1957: The first "neural network" capable of being trained was called the "Perceptron," developed by a Cornell University psychologist, Frank Rosenblatt.
- 1961: Creation of one of the first functioning generative AI - ELIZA Chatbot.
- 2014: The concept of the Generative Adversarial Network (GAN) was introduced which lay the foundation for the Large Language Models (LLMs) today [6–8].

Gen AI, which we see today, is an emerging general AI-based technology that enables machines to carry out a wide range of non-physical tasks, including meta-cognitive abilities like learning new skills [9, 10]. With the advent of ChatGPT [11], Gemini, and Llama 2, the power of LLMs [2] is now available to laymen with stable internet connectivity and technological literacy.

With the aid of computationally intensive predictive modelling approaches applied to trillions of bytes of data available in the public domain, Gen AI has the potential to revolutionize the healthcare sector [12]. It can analyse large volumes of medical data and create entirely new content, which is technically synthetic or simulated data. This technology can improve the quality of care, make it more accessible and affordable, reduce inequities in research and care delivery, and help companies unlock business value in new ways [13, 14]. For example, a new generative AI technology, enabled by GPT-4, modelled how a healthcare clinician might use new platforms to turn a patient interaction into clinician notes in seconds or diagnose a disease in minutes, thus lowering the cost of care without compromising quality [15]. This near-instantaneous process makes the manual, time-consuming, and administrative work that a clinician must complete for every patient interaction, hassle-free. With advances in clinical trials for drug/device/vaccine development, entities can now leverage the benefits of Gen AI and fasten the pace of quality research to improve the public health landscape.

Gen AI in healthcare has several strengths. It can automate tedious and error-prone operational work, bringing years of data to a researcher's fingertips in seconds. It can improve the quality of care, and make it more accessible and affordable. It can take unstructured data sets and analyze them, representing a potential breakthrough for healthcare operations [16]. However, there are also weaknesses. Patient healthcare information is particularly sensitive, making data security paramount. Given the frequency with which Gen AI produces incorrect responses, healthcare practitioner facilitation and monitoring will be required. Gen AI heavily relies on user feedback, and hence, can be

Table 1. SWOC analysis to assess the impact of Gen AI in healthcare

Strengths	Weaknesses
• Increased access to healthcare information and resources (improved literacy) • Potential cost and time savings through automation of day-to-day tasks (improved productivity and outcomes) • Ability to generate customized and contextualized healthcare content • Augments human expertise into decision-making • Evidence-based findings as the results rely on historical data • Improved diagnostics due to the ability to generate synthetic data mimicking real-life scenarios • Code-free data analytics	• Algorithmic biases leading to potential harm to users • Lack of transparency and interpretability in the decision-making process • Subjectivity in responses • Dependence on quality and diversity of training data • High implementation costs and infrastructural needs for effective use • Requires skills in prompting • Data dependence • Explainability and Interpretability Challenges • Data privacy and data sharing
Opportunities	Threats
• Encourages continuous learning from data leading to improved outcomes • Accelerated clinical trials and development of drugs/devices/applications • Faster penetration of digital health applications • Enhanced pace of research	• Resistance to Adoption and Acceptance • Cybersecurity concerns, and data breaches • Regulatory challenges and absence of policies to incorporate Gen AI • Job displacement and disruption of existing healthcare workflows • Over-dependence on Gen AI-based systems and deskilling • Ethical and legal liabilities post decision-making based on Gen AI • Risk of perpetuating biases and discrimination in healthcare

misguided as well [17, 18]. Looking at the opportunities, Gen AI represents a meaningful new tool that can help unlock a piece of the unrealized $1 trillion of improvement potential present in the industry. It can modernize health systems infrastructure. On the other hand, there are threats.

One of the primary potential threats of Gen AI is the abuse of patient privacy. There could be overreliance among patients on AI-generated guidance. While generative AI holds great promise for the healthcare industry, it is important to navigate its application carefully, considering both its potential benefits and risks [19–21]. Table 1 presents the SWOC (strengths, weaknesses, opportunities, and challenges associated with Gen AI in healthcare.

Data privacy concerns associated with Gen AI are one of the biggest challenges for all the stakeholders of healthcare. This must be perceived in two ways. Firstly, there is no way to undo or delete any form of data including prompts, uploaded data, and results generated by LLMs. Secondly, the definition of publicly available data is unclear and there is a lack of transparency in understanding the user consent for the data used by the models used by Gen AI.

The present research uses the state-of-the-art review methodology to explore the following research questions.

a) What are the ethical frameworks applicable to Gen AI in healthcare?
b) What are the methods used to address data privacy challenges in Gen AI in healthcare?

2 Materials and Methods

To further understand the ethical frameworks and data privacy aspects applicable to Gen AI in healthcare, we make use of a state-of-the-art review framework which has been extensively used in the medical education sector to understand the current state of an underlying phenomenon of interest. State-of-the-art (SotA) reviews are recommended when there is a need to synthesize large bodies of knowledge on a specific phenomenon. SotA reviews provide a comprehensive overview of the latest advancements, trends, and developments in a particular sphere of research. SotA reviews are undertaken to create a three-part argument about the current state of knowledge for a specific phenomenon: This is where we are now, this is how we got here, and this is where we could go next [21–23]. Considering the multidisciplinary nature of Gen AI research in healthcare, SotA reviews provide information on the current understanding, the historical roots that shaped the understanding, and potential next directions for future research in the context of privacy and ethics of Gen AI in healthcare. The following table (see Table 2) gives a summary of the steps associated with SotA reviews.

Table 2. Steps in the SotA review process.

Sl. No	Step	Description
1	Define Research Questions	Identify the specific knowledge gaps one aims to address through the review. What are the key areas of inquiry within the field?
2	Develop Search Strategy	Determine relevant keywords, databases, and search filters to locate high-quality research articles
3	Conduct Literature Search	Systematically search for scholarly articles based on the defined search strategy
4	Screen and Select Studies	Establish inclusion and exclusion criteria to evaluate the relevance and quality of identified studies. Apply these criteria to select the most pertinent articles
5	Data Extraction and Synthesis	Extract key information from the selected studies, including research methods, findings, and conclusions. Analyze and synthesize this information to identify trends, gaps, and areas for future research
6	Write and Structure the Review	Organize and present the findings in a clear and concise manner. Typically, this includes an introduction, background on the topic, discussion of key findings, identification of research gaps, and a conclusion summarizing the state of the art in this format: This is where we are now, this is how we got here, and this is where we could go next

3   Key Findings

This section covers the three phases of SotA review. The first section discusses the current updates in the domains of ethical frameworks and data privacy in the context of Gen AI in healthcare. In the second section, the key frameworks for ethics and privacy in AI which provide the roadmap for the development of similar methodologies for Gen AI are discussed. This enables us to identify the future steps that will enable the stakeholders of healthcare to incorporate suitable changes to the existing frameworks to fit the needs of Generative AI applications in healthcare.

An extensive literature search was carried out as part of the study with the keywords "ethical framework", "privacy", "data privacy", "Generative AI/Gen AI/GAI", and "healthcare" with Boolean operator combinations (AND/OR) in the Scopus and PubMed databases. The filters in the search include Language: English, and Article: Full-text only across all article types. The search generated 10 articles on Scopus and 8 articles on PubMed. All articles were published during 2022–24 indicating the novelty of the topic, and highlighting the need to document the literature and summarize the findings expanding the scope for further research. The study was carried out from January 1, 2024–April 10, 2024.

3.1 Where We Are Now

Table 3. Ethical aspects of Generative AI in healthcare

Year	Step	Description
2024	Implementation Science Informed Translational Path [16]	This framework emphasizes the need for careful planning, execution, and management of expectations in adopting generative AI in clinical medicine, considering factors such as data privacy, security, and the irreplaceable role of clinicians' expertise
2024	WHO Guidance on Ethics and Governance [24]	The World Health Organization provides over 40 recommendations for the ethical use of large multi-modal models in healthcare, addressing risks and promoting health equity
2024	Inclusive Ethical Frameworks [25]	This set of best practices includes the development of inclusive ethical frameworks, regular ethical audits, and comprehensive training and education programs for the deployment of generative AI in healthcare
2023	GREAT PLEA Ethical Principles [26]	The GREAT PLEA ethical principles, namely Governability, Reliability, Equity, Accountability, Traceability, Privacy, Lawfulness, Empathy, and Autonomy, are proposed for generative AI in healthcare
2023	Harrer's Regulatory Framework [27]	Dr. Harrer's regulatory framework comprises ten principles aimed at mitigating the risks associated with generative AI in healthcare, including human oversight, data transparency, and privacy protection

Based on research specific to ethical aspects of Gen AI in healthcare, as tabulated in Table 3, it is observed that the existing research agrees with the fact the ethical framework for Gen AI needs to step up to cater to the demands for data privacy in the context of the ever-growing needs of the LLMs which continuously consume data which is not only publicly available as of a specific date (for instance, ChatGPT 3.5 uses data up to September 2021) but also the data generated through continuous user input and feedback. Among the available literature, the recently released WHO Guidance document [24] focuses more on the risk management aspects of the use of LLMs among the stakeholders of healthcare with a special focus on fragile populations (children/adolescents/elderly/disabled population). There is limited research on how data privacy and ethics can be comprehensively implemented in the context of using Generative AI in healthcare.

Privacy-by-design is another aspect that must be seen in the light of Generative AI in healthcare [28]. This is of great importance in designing digital health applications (websites, mobile applications, devices, extended reality-based applications). Privacy-by-design methods ensure that generative AI technologies are developed and deployed with privacy considerations at the forefront. Privacy-by-design approaches encourage transparency and user awareness and promote the use of synthetic (or simulated) data, and machine-learning algorithms that enhance privacy. It values individual consent, limits data use, and enables data minimization and access control [29]. While there are concerns about the transparency associated with the intricacies of privacy-by-design algorithms, the principles promote data privacy right from designing the technology to data collection and dissemination of findings from analytics on the data [24–26, 30, 31].

3.2   This is How We Got Here

Approximately 137 out of 194 countries have legislations to secure data and privacy protection. Africa and Asia show varying levels of adoption, with 61% and 57% of countries having adopted suitable regulations at the national level [27]. Table 4 summarizes the key regulations regarding the protection of citizen data across countries with a special focus on health. In addition, several entities including OECD, WHO, and ICMR have released guidance documents to address ethical aspects of the use of AI in healthcare.

However, it is pertinent to note that many of these regulations do not specifically address the dynamic needs of the LLM-led Gen AI. Furthermore, several researchers have introduced AI frameworks; the details of which have been summarized in Table 5.

Table 4. Countries and Regulations specific to healthcare data

Sl. No.	Data Regulations	Country/Region	Year
1	General Data Protection Regulation (GDPR)	European Union and European Economic Area	2018
2	Personal Information Protection Law (PIPL)	China	2021
3	California Consumer Privacy Act (CCPA) and Health Insurance Portability and Accountability Act (HIPAA)	United States	2018, 1996
4	Data Protection Directive 95/46/EC (replaced by GDPR)	European Union (superseded by GDPR)	1995
5	UK General Data Protection Regulation (UK GDPR)	United Kingdom	2021
7	Privacy Act (1988)	Australia	1988
8	Digital Personal Data Protection Act (2023)	India	2023

Table 5. Notable AI Frameworks for healthcare

Sl. No	Framework	Description	Focus Areas	Year
1	AI4Health (European Union Commission)	High-level principles for trustworthy AI in healthcare	Transparency, fairness, accountability, human-centricity, safety and well-being, privacy and security	2022
2	Montreal Declaration for Responsible AI Development	General principles for ethical development and use of AI	Transparency, accountability, fairness, non-maleficence, human well-being, privacy, security, sustainability, and societal well-being	2018
3	Utilitarian Framework [32]	Focuses on maximizing overall well-being through AI use	Maximizing benefits for the greatest number of people	18th Century
4	Rights-Based Framework	Emphasizes protecting fundamental human rights in AI development and deployment	Privacy, autonomy, non-discrimination, access to AI benefits	1948
5	Principalist Framework	Focuses on four core ethical principles: autonomy, beneficence, non-maleficence, and justice	Respect for user autonomy, maximizing benefit, avoiding harm, and ensuring fair access to and distribution of AI	1971
6	ACLS-HAI (American College of Clinical Leaders Healthcare Artificial Intelligence)	Framework for responsible development and use of AI in healthcare delivery	Safety, effectiveness, fairness, accountability, patient privacy, and clinician support	2019

3.3 This is Where We Could Go Next

Tracing the historic milestones in the context of data privacy, and ethical frameworks in Gen AI in healthcare, it is pertinent to note that there is a lacuna in literature of privacy and ethics in Gen AI. While deliberations on privacy impact assessment and privacy risk assessment find a mention in the guidance from WHO, these measures focus on methods that could be used in the post-implementation phase of a digital health technology that uses Gen AI. There is a growing need to ensure that ethics audits are regularly conducted among all stakeholders of any technology that uses Gen AI. It is important to ensure that the synthetic data generated by Gen AI based on publicly available data does not lead to any form of data security, confidentiality, or privacy violations.

While the IEEE P7003 Standard for Algorithmic Bias Considerations [33], focuses on minimizing the biases in the algorithms underlying LLMs, informed consent and privacy violations continue to threaten Gen AI-based data. Gen AI could integrate the principles of cooperative AI and explainable AI while prioritizing well-being, safety, and positive outcomes in public health.

4   Conclusion

The present study highlights the importance of addressing the privacy and ethical aspects of Gen AI in healthcare. While this state-of-the-art review is subjective in nature, it emphasizes the need for the development of a customized framework specific to each of the healthcare stakeholders that addresses privacy and ethics in Gen AI. This will enhance trust, and transparency in data analytics integrated into Gen AI. While the currently available guidelines and frameworks provide valuable assistance, they do not fully address ethical and legal implications. This calls for an extensive need to integrate ethical aspects, such as bias mitigation, privacy protection, and human oversight into the Gen AI design.

Acknowledgments. The authors express sincere gratitude to the reviewers for their constructive comments which have considerably improved the quality of this research. The authors also thank the organizers of the event for the opportunity to present the work at the Conference and their affiliated institutions for their support.

Disclosure of Interests. The authors have no competing interests. This research received no specific grant from any funding agency in the public, commercial, or not-for-profit sectors. However, the authors are open to collaborating or receiving funding to further contribute to the application/technology aspects of this research.

References

1. Natale, S.: If software is narrative: Joseph Weizenbaum, artificial intelligence and the biographies of ELIZA. New Media Soc. **21**(3), 712–728 (2019). https://doi.org/10.1177/146144481 8804980
2. Shashank, B., Damien, B., Jessica, L., George, S.: Tackling healthcare's biggest burdens with generative AI. https://www.mckinsey.com/industries/healthcare/our-insights/tackling-health cares-biggest-burdens-with-generative-ai. Accessed 10 July 2023
3. Matthew, H., Josh, K., Krishna, S., Krishna, D., Daniel, M.: Generative AI Will Transform Health Care Sooner Than You Think. https://www.bcg.com/publications/2023/how-genera tive-ai-is-transforming-health-care-sooner-than-expected. Accessed 22 June 2023

4. Hemachandran, K.: The Impact of Generative AI on healthcare industry in India. Ministry of Information and Technology, Government of India. https://indiaai.gov.in/article/the-impact-of-generative-ai-on-healthcare-industry-in-india. Accessed 11 Apr 2023
5. Sudeep, S.: How Generative AI is Reshaping the Healthcare Industry – 10 Applications and Use Cases. Appinventiv. https://appinventiv.com/blog/generative-ai-in-healthcare/. Accessed 20 May 2024
6. Michelle, H.: Generative AI Timeline: 9 Decades of Notable Milestones. Cmswire. https://www.cmswire.com/digital-experience/generative-ai-timeline-9-decades-of-notable-milestones/. Accessed 28 June 2023
7. Pat, L., Jerry, C.: The rise of generative AI: A timeline of breakthrough innovations. Qualcomm. https://www.qualcomm.com/news/onq/2024/02/the-rise-of-generative-ai-timeline-of-breakthrough-innovations. Accessed 12 Feb 2024
8. Toloka. History of generative AI. https://toloka.ai/blog/history-of-generative-ai/. Accessed 23 Aug 2023
9. Li, H., Zhang, R., Lee, Y.-C., Kraut, R.E., Mohr, D.C.: Systematic review and meta-analysis of AI-based conversational agents for promoting mental health and well-being. npj Digit. Med. **6**(1), 236 (2023). https://doi.org/10.1038/s41746-023-00979-5
10. Lv, Z.: Generative artificial intelligence in the metaverse era. Cogn. Robot. **3**, 208–217 (2023). https://doi.org/10.1016/j.cogr.2023.06.001
11. Lindsey, W.: The rise of generative AI: a timeline of triumphs, hiccups and hype. Cio Dive. https://www.ciodive.com/news/generative-ai-one-year-chatgpt-openai-timeline/698110/. Accessed 22 Nov 2023
12. Kuzlu, M., Xiao, Z., Sarp, S., Catak, F.O., Gurler, N., Guler, O.: The rise of generative artificial intelligence in healthcare. In: 2023 12th Mediterranean Conference on Embedded Computing (MECO), 6–10 June 2023, pp. 1–4 (2023). https://doi.org/10.1109/MECO58584.2023.10155107
13. Singh, P., Tiwari, S.: Chapter 9 Machine learning models for cost-effective healthcare delivery systems. In: Rishabha, M., Sonali, S., Rajesh Kumar, D., Seifedine, K. (eds.) Digital Transformation in Healthcare 5.0, pp. 245–276. De Gruyter, Berlin (2024)
14. Thethi, S.K.: Chapter 8 Machine learning models for cost-effective healthcare delivery systems: a global perspective. In: Rishabha, M., Sonali, S., Rajesh Kumar, D., Seifedine, K. (eds.) Digital Transformation in Healthcare 5.0, pp. 199–244. De Gruyter, Berlin (2024)
15. Khan, Z.F., Alotaibi, S.R.: Applications of artificial intelligence and big data analytics in m-health: a healthcare system perspective. J. Healthc. Eng. **2020**(1), 8894694 (2020). https://doi.org/10.1155/2020/8894694
16. Reddy, S.: Generative AI in healthcare: an implementation science informed translational path on application, integration and governance. Implement. Sci. **19**(1), 27 (2024). https://doi.org/10.1186/s13012-024-01357-9
17. Kocielnik, R., Amershi, S., Bennett, P.N.: Will you accept an imperfect AI? Exploring designs for adjusting end-user expectations of AI systems. Presented at the Proceedings of the 2019 CHI Conference on Human Factors in Computing Systems, Glasgow, Scotland UK (2019). https://doi.org/10.1145/3290605.3300641
18. Henman, P.: Improving public services using artificial intelligence: possibilities, pitfalls, governance. Asia Pac. J. Public Adm. **42**(4), 209–221 (2020)
19. Nicole, C.: Towards an AI Integrated Healthcare Ecosystem: A SWOT Analysis. The Medium. https://medium.com/@TheImmersiveNurse/toward-an-ai-integrated-healthcare-ecosystem-a-swot-analysis-7ac90f2e660f. Accessed 6 Dec2023
20. Ricardo, B., Matt, M., Spencer, R., Nick, B.: The Power of Prediction: How Generative AI Can Drive Biopharma Strategy. https://www.lek.com/insights/hea/us/ei/power-prediction-how-generative-ai-can-drive-biopharma-strategy. Accessed 30 May 2023

21. Barry, E.S., Merkebu, J., Varpio, L.: State-of-the-art literature review methodology: a six-step approach for knowledge synthesis. Perspect. Med. Educ. **11**(5), 281–288 (2022). https://doi.org/10.1007/s40037-022-00725-9

22. Barry, E.S., Merkebu, J., Varpio, L.: How to conduct a state-of-the-art literature review. J. Grad. Med. Educ. **14**(6), 663–665 (2022). https://doi.org/10.4300/jgme-d-22-00704.1

23. El Kettaneh, J.: State of the Art: What is it and how to conduct it? The Medium https://josephkettaneh.medium.com/state-of-the-art-what-is-it-and-how-to-conduct-it-e1b913f72f01. Accessed 16 Mar 2023

24. SCI Chief Scientist and Science Division and H. H. E. a. Governance, Ethics and governance of artificial intelligence for health: Guidance on large multi-modal models, p. 98 (2024)

25. Ijiga, A., et al.: Ethical considerations in implementing generative AI for healthcare supply chain optimization: a cross-country analysis across India, the United Kingdom, and the United States of America. Int. J. Biol. Pharm. Sci. Arch. **7**, 048–063 (2024). https://doi.org/10.53771/ijbpsa.2024.7.1.0015

26. Francisco, D.S.: 'GREAT PLEA' system proposed for responsible use of generative AI in healthcare. https://www.news-medical.net/news/20231205/GREAT-PLEA-system-proposed-for-responsible-use-of-generative-AI-in-healthcare.aspx#:~:text=We%20propose%20the%20%E2%80%9CGREAT%20PLEA,Traceability%2C%20Empathy%2C%20and%20Autonomy. Accessed 5 Dec 2023

27. Esposito, M., Tse, T.: Mitigating the risks of generative AI in government through algorithmic governance. Presented at the Proceedings of the 25th Annual International Conference on Digital Government Research, Taipei, Taiwan (2024). https://doi.org/10.1145/3657054.3657124

28. Davida, Z., Lubasz, D.: Privacy by design – searching for the balance between privacy, personal data protection and development of artificial intelligence systems In: Szostek, D., Załucki, M. (eds.) Internet and New Technologies Law: Perspectives and Challenges, 1st edn., pp. 337–360. Nomos Verlagsgesellschaft mbH & Co. KG, Baden-Baden (2021)

29. Pedraza, J., Patricio, M.A., de Asís, A., Molina, J.M.: Privacy-by-design rules in face recognition system. Neurocomputing **109**, 49–55 (2013). https://doi.org/10.1016/j.neucom.2012.03.023

30. Katharina, K.: Generative AI: Privacy and tech perspectives. https://iapp.org/news/a/generative-ai-privacy-and-tech-perspectives. Accessed

31. Sean, F.: Privacy in the age of generative AI. https://stackoverflow.blog/2023/10/23/privacy-in-the-age-of-generative-ai/. Accessed 23 Oct 2023

32. Beauchamp, T.L., Rauprich, O.: Principlism. In: ten Have, H. (eds.) Encyclopedia of Global Bioethics, pp. 2282–2293. Springer, Cham (2016). https://doi.org/10.1007/978-3-319-09483-0_348

33. Koene, A., Dowthwaite, L., Seth, S.: IEEE P7003TM standard for algorithmic bias considerations. In: 2018 IEEE/ACM International Workshop on Software Fairness (FairWare), 29–29 May 2018, pp. 38–41 (2018). https://doi.org/10.23919/FAIRWARE.2018.8452919

Explainable Machine Learning: Predicting Clinical Outcomes in Welsh Emergency Departments

Megan Lind Morgan[1]($\boxtimes$), Alma Rahat[1], Gareth Jenkins[2], and Jiaxiang Zhang[1]

[1] Department of Computer Science, Swansea University, Swansea, Wales
{2142745,a.a.m.rahat,jiaxiang.zhang}@swansea.ac.uk
[2] Hywel Dda University Health Board, Data Science Department, NHS, Carmarthen, Wales
gareth.jenkins3@wales.nhs.uk

Abstract. The UK NHS emergency departments (EDs) are the front-line for patient care, with a wide range of patient presentations but limited resources. Using over 1.5 million ED data entries collected during 2015–2023 from a health board in Wales, we explored the application of machine learning models in predicting clinical outcomes. The features in the models included age, sex, incident type, the reason for attendance, method of arrival, and the County of the ED. First, five supervised learning models were trained and evaluated on data collected before the 3rd quarter of 2019, and the Random Forest classifier outperformed other models with a weighted F1 score of 0.78. The same classifier yielded similar performance on subsequent data collected during 2019–2023. We then evaluated the stability of the classification performance by conducting cross-classification, using quarterly data before, during and after the COVID-19 pandemic (2019–2023). Predictive classification from models trained with historical data is stable during this period. Furthermore, we examined the feature importance (quantified by the mean decrease impurity score) of the fitted model. As expected, incident type (major vs minor) is the most important feature. Interestingly, the importance of age in predicting clinical outcomes varies substantially before and after the 4th quarter of 2019. Together, these results demonstrate the capacity of machine learning and its explainability in predicting ED clinical outcomes from simple features.

Keywords: Machine learning · Explainable data mining · Emergency departments · Clinical outcomes

1 Introduction

In the UK National Health Service (NHS), emergency departments (EDs) are a crucial element of healthcare, with consistent staffing and no requirement for appointments, meaning patients arrive daily, at any time, for accidents or health

X. Xie et al. (Eds.): AIiH 2024, LNCS 14976, pp. 290–301, 2024.
https://doi.org/10.1007/978-3-031-67285-9_21

issues. Some ED units specialise in minor injuries (i.e., minor injuries units), such as fractures or cuts, whereas others provide general emergency care [9]. In the ED, patients are first triaged, and their clinical notes are taken. Depending on the nature and severity of the medical condition, patients could undergo additional checks and lab tests. After necessary treatments, patients with non-urgent conditions may be discharged or booked with outpatient appointments. Other times, patients with more severe conditions will need to be monitored, or their treatments may involve complicated procedures. In those cases, the patients will be admitted to a ward for around-the-clock care. Unfortunately, patients with life-threatening conditions may die in the ED, although this is rare at the pre-admission stage [25].

The purpose of the ED is to treat urgent and potentially life-threatening conditions. However, over 16% of attendances in the ED were subsequently categorised as non-urgent, and nearly 20% of non-urgent attendees arrived by ambulance, which places additional demands on NHS resources that are already stretched thin [21]. This could indicate that messaging around the purpose of the ED is unclear, or that a more effective method of predicting demand early could lead to better resource allocation within the ED itself.

Recently, machine learning (ML) analysis on healthcare data is gaining interest in the healthcare sector [27]. For example, Assaf et al. showed that ML models can accurately predict critical diseases among COVID-19 patients [2]. Work by Elhaj et al. compared several supervised classifiers and identified that the random forest classifier is efficient in predicting triage outcomes for patients in the ED. This is strengthened by Kim et al.s' study in predicting septic shock in the ED, which found that ensemble classifiers outperformed other models and successfully identified at-risk patients [13]. Sbudhi et al. also demonstrate that ensemble classifiers are best when predicting ICU admission among COVID-19 patients [24]. These studies demonstrate that ensemble classifiers, particularly Random Forest, are appropriate ML models to extract information from healthcare records. Beyond clinical outcomes, several studies aimed to predict patients' length of stay in ED, for which natural language processing, ensemble classifiers and deep neural networks yield good results [3,7,16].

By analysing patient profiles through ML and deducing the risk factors associated with both demographic and ailment types, our goal is to identify higher-risk patients in the ED, and consequently help in managing demand. Here, we examined whether ML models trained on the data gathered upon entry to the department, such as patient demographics and the nature of the visit, could provide an early indication as to whether the patient is likely to be admitted, discharged, or die. At this stage, the work is proof-of-concept.

Specifically, the current study considered ED data collected between 2015 and 2023 from a NHS health board in Wales. First, we trained five ML classifiers (Random Forest, Gradient Boosting, AdaBoost, Support Vector Machine, and Logistic Regression) to predict patients' clinical outcomes from the data between Q3-2015 and Q3-2019. All models used the same set of data features, including patients' age and sex, and the nature of the patient's visit, such as their methods of arrival. Second, the best-performing model was trained and validated using aggregated and quarterly data from Q4-2019 to Q4-2023, which includes the period of the COVID-19 pandemic. Third, we investigated the importance of data features in the ML model, providing explainable information that is critical to patients' risks. Our results support the possibility of ML as a valuable tool in predicting clinical outcomes within the ED. Finally, we discussed the implications of our results in improving efficiency in EDs.

2   Methods

2.1   The ED Dataset

We conducted secondary analyses on an ED dataset collected by Hywel Dda University Health Board (HDUHB). HDUHB is one of the seven NHS health boards in Wales, UK. It is the planner and provider of NHS healthcare services for over 385,000 residents in a large part of middle and west Wales, including three main counties; Carmarthenshire, Ceredigion, and Pembrokeshire.

The ED dataset has been routinely updated by HDUHB and securely provided to the researchers. Each entry of the dataset represents an event of a patient presenting at one of the emergency departments of HDUHB. Here, we considered a total of 1,543,124 data entries that occurred between 2015 and 2023. The dataset is anonymized, including demographic information (e.g., age, sex, county) and specific features relating to the event. The additional features include the method of arrival at the ED (e.g., by private transport or by ambulance), incident type, incident reason (e.g., non-traumatic injury or fall), and the county of the ED. Table 1 lists all the features considered in the current study and their possible values. For each ED event, one of three possible outcomes was recorded: discharged, admitted, or died. Additional information, such as administrative details, was not considered in the current study due to irrelevance. The study was approved by Swansea University's Research Ethics Committee.

2.2   Data Pre-processing

The six chosen features (Table 1) were extracted from the NHS SQLServer database and imported in Python. Rows containing missing values were removed from subsequent analyses (0.5% of all events). To correct occasional deviations and irregularities in data entries, text-based features were carefully checked and re-coded into integer values, corresponding to their contextual categories. For example, events with the outcome of "became outpatient" were re-coded in the same category as "discharged", as patients in those events were not admitted following clinical assessments or treatments in the ED. In subsequent analyses, based on patients' arrival time recorded in the dataset, we further split the data entries into quarterly data across the whole time range (2015–2023), with each batch of quarterly data consisting of 3 months of patients' records.

Table 1. The features and values of the ED dataset. The percentages denote the top three prevalence rates of each feature.

Feature	Values
Sex	Male (49.6%), Female (50%), Undetermined (0.4%)
Age	Range: 0 - 120 years (mean: 44 years; standard deviation: 26 years)
Department County	Carmarthenshire (50%), Pembrokeshire (28%), Ceredigion (22%)
Incident Type	Major (42%), Minor (58%)
Incident Reason	18 Categories, including non-traumatic injury (70%), emergency (10%), falls from low height (8%), falls from tall heights, sports injury, self-harm and more
Arrival Method	Private transport (79%), Ambulance (9%), 999 Emergency (8%), Police transport, Public transport, On foot, Air support, Other
Clinical Outcome (Target Prediction)	Discharged (74%), Admitted (25%), Died (1%)

2.3 Model Specification

We considered five supervised ML models: Random Forest (RF), Gradient Boosting (GB), AdaBoost (AB), Support Vector Machine (SVM) and Logistic Regression (LR). The first three models considered here are ensemble classifiers, with multiple estimators used to vote on the most likely class [4,5].

All models were tested in Python (version 3.11.7) and scikit-learn (version 1.2.1). 200 estimators were used for RF, GB and AB, with a maximum depth of 6. Stochastic Gradient Descent optimization was used for the SVM. Other model parameters retained their default values. Hence, we seek to demonstrate that standard applications of ML models are capable of detecting patterns in a large ED dataset, such as the one considered here.

2.4 Model Training and Testing

The ML model was first trained and tested using the pre-processed ED data. Stratified 10-Fold cross-validation procedure was used, which preserves the distribution of each class in each fold. The models were trained to classify ED events into the three clinical outcomes (discharged, admitted, or died). Because the three outcomes are imbalanced (Table 1), we assessed model performance by using weighted F1 score and weighted Area Under the ROC Curve (AUC), averaged from all cross-validation folds.

We first trained and tested all five ML models using the data dated between Q3-2015 and Q3-2019. The best-performing model was then used to train and test new data from a non-overlapping interval, between Q4-2019 and Q4-2023. This data split at Q4-2019 allowed us to evaluate the robustness of our results in the context of the COVID-19 pandemic [18], during which EDs across the world were heavily affected [8,20]

2.5   Cross-Classification on Quarterly Data

To provide a more granular evaluation of the robustness of our result, we used the best-performing model in the previous analysis to conduct cross-classification on quarterly data from Q4-2019 to 2023. For quarterly data, we first trained the ML model and then evaluated its performance (weighted F1 score) on all subsequent unseen quarterly data. This approach allowed us to examine to what extent the COVID-10 pandemic impacted the performance of the trained model in predicting clinical outcomes in the ED.

2.6   Feature Importance

Identifying important features within the dataset gives us an insight into which features influence model performance, which is a vital aspect of Explainable AI [1, 23]. The best-performing model's significant features were identified separately for the 2015–2019 and 2019–2023 periods. Specifically, we calculated the Mean Decrease in Impurity (MDI) values (i.e., the Gini importance) of the trained random forest classifiers, which quantifies the contribution of individual features to the classifier and is often used as an interpretable measure for Random Forest [6, 15]. In the current study, all features represent primary information on ED visits. Therefore, their MDI values provide insights into how important the demographical and clinical features are in predicting the outcome of ED events.

3   Results

3.1   Robust Prediction of ED Clinical Outcomes

We examined the performance (weighted F1 score and weighted AUC) of 5 supervised classifiers using stratified 10-fold cross-validation. For data between 2015 and Q3-2019, the random forest classifier was the best-performing model (Table 2, weighted F1 score: 0.78; weighted AUC: 0.76) in predicting the clinical outcomes of ED patients (discharged, admitted, or died).

As Random Forest performed best on the data between 2015 and Q3-2019, it was evaluated further on the data from Q4-2019 to Q4-2023. Following the same stratified cross-validation procedure, the random forest classifier achieved a mean weighted F1 score of 0.80 and a mean weighted AUC value of 0.77. These results demonstrated that, for ED data within the last decade, Random Forest is a robust model for predicting ED clinical outcomes.

3.2   Feature Importance in Predicting ED Clinical Outcomes

We used the mean decrease in impurity (MDI) as a feature importance metric to quantify the improvement in model predictability due to each feature. For the random forest classifiers trained on the two non-overlapping time intervals, Incident type is the most important feature influencing the model performance (Fig. 1A, 2015 to Q3-2019; Fig. 1B, Q4-2019 to Q4-2023). This result is expected

Table 2. Mean weighted F1 Scores and mean weighted AUC values from 10-fold cross-validation, with range of results across the 10 folds. All models were trained and tested using data from 2015 to Q3-2019.

Model	Mean and range of F1	Mean and range of AUC
Random Forest	0.78 [0.74 - 0.81]	0.76 [0.73 - 0.78]
AdaBoost	0.75 [0.72 - 0.78]	0.74 [0.72 - 0.77]
Support Vector Machine	0.74 [0.70 - 0.76]	0.74 [0.71 - 0.76]
Gradient Boosting	0.71 [0.67 - 0.74]	0.72 [0.66 - 0.73]
Logistic regression	0.70 [0.66 - 0.72]	0.69 [0.64 - 0.71]

because Incident Type is directly linked to the severity of the patient upon arrival (i.e., major vs. minor). Both Incident Reason and Age strongly influence the model performance. Incident Reason describes the purpose of the patient's visit to the ED, which indirectly relates to the severity of the event. Interestingly, although the age distribution remains similar from 2015 to 2023, the importance of age to clinical outcome prediction becomes more apparent for data between Q4-2019 and 2023 (Fig. 1B).

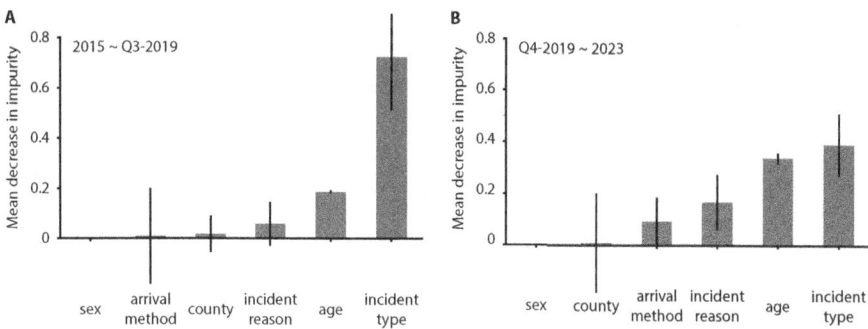

Fig. 1. The mean decrease in impurity (MDI) of the random forest classifiers. (A) The MDI from the ED data between 2015 and Q3-2019. (B) The MDI from the ED data between Q4-2019 and 2023. Error bars denote inter-trees variability.

To further examine the effect of age on clinical outcomes, we plotted age distributions separately for each clinical outcome (Fig. 2). Distribution of age leans towards the older end of the range when the outcome is 'died' or 'admitted' with most young patients 'discharged'. Compared with ED data from 2015 to Q3-2019, for events that occurred during Q4 2019 and 2023, older patients (e.g., over 70 years old) are more likely to be admitted. These results suggest that the importance of certain features to outcome prediction varies over time.

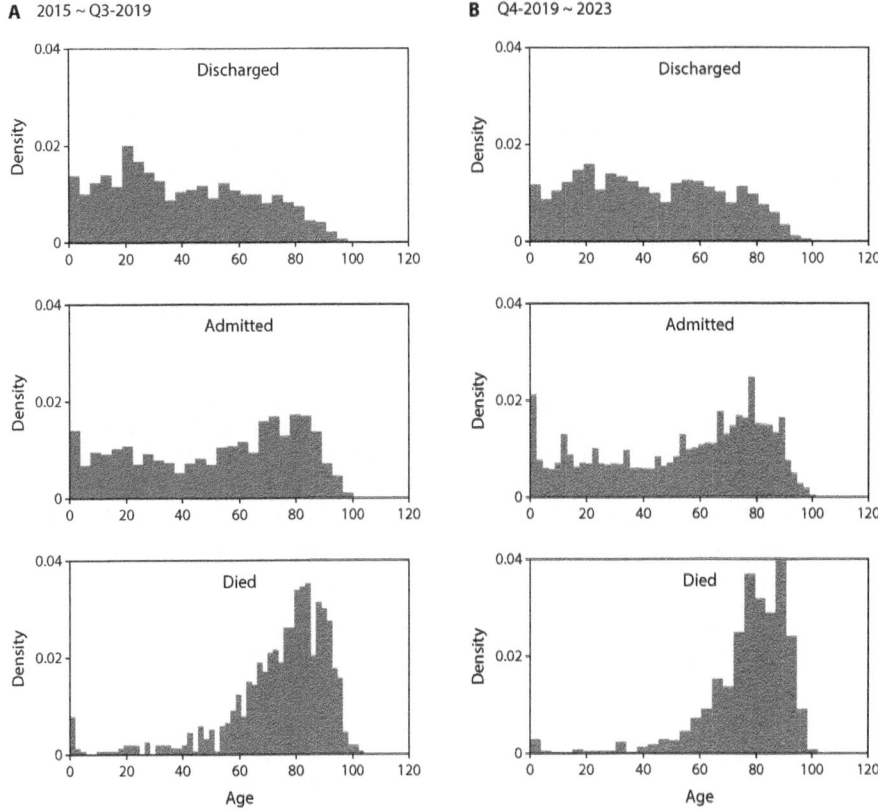

Fig. 2. Age distribution density grouped by ED clinical outcomes from (A) data between 2015 and Q3-2019, and (B) data between Q4-2019 and 2023.

3.3   Cross-Classification on Quarterly Data

We trained the Random Forest model on the ED data from each quarter between Q4-2019 and Q4-2023. The trained model was then evaluated on the current season used for training, and all subsequent quarterly data. This cross-classification analysis showed a minor decrease in the model performance (weighted F1 score) in Q4 2020 and Q1 2021 Fig. 3, the period that includes the first winter of the COVID-19 pandemic. In most other quarters, the model yielded stable performance in predicting clinical outcomes with weighted F1 scores above 80%. These results indicate that despite feature importance varying over time, the same set of features provides consistent predictive performance.

4   Discussion

The current study highlighted two key findings in applying ML models to predict ED clinical outcomes: (1) the significant features influencing the model

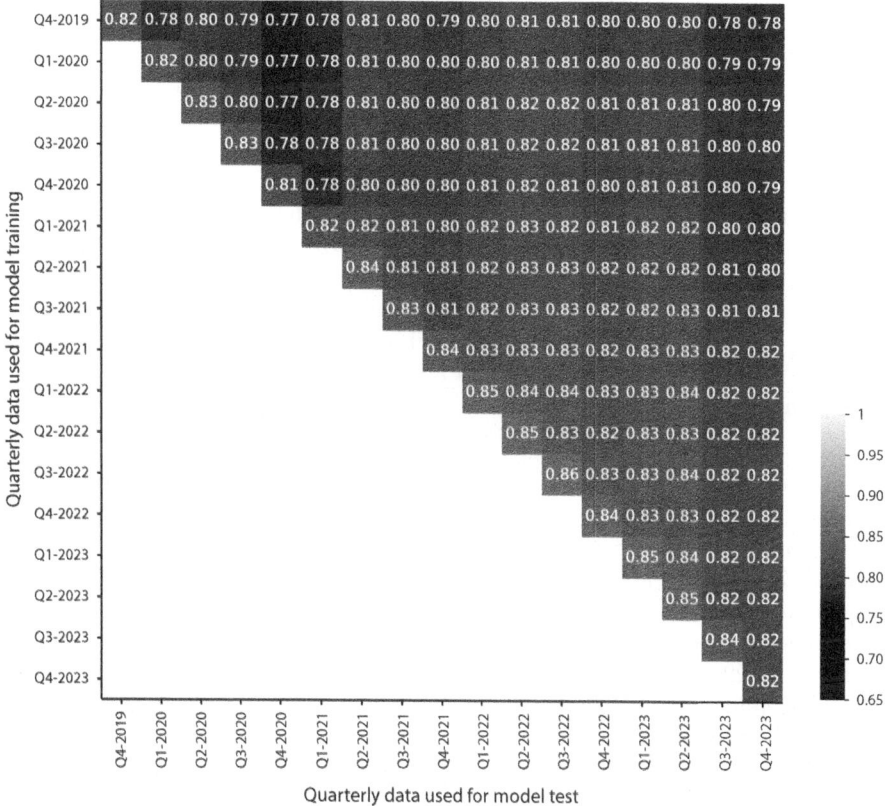

Fig. 3. Weighted F1 Scores from the cross-classification analysis. For each quarter between Q4-2019 and Q4-2023, a random forest model is trained on the ED data from that quarter (as indicated on the vertical axis), and then tested on each of the subsequent quarterly data (as indicated on the horizontal axis). Minimum F1 score: 0.77. Maximum F1 score: 0.86.

performance, and (2) the consistency of the model performance throughout the COVID pandemic. Below, we will discuss these results in detail, including their implications.

Impact of Important Features on Model performance. Feature importance quantified by MDI allows researchers and practitioners to identify features predominantly influencing clinical outcomes, which would otherwise be difficult to detect. Our results showed that the combination of demographic and clinical features provides stable and robust prediction of clinical outcomes in the ED.

Based on the MDI values, the most important features when classifying outcomes are incident type, incident reason, and age. Age is commonly seen as an important feature when considering patient risk, due to an increased likelihood of chronic illness, frailty and reduced immunity in older age. There is also a increased likelihood of older patients taking medication that may put them at higher risk of bleeding, falls or other accidents [11]. On the other hand, old age is not always a necessary condition that determines clinical outcomes, as younger patients also present with chronic health issues, and very young children and babies can also be at an elevated risk of hospital admission [19]. Our results show that the impact of age becomes more prominent during the 2019–2023 interval, suggesting that factors such as COVID may have been affecting the ED outcomes of different age groups. This is likely why incident type is the most important feature, as the classification of major or minor once at the ED gives a strong suggestion as to whether the patient is at high risk of further complication. Together, our results could provide an early indication (at the point of entry to the ED) of which patients are likely to need more care, and as a consequence, greater resources.

Impact of the COVID-19 Pandemic on Model performance. The COVID-19 pandemic was a global crisis, unexpected and devastating to health efforts worldwide. The model performance in predicting ED clinical outcomes maintained a steady level during this period (2019–2023), with small changes across quarters in the cross-classification analysis. This may appear to be counterintuitive, as the pandemic severely affected many NHS departments, including the ED [22]. Nevertheless, statistical records showed that ED attendance dropped significantly during the COVID-19 pandemic, particularly in the earlier months [14]. This pattern was especially true for Minor Injuries Units, which is one of the main departments of the Welsh NHS health board considered here. It is possible that, although the length of stay in the ED was negatively impacted during the COVID-19 pandemic [3], the relationship between patients' clinical outcomes and the combination of features considered here did not vary substantially, even the contribution of individual features (e.g., age) may vary. Further research is required to replicate our findings in other NHS health boards.

Implications and Future Work. The models developed within this work followed a simple implementation to assess the capability of ML in analysing trends within NHS EDs, as solutions with low requirements on computational resources are more likely to be useful in practice. We demonstrated that simple models trained with a limited number of features are sufficient in predicting clinical outcomes with reasonable accuracy. To achieve higher accuracy, more sophisticated models could be developed within future work, although the obtained results demonstrate that complexity is not always needed to obtain adequate results.

Furthermore, explainable ML metrics such as the MDI provided further insights into which features influence clinical outcomes, which is valuable information within the ED. The prediction of severe outcomes such as death could assist in providing early intervention and treatment, and the prediction of admission could improve resource allocation. This technique can also identify variations in significant features, which indicates changes in the population's health and the presentation of patients at the ED. MDI is a measure used when Random Forest is the chosen classifier, and while there are many other valuable measures of feature importance, such as SHAP values and Local Interpretable Model-Agnostic Explanations (LIME) [10,17], MDI is a useful and simple analysis of feature relevance within Random Forests' decision making [15]. Future work should consider other explainability measures and compare their output to MDI.

Future work could include additional features to improve model performance. For example, one could utilize the patient's postcode by linking each postcode to the UK's deprivation index [12], which will provide additional insight into the socioeconomic status (SES) of patients, as low SES is associated with a heightened risk of hospitalization among ED attendees [26]. Second, integrating ED data with health information from patients' primary care could lead to a personalized predictive model, which, at the population level, offers an accurate forecast of ED demands.

5   Conclusion

This work used simple ML models to predict ED clinical outcomes from a long-term and large-scale NHS dataset, covering the 2015–2023 period. Simple supervised classifiers provided robust and stable prediction performance. By comparing model performance over two intervals before and during the COVID-19 pandemic, as well as quarterly cross-classification during the pandemic, we observed that the model yielded reliable performance. Feature importance analysis allowed us to further highlight the incident type and age as the two preliminary features that influence model predictions. In summary, we demonstrated an explainable ML workflow to inform predictive analysis in the ED outcomes. The novelty of this stems from an applied experimental approach using NHS ED data, meaning these results are a true reflection of current NHS trends. This work can also serve as a starting point for further development into a holistic approach encompassing early intervention and management of resources throughout hospital departments.

Acknowledgement. This project was funded by the EPSRC Centre for Doctoral Training in *Enhancing Human Interactions and Collaborations with Data and Intelligence-Driven Systems* (EP/S021892/1) based at Swansea University. The industry partner for this co-funded PhD project is Hywel Dda University Health Board, Wales.

References

1. Angelov, P.P., Soares, E.A., Jiang, R., Arnold, N.I., Atkinson, P.M.: Explainable artificial intelligence: an analytical review. Wiley Interdiscip. Rev. Data Mining Knowl. Discov. **11**(5), e1424 (2021)
2. Assaf, D., et al.: Utilization of machine-learning models to accurately predict the risk for critical Covid-19. Intern. Emerg. Med. **15**, 1435–1443 (2020)

3. Bacchi, S., Tan, Y., Oakden-Rayner, L., Jannes, J., Kleinig, T., Koblar, S.: Machine learning in the prediction of medical inpatient length of stay. Intern. Med. J. **52**(2), 176–185 (2022)
4. Bentéjac, C., Csörgő, A., Martínez-Muñoz, G.: A comparative analysis of gradient boosting algorithms. Artif. Intell. Rev. **54**, 1937–1967 (2021)
5. Biau, G., Scornet, E.: A random forest guided tour. TEST **25**, 197–227 (2016)
6. Breiman, L.: Random forests. Mach. Learn. **45**, 5–32 (2001)
7. Chrusciel, J., Girardon, F., Roquette, L., Laplanche, D., Duclos, A., Sanchez, S.: The prediction of hospital length of stay using unstructured data. BMC Med. Inform. Decis. Mak. **21**(1), 351 (2021)
8. Chun, S.Y., Kim, H.J., Kim, H.B.: The effect of Covid-19 pandemic on the length of stay and outcomes in the emergency department. Clin. Experiment. Emerg. Med. **9**(2), 128 (2022)
9. Cowling, T.E., Soljak, M.A., Bell, D., Majeed, A.: Emergency hospital admissions via accident and emergency departments in England: time trend, conceptual framework and policy implications. J. R. Soc. Med. **107**(11), 432–438 (2014)
10. Dieber, J., Kirrane, S.: Why model why? assessing the strengths and limitations of lime. arXiv preprint arXiv:2012.00093 (2020)
11. Franchi, C., et al.: Risk factors for hospital readmission of elderly patients. Eur. J. Intern. Med. **24**(1), 45–51 (2013)
12. Gordon, D.: Census based deprivation indices: their weighting and validation. J. Epidemiol. Commun. Health **49**(Suppl 2), S39–S44 (1995)
13. Kim, J., Chang, H., Kim, D., Jang, D.H., Park, I., Kim, K.: Machine learning for prediction of septic shock at initial triage in emergency department. J. Crit. Care **55**, 163–170 (2020)
14. Leow, S.H., Dean, W., MacDonald-Nethercott, M., MacDonald-Nethercott, E., Boyle, A.A.: The attend study: a retrospective observational study of emergency department attendances during the early stages of the Covid-19 pandemic. Cureus **12**(7) (2020)
15. Louppe, G., Wehenkel, L., Sutera, A., Geurts, P.: Understanding variable importances in forests of randomized trees. In: Advances in Neural Information Processing Systems **26** (2013)
16. Ma, F., Yu, L., Ye, L., Yao, D.D., Zhuang, W.: Length-of-stay prediction for pediatric patients with respiratory diseases using decision tree methods. IEEE J. Biomed. Health Inform. **24**(9), 2651–2662 (2020)
17. Marcílio, W.E., Eler, D.M.: From explanations to feature selection: assessing shap values as feature selection mechanism. In: 2020 33rd SIBGRAPI Conference on Graphics, Patterns and Images (SIBGRAPI), pp. 340–347. IEEE (2020)
18. Murray, C.J.: Covid-19 will continue but the end of the pandemic is near. The Lancet **399**(10323), 417–419 (2022)
19. Network, T.I.N.: The crib (clinical risk index for babies) score: a tool for assessing initial neonatal risk and comparing performance of neonatal intensive care units. Lancet **342**(8865), 193–198 (1993)
20. Nguyen, J., Liu, A., McKenney, M., Liu, H., Ang, D., Elkbuli, A.: Impacts and challenges of the Covid-19 pandemic on emergency medicine physicians in the united states. Am. J. Emerg. Med. **48**, 38–47 (2021)
21. O'Keeffe, C., Mason, S., Jacques, R., Nicholl, J.: Characterising non-urgent users of the emergency department (ed): a retrospective analysis of routine ed data. PloS one **13**(2), e0192855 (2018)
22. Propper, C., Stoye, G., Zaranko, B.: The wider impacts of the coronavirus pandemic on the NHS. Fisc. Stud. **41**(2), 345–356 (2020)

23. Saarela, M., Jauhiainen, S.: Comparison of feature importance measures as explanations for classification models. SN Appl. Sci. **3**(2), 272 (2021)
24. Subudhi, S., et al.: Comparing machine learning algorithms for predicting ICU admission and mortality in Covid-19. NPJ Digital Med. **4**(1), 87 (2021)
25. Sun, B.C., Burstin, H.R., Brennan, T.A.: Predictors and outcomes of frequent emergency department users. Acad. Emerg. Med. **10**(4), 320–328 (2003)
26. Wachelder, J.J., et al.: Association of socioeconomic status with outcomes in older adult community-dwelling patients after visiting the emergency department: a retrospective cohort study. BMJ Open **7**(12), e019318 (2017)
27. Wiens, J., Shenoy, E.S.: Machine learning for healthcare: on the verge of a major shift in healthcare epidemiology. Clin. Infect. Dis. **66**(1), 149–153 (2018)

Enhancing Performance for Highly Imbalanced Medical Data via Data Regularization in a Federated Learning Setting

Georgios Tsoumplekas[1]([⊠]) [ID], Ilias Siniosoglou[1,2] [ID], Vasileios Argyriou[3] [ID], Ioannis D. Moscholios[4] [ID], and Panagiotis Sarigiannidis[1,2] [ID]

[1] MetaMind Innovations P.C., Kozani, Greece
{gtsoumplekas,isiniosoglou,psarigiannidis}@metamind.gr

[2] Department of Electrical and Computer Engineering, University of Western Macedonia, Kozani, Greece
{isiniosoglou,psarigiannidis}@uowm.gr

[3] Department of Networks and Digital Media, Kingston University, Kingston upon Thames, UK
vasileios.argyriou@kingston.ac.uk

[4] Department of Informatics and Telecommunications, University of Peloponnese, Tripolis, Greece
idm@uop.gr

Abstract. The increased availability of medical data has significantly impacted healthcare by enabling the application of machine/deep learning approaches in various instances. However, medical datasets are usually small and scattered across multiple providers, suffer from high class-imbalance, and are subject to stringent data privacy constraints. In this paper, the application of a data regularization algorithm, suitable for learning under high class-imbalance, in a federated learning setting is proposed. Specifically, the goal of the proposed method is to enhance model performance for cardiovascular disease prediction by tackling the class-imbalance that typically characterizes datasets used for this purpose, as well as by leveraging patient data available in different nodes of a federated ecosystem without compromising their privacy and enabling more resource sensitive allocation. The method is evaluated across four datasets for cardiovascular disease prediction, which are scattered across different clients, achieving improved performance. Meanwhile, its robustness under various hyperparameter settings, as well as its ability to adapt to different resource allocation scenarios, is verified.

Keywords: Federated Learning · Imbalanced Learning · Balanced Mixup · Medical Data · Cardiovascular Disease Prediction

1 Introduction

The modern era of Big Data has brought about tremendous changes in various domains that impact people's everyday lives, including healthcare. Specifically,

X. Xie et al. (Eds.): AIiH 2024, LNCS 14976, pp. 302–315, 2024.
https://doi.org/10.1007/978-3-031-67285-9_22

the advent of medical software and devices has enabled the generation of large amounts of assorted data regarding patient records. Consequently, such large quantities of medical data have greatly facilitated the application of machine learning (ML) and deep learning (DL) solutions in the medical field. In many cases, these applications aim to complement conventional medical diagnosis methods by reducing the time needed to process large quantities of data, assisting in better decision-making, and enabling the timely prediction of diseases.

However, real-world medical datasets pose several challenges due to their inherent nature [10]. One common problem that typically arises in medical datasets for disease classification is that they tend to be highly skewed since most available data refer to healthy individuals while there is only a limited number of data related to patients suffering from a particular disease. This extreme class-imbalance, however, can hinder the practical application of ML methods since these algorithms fail to identify patients with a disease accurately due to the lack of available data for that class.

At the same time, medical datasets are typically small and scattered across different healthcare providers, making it challenging to train ML models, especially when they are highly imbalanced. Combining datasets to train larger models is also challenging due to privacy constraints imposed on medical data. In recent years, federated learning (FL) has gained popularity for such applications due to its inherent characteristics that ensure data privacy by design since it obviates the need for exchanging sensitive data. However, in such critical cases, it is also crucial to consider the computational cost of these decentralized applications and their ability to adapt to different resource allocation scenarios.

This paper aims to tackle data imbalance and privacy considerations in medical datasets by combining imbalanced learning via data regularization with FL. The proposed method is evaluated using four real-world datasets, leading to improved results across all cases compared to methods that do not incorporate the imbalanced and FL criteria. At the same time, it demonstrates robustness under various hyperparameter settings, while it can also maintain high performance under limited available communication resources. The overall contributions of this paper can be summarized as follows:

- Proposes the utilization of Balanced-MixUp [5] to deal with imbalanced learning for cardiovascular disease prediction using tabular data.
- Applies Balanced-MixUp in a FL setting, enhancing model performance across all clients' datasets while also ensuring data privacy of sensitive patient information.
- Presents a thorough evaluation of the proposed method under various experimental settings, demonstrating its robustness and resource efficiency.

The rest of this paper is organized as follows: the related work is discussed in Sect. 2, followed by an overview of the methodology in Sect. 3. Section 4 provides a comprehensive analysis of the available data and the models' performance under imbalanced learning in a federated setting, and finally, Sect. 5 concludes the paper.

2   Related Work

2.1   Federated Learning

FL has increasingly been seen in the medical sector due to its innate attributes, namely privacy-by-design and resource allocation on the edge, but also due to its ability to optimize models by combining the distributed knowledge of decentralized data. This is also the case with the model fusion algorithms employed to merge the decentrally trained models into an optimized global model, that contains the shared knowledge from the remote data. In particular, in [19] the authors develop an FL system to address the issue of data privacy for Health Service Provider (HSP) systems. The paper utilizes a modified version of the FedMA [18] model fusion algorithm to ensure the privacy of heart disease data while also showing optimized results for the utilized data. In [17], the authors propose an improved FL framework that enhances the security of multi-party collaboration in the sensitive context of healthcare data. The work employs this framework to optimize a decentralized AI model for the prediction of Diabetes Mellitus risk, demonstrating enhanced model accuracy, while providing scalability and efficiency. The authors in [20] propose a privacy-aware FL framework for heart disease prediction also leveraging the FedMA algorithm. The work employs a proposed Modified Artificial Bee Colony (M-ABC) optimizer at the client end for optimal feature selection of heart disease data, presenting enhanced accuracy of results. This work is further advanced in [7] where the authors propose an asynchronous FL (Async-FL) technique for predicting heart diseases. In particular, they employ a temporally weighted aggregation method on the server to enhance the convergence of the global model, using locally trained models from the decentralized nodes. The work shows high model accuracy while addressing privacy concerns and computational efficiency.

2.2   Imbalanced Learning

One of the main challenges that arise in classification tasks within the medical domain is the high class-imbalance that typically discerns the available data [10]. Over the years, various approaches have been proposed to handle class-imbalance, ranging from simple techniques such as random oversampling/undersampling to more sophisticated ones such as synthetic sampling with data generation, e.g., SMOTE and its variants. In addition to data manipulation techniques, other approaches have focused on the algorithms used to train the classifier on the imbalanced dataset. Some standard methods include cost-sensitive learning [8] and using different weights for the contribution of each sample during training [22]. More recently, various techniques extending data regularization approaches, such as MixUp [21], have also been successfully applied to deal with class-imbalance. Examples of these techniques include Remix [3], which assigns the synthetic sample label in favor of the minority class, and Balanced-MixUp [5], which introduces a sampling mechanism favoring the creation of synthetic samples near the minority class samples.

2.3 Cardiovascular Disease Prediction

While traditionally, cardiovascular disease prediction has been considered a medical task typically performed by physicians, the availability of consolidated data from various patients has enabled the application of ML methods for this task [12]. For instance, in [14], an ensemble of K-Nearest Neighbors (KNN) and logistic regression models is used to perform early diagnosis of cardiovascular diseases in the Framingham [1] and Cleveland [6] datasets. Ensembling has also been utilized in [15], where the proposed stacking ensemble model outperforms all individual models in the Framingham dataset, and in [13], where an accuracy-based weighted aging classifier ensemble that contains decision trees trained on random splits of the Cleveland and Framingham datasets is proposed. Finally, in [4], integrating different datasets by extracting a shared set of features using decision trees is proposed. The final predictions are then obtained using a decision tree in the total unified dataset. Our approach also focuses on merging different datasets. However, this is done in a FL setting that ensures data privacy of sensitive patient information while, at the same time, we tackle class-imbalance via data regularization. It is also worth noting that while most of the approaches above aim to tackle class-imbalance using SMOTE or its variants, a direct comparison of our approach to these methods would be unjust since the reported metrics in these works refer to the balanced versions of these datasets.

3 Methodology

3.1 Imbalanced Learning with Data Regularization

To deal with the high class-imbalance that characterizes many cardiovascular disease prediction datasets, Balanced-MixUp [5], a data regularization technique suitable for imbalanced learning, is utilized.

Before delving into the specifics of Balanced-MixUp, it is crucial to provide a brief overview of MixUp [21], which constitutes the basis of the examined method. MixUp is a data regularization technique initially proposed to enhance deep learning performance by reducing overfitting. It relies on composing novel synthetic samples by taking convex combinations of existing training samples and their corresponding labels. In particular, given a dataset $\mathcal{D} = \{(x_i, y_i)\}_{i=1}^{N}$ with N samples, where $x_i \in \mathbb{R}^M$ is the i-th input sample and y_i is its corresponding label, MixUp replaces $\mathcal{D}$ with a novel synthetic dataset $\tilde{\mathcal{D}} = \{(\tilde{x}_k, \tilde{y}_k)\}_{k=1}^{N}$, where:

$$\tilde{x}_k = \lambda x_i + (1 - \lambda)x_j, \quad \tilde{y}_k = \lambda y_i + (1 - \lambda)y_j \tag{1}$$

In this case, $(x_i, y_i), (x_j, y_j)$ are randomly drawn from $\mathcal{D}$, with $i \neq j$, and $\lambda \in [0, 1]$ is drawn from a Beta distribution, $\lambda \sim Beta(\alpha, \alpha)$, with $\alpha > 0$.

While MixUp has successfully been applied to various domains, increasing model generalization, one noticeable drawback is that randomly selecting samples to create $\tilde{\mathcal{D}}$ does not account for any differences in the number of samples in the dataset's classes. Subsequently, Balanced-MixUp was proposed as an extension of MixUp that considers any class-imbalances in $\mathcal{D}$ and induces over-sampling of the minority classes within the MixUp formulation. In particular, instead of combining randomly drawn samples from $\mathcal{D}$, Balanced-MixUp combines randomly sampled (x_i, y_i) with (x_j, y_j) that are uniformly sampled from each class. More formally, given C non-overlapping classes in $\mathcal{D}$, each containing n_c samples so that $\sum_{c=0}^{C-1} n_c = N$, the probability of (x_i, y_i) belonging to class c is $p_{c,i} = \frac{n_c}{N}$, while the probability of (x_j, y_j) belonging to class c is $p_{c,j} = \frac{1}{C}$. As a result, for (x_j, y_j), the probability of sampling from a minority class is increased while the probability of sampling from a majority class is reduced compared to (x_i, y_i). This difference in the sampling mechanisms applied to select the original samples in (1) leads to the creation of novel synthetic samples closer to the areas where the minority class samples lie, consequently increasing model performance in these areas. Additionally, while Balanced-MixUp's λ is also drawn from a Beta distribution, the distribution is now parameterized as $\lambda \sim Beta(\alpha, 1)$, with $\alpha > 0$, so that the drawn λ values are small and the created synthetic samples lie closer to the minority class samples.

Although Balanced-MixUp was initially proposed for medical image classification, in Sect. 4, we show that it can also be effectively applied in the context of cardiovascular disease prediction using tabular data.

3.2 Federated Learning

Federated Learning (FL) has recently flourished as a widespread tool for distributed ML/DL implementations, as it is a technique aimed at privacy preservation. This methodology takes over the orchestration, distribution, learning, and aggregation of DL models coming from a large amount of distributed edge devices or remote workers [2] that possess local data not available to other devices or the network, as can be seen in Fig. 1. Models are trained locally on each device's collected data while the trained model weights are transmitted to a centralized unit where they are subsequently aggregated to produce a mutual global model using a fusion algorithm like Federated Averaging [11]. The fused mutual model is then disbursed back to the edge nodes, updating the previous one.

Delving deeper into the FL process, the central server disseminates an initial global model w_{global}^0 along with metadata about the training procedure to a federated population of $P_f \geq 1$ nodes. Each node holds a set of local data $\mathcal{D}_p$, with $p = 1, 2, .., P_f$, and a local model $w_{local,0}^p$. After transforming each node's dataset to $\tilde{\mathcal{D}}_p$ using Balanced-MixUp, the distributed models are then trained on the transformed datasets, and the model weights w_{global}^e are retrieved by the central server to be fused utilizing the Federated Averaging algorithm. Here $e = 1, 2, ..., E_{FL}$ refers to the current communication round, and E_{FL} is the total number of communication rounds. After each communication round, a new global model w_{global}^e [16] containing the newly collected knowledge is produced based on:

$$w_{global}^e = \frac{1}{\sum_{p=1}^{P_f} \tilde{\mathcal{D}}_p} \sum_{p=1}^{P_f} \tilde{\mathcal{D}}_p w_{local,e}^p \tag{2}$$

where, w^e_{global} is the global model on the e_{th} communication round and $w^p_{local,e}$ is the p-th remote model at that round.

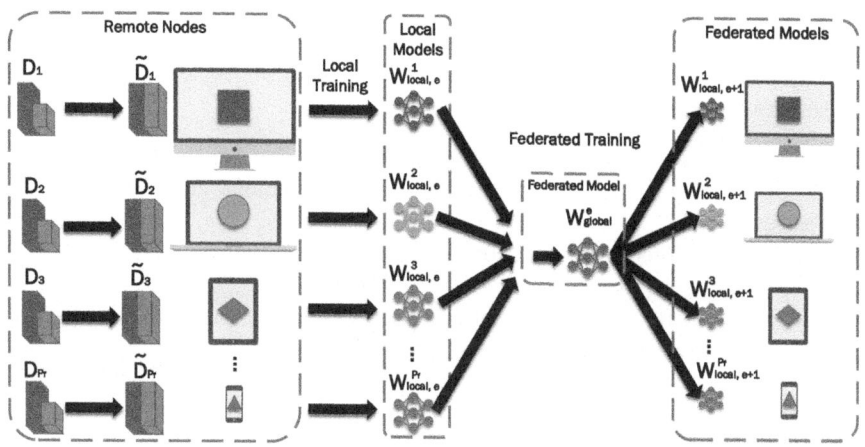

Fig. 1. Model training process including employing Balanced-Mixup to deal with class-imbalance and training in a federated learning setting.

4   Experimental Results

4.1   Experimental Setting

Regarding imbalanced learning evaluation, in each of the following experiments, apart from Balanced-MixUp, denoted as *Bal-MixUp*, standard MixUp, denoted as *MixUp*, and training without any data regularization, denoted as *No MixUp*, are also examined for comparison purposes. Additionally, the advantages of leveraging a FL approach, denoted as *FL* in subsequent experiments, are demonstrated by comparing the relevant results with those obtained in a local training setting, denoted as *Local*. To ensure a fair comparison among these methods, we use the same multilayer perceptron (MLP) network model consisting of two hidden layers with 128 neurons per layer. The models are optimized using Adam [9], and the batch size is set to 24. For *No MixUp* and *MixUp*, we apply a learning rate of 0.004, while for *Bal-MixUp* the learning rate is set to 0.034. For *MixUp*, optimal results are obtained for $\alpha = 0.1$, while for *Bal-MixUp* optimal performance is achieved with $\alpha = 0.3$. Finally, in the local training scenario, each model is trained for 100 epochs. In the FL scenario, we set the number of communication rounds to 5. However, to ensure a fair comparison between the two scenarios, the number of local epochs in the FL scenario is reduced to 20 so that the number of minibatch gradient calculations remains the same across both settings.

4.2   Datasets

For the following experiments, four different tabular datasets related to cardiovascular disease prediction are examined. Specifically, these data represent
different patients' records, and the problem is formulated as a binary classification task where the goal is to predict whether a given patient will suffer from
cardiovascular disease after 10 years. For all datasets, an 80/20 train-test split
ratio was used. The specific datasets are:

- Framingham [1]: Consists of 4240 health record samples from different
  patients, of which 15.19% have suffered from cardiovascular disease after
  10 years.
- Cleveland [6]: Consists of 282 records from different patients, with 44.33%
  suffering from cardiovascular disease after 10 years.
- Long Beach [6]: It contains 200 samples, and 74.5% of them are classified as
  suffering from cardiovascular disease after 10 years.
- Switzerland [6]: It consists of 123 different patient samples, of which 95.5%
  have been diagnosed with cardiovascular disease after 10 years.

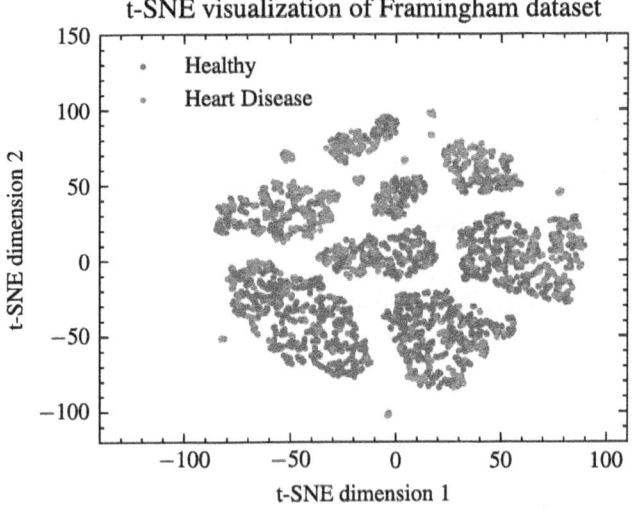

Fig. 2. Two-dimensional t-SNE representations of Framingham's samples.

Overall, it is evident that all examined datasets are small and demonstrate high
class-imbalance, rendering model training in them a nontrivial task. The difficulty of training efficient models in these datasets is also illustrated in Fig. 2,
which shows that there is no clear decision boundary for the t-SNE representations of Framingham's samples. Additionally, while all four of the aforementioned
datasets contain tabular data, including demographic and behavioral patient

characteristics as well as patients' medical history and current medical conditions, their included features are not identical. Consequently, to allow their utilization in a homogeneous FL setting, we only consider a subset of 10 features available in all four datasets. Table 1 contains a short overview of these features. Finally, before being used for training and evaluation, all features are normalized and mean value interpolation is used to fill any missing values.

Table 1. Description of the shared features across the examined datasets.

Feature	Type	Description
age	Continuous	Patient age
male	Binary	Patient gender
hyp	Binary	Patient suffers from hypertension
smoker	Binary	Patient is a smoker
cigsperday	Continuous	Number of cigarettes smoked per day
diabetes	Binary	Patient has diabetes
chol	Continuous	Total cholesterol level
heartRate	Continuous	Patient heart rate
sysBP	Continuous	Systolic blood pressure
diaBP	Continuous	Diastolic blood pressure

4.3   Evaluation Metrics

Since the problem at hand is formulated as a binary classification task, the following metrics have been leveraged to evaluate model performance:

- **Binary Cross-Entropy:** It is used as the loss that is minimized during training, but we also report its values during model evaluation. It is formulated as:

$$\mathcal{L}_{BCE} = -\frac{1}{N} \sum_{i=1}^{N} (y_i \log(\hat{y}_i) + (1 - y_i) \log(1 - \hat{y}_i)) \tag{3}$$

  where y_i are the true and $\hat{y}_i$ are the predicted values for N test data points.
- **Accuracy:** Accuracy refers to the fraction of correct model predictions over all predictions made. Given a confusion matrix containing the number of True Positive (TP), True Negative (TN), False Positive (FP), and False Negative (FN) values, accuracy (Acc) can be formulated as:

$$Acc = \frac{TP + TN}{TP + TN + FP + FN} \tag{4}$$

– **F-Score:** It is defined as the harmonic mean between the model's precision and recall, consolidating and striking a balance between these two metrics. It can also be formulated as:

$$F\text{-}Score = \frac{2TP}{2TP + FP + FN} \tag{5}$$

It is worth noting that due to the high class-imbalance that discerns the examined datasets, *Acc.* can lead to misleading results. Consequently, our primary focus is towards models that achieve higher *F-Score* values, which is inherently less biased under class-imbalance.

Table 2. Model performance metrics for each dataset in the local training and federated learning setting.

Dataset	Model	Local			FL, 5 rounds		
		Loss	Acc	F-Score	Loss	Acc	F-Score
Framingham	No MixUp	0.408	84.52	50.63	**0.396**	**84.64**	45.84
	MixUp ($\alpha = 0.1$)	**0.402**	**84.76**	47.38	0.398	**84.64**	49.41
	Bal-MixUp ($\alpha = 0.3$)	0.585	69.52	**56.95**	0.537	74.05	**59.08**
Cleveland	No MixUp	0.720	62.50	61.90	0.670	54.17	35.14
	MixUp ($\alpha = 0.1$)	0.581	**72.92**	**72.62**	0.632	58.33	49.58
	Bal-MixUp ($\alpha = 0.3$)	**0.560**	66.67	66.61	**0.582**	**70.83**	**70.78**
Long Beach	No MixUp	0.685	62.50	46.93	0.845	20.83	17.24
	MixUp ($\alpha = 0.1$)	**0.623**	66.67	49.47	0.720	50.00	48.57
	Bal-MixUp ($\alpha = 0.3$)	0.730	**75.00**	**69.75**	**0.555**	**79.17**	**70.52**
Switzerland	No MixUp	0.696	**83.33**	45.45	0.851	12.50	11.11
	MixUp ($\alpha = 0.1$)	**0.635**	**83.33**	45.45	0.729	45.83	40.80
	Bal-MixUp ($\alpha = 0.3$)	0.665	70.83	41.46	**0.440**	**91.67**	**72.73**

4.4   Experimental Results

Main Results. Table 2 shows the performance results of the three examined models for both local and FL settings in each dataset. Initially, it is worth noting that the *Loss* and *Acc.* values fail to provide a clear view of which model performs best, especially in the local setting where, depending on the dataset, optimal results are either obtained using *MixUp* or *Bal-MixUp*. However, using a data regularization technique in all four datasets leads to better or at least equivalent results compared to *No-MixUp*. This is also true for *F-Score* in the local training setting. In the federated setting, it is evident that *Bal-MixUp* outperforms all other methods, demonstrating the best *F-Score* in all four datasets. Although *Bal-MixUp*'s *Loss* and *Acc.* are worse than those of the other two models for the Framingham dataset, these values can be misleading due to the high class-imbalance. As a result, *F-Score* is used as a more reliable performance indicator. Additionally, when moving to the FL setting, while *No MixUp* and *MixUp* show worse *F-Score* performance, *Bal-MixUp*'s performance is improved, showing a 2.13% improvement for Framingham, 4.17% for Cleveland, 0.77% for Long Beach, and 31.27% for Switzerland. Overall, it is clear that the combination of using data regularization techniques, especially when dealing with high class-imbalance, as in *Bal-MixUp*, as well as leveraging additional data during training, as in the case of FL, can improve overall performance in all datasets involved.

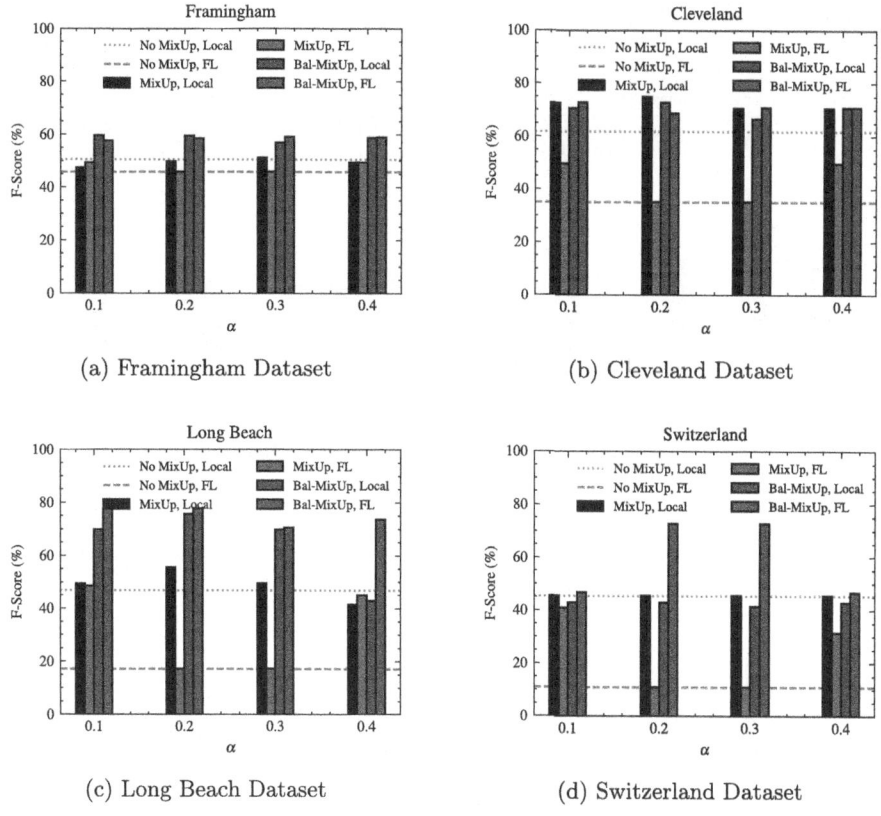

Fig. 3. F-Score of examined methods for varying values of α in each dataset.

Effect of Data Regularization. In general, the α hyperparameter used in *MixUp* and *Bal-MixUp* influences the shape of the Beta distribution from which the λ coefficients in (1) are obtained, with lower α values leading to synthetic samples that are more likely to be close to the original samples used. Following [5,21] we test different α values in the range of [0.1, 0.4]. Figure 3 illustrates the effect of α on model performance in the local and FL setting. In the Framingham and Long Beach datasets, *Bal-MixUp* consistently outperforms all other methods. As for the Switzerland dataset, while *Bal-MixUp, FL* still outperforms all other methods, *Bal-MixUp, Local*'s performance is not optimal, pinpointing the need for leveraging additional data in an FL setting, especially when data is scarce. Finally, in the Cleveland dataset, the best results are achieved using *MixUp, Local*. However, its performance on the rest of the datasets is generally worse compared to *Bal-MixUp*. On the other hand, *Bal-MixUp*'s performance in the Cleveland dataset is still on par compared to *MixUp*. Consequently, *Bal-MixUp* demonstrates the best overall performance irrespective of the α value chosen.

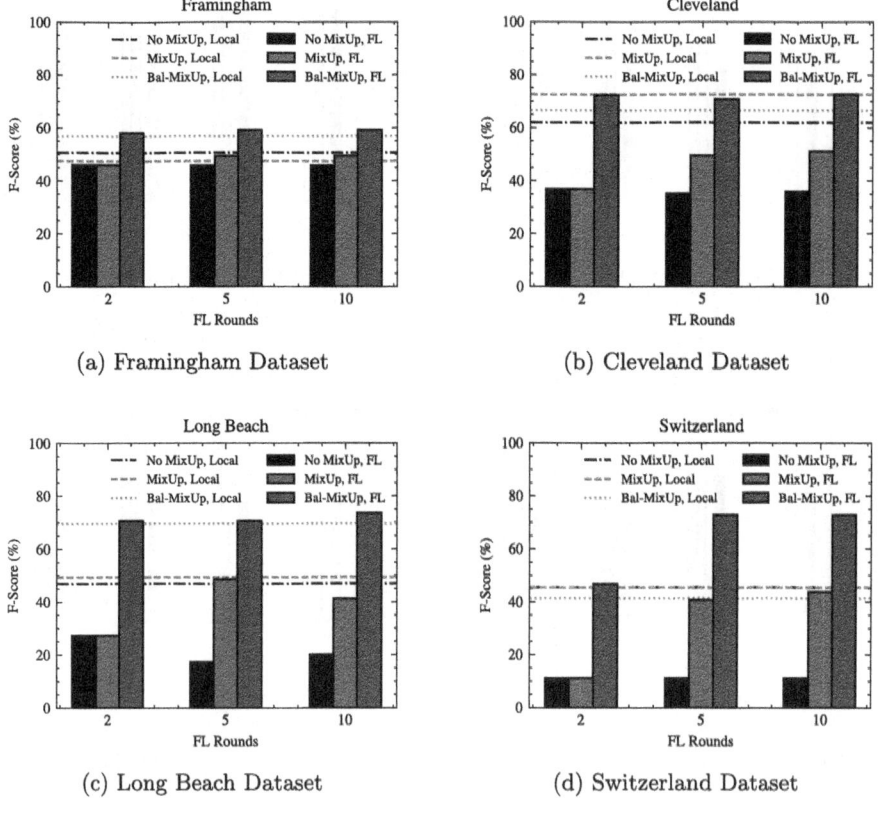

(a) Framingham Dataset

(b) Cleveland Dataset

(c) Long Beach Dataset

(d) Switzerland Dataset

Fig. 4. F-Score of examined methods for a varying number of communication rounds in each dataset.

Effect of Federated Learning. While increasing the number of communication rounds in the FL setting can lead to better generalization performance across all clients, it can also lead to increased communication overhead, negatively impacting the model's time efficiency. In this set of experiments, we examine how varying the number of communication rounds in FL affects performance. To ensure a fair comparison across different numbers of communication rounds, we keep the number of gradient calculations constant across all settings by setting $E_{FL} \times E_{local} = 100$, where E_{FL} is the number of communication rounds and E_{local} is the number of local epochs within each round. Figure 4 illustrates the F-Score achieved by each method for 2, 5, and 10 communication rounds. Initially, *Bal-MixUp* outperforms all other methods in all datasets except Cleveland. However, its performance is still on par with the best-performing model, *MixUp, Local.* Additionally, *Bal-MixUp* exhibits robustness in its performance even when the number of communication rounds is reduced, which is desirable as it allows reducing the communication rounds without negatively impacting the model's performance. However, this is not true for the rest of the models, which are more sensitive to this hyperparameter. Specifically, *MixUp*'s performance generally increases when increasing the number of communication rounds. However, it still underperforms compared to *Bal-MixUp*. Overall, the positive impact of the synergies between imbalanced learning via data regularization and FL is also manifest in this setting by the superior performance of the *Bal-MixUp* model.

5 Conclusions

One of the most challenging points when deploying ML models in healthcare domain applications is dealing with the imbalance that typically characterizes medical data. At the same time, the need to ensure data privacy of sensitive patient information has led to the increased utilization of FL approaches in this domain. One medical application where meeting both these requirements is crucial is cardiovascular disease prediction. In this paper, we propose employing Balanced-MixUp, a data regularization method suitable for dealing with class-imbalance, in a FL setting that enforces data privacy by design for cardiovascular disease prediction. The proposed method was evaluated in a realistic setting with multiple nodes, outperforming all methods that failed to address both imbalanced and FL needs. Finally, further experiments were conducted to demonstrate the proposed method's robustness under different hyperparameter values and resource efficiency under limited resource allocation in the federated setting.

Acknowledgments. This project has received funding from the European Union's Horizon Europe research and innovation programme under grant agreement No. 101095435 (REALM).

Disclosure of Interests. The authors have no competing interests to declare that are relevant to the content of this article.

References

1. Bhardwaj, A.: Framingham heart study dataset (2022). https://doi.org/10.34740/KAGGLE/DSV/3493583
2. Bonawitz, K., et al.: Towards federated learning at scale: System design (02 2019)
3. Chou, H.-P., Chang, S.-C., Pan, J.-Y., Wei, W., Juan, D.-C.: Remix: rebalanced mixup. In: Bartoli, A., Fusiello, A. (eds.) Computer Vision – ECCV 2020 Workshops: Glasgow, UK, August 23–28, 2020, Proceedings, Part VI, pp. 95–110. Springer International Publishing, Cham (2020). https://doi.org/10.1007/978-3-030-65414-6_9
4. El-Bialy, R., Salamay, M.A., Karam, O.H., Khalifa, M.E.: Feature analysis of coronary artery heart disease data sets. Proc. Comput. Sci. **65**, 459–468 (2015)
5. Galdran, A., Carneiro, G., González Ballester, M.A.: Balanced-mixup for highly imbalanced medical image classification. In: de Bruijne, M., Cattin, P.C., Cotin, S., Padoy, N., Speidel, S., Zheng, Y., Essert, C. (eds.) Medical Image Computing and Computer Assisted Intervention – MICCAI 2021: 24th International Conference, Strasbourg, France, September 27 – October 1, 2021, Proceedings, Part V, pp. 323–333. Springer International Publishing, Cham (2021). https://doi.org/10.1007/978-3-030-87240-3_31
6. Janosi, A., Steinbrunn, W., Pfisterer, M., Detrano, R.: Heart Disease. UCI Machine Learning Repository (1988). https://doi.org/10.24432/C52P4X
7. Khan, M.A., et al.: Asynchronous federated learning for improved cardiovascular disease prediction using artificial intelligence. Diagnostics **13**(14) (2023)
8. Khan, S.H., Hayat, M., Bennamoun, M., Sohel, F.A., Togneri, R.: Cost-sensitive learning of deep feature representations from imbalanced data. IEEE Trans. Neural Netw. Learn. Syst. **29**(8), 3573–3587 (2017)
9. Kingma, D.P., Ba, J.: Adam: A method for stochastic optimization. arXiv preprint arXiv:1412.6980 (2014)
10. Mazurowski, M.A., Habas, P.A., Zurada, J.M., Lo, J.Y., Baker, J.A., Tourassi, G.D.: Training neural network classifiers for medical decision making: the effects of imbalanced datasets on classification performance. Neural Netw. **21**(2–3), 427–436 (2008)
11. McMahan, B., Moore, E., Ramage, D., Hampson, S., y Arcas, B.A.: Communication-efficient learning of deep networks from decentralized data. In: Artificial Intelligence and Statistics, pp. 1273–1282. PMLR (2017)
12. Miao, L., Guo, X., Abbas, H.T., Qaraqe, K.A., Abbasi, Q.H.: Using machine learning to predict the future development of disease. In: 2020 International Conference on UK-China Emerging Technologies (UCET), pp. 1–4. IEEE (2020)
13. Mienye, I.D., Sun, Y., Wang, Z.: An improved ensemble learning approach for the prediction of heart disease risk. Inform. Med. Unlocked **20**, 100402 (2020)
14. Rahim, A., Rasheed, Y., Azam, F., Anwar, M.W., Rahim, M.A., Muzaffar, A.W.: An integrated machine learning framework for effective prediction of cardiovascular diseases. IEEE Access **9**, 106575–106588 (2021)
15. Rustamov, Z., Rustamov, J., Sultana, M.S., Ywei, J., Balakrishnan, V., Zaki, N.: Cardiovascular disease prediction using ensemble learning techniques: a stacking approach. In: 2023 19th IEEE International Colloquium on Signal Processing and Its Applications (CSPA), pp. 93–98. IEEE (2023)

16. Siniosoglou, I., Argyriou, V., Lagkas, T., Moscholios, I., Fragulis, G., Sarigiannidis, P.: Unsupervised bias evaluation of dnns in non-iid federated learning through latent micro-manifolds. In: IEEE INFOCOM 2022 - IEEE Conference on Computer Communications Workshops (INFOCOM WKSHPS), pp. 1–6 (2022), https://doi.org/10.1109/INFOCOMWKSHPS54753.2022.9798157

17. Su, Y., Huang, C., Zhu, W., Lyu, X., Ji, F.: Multi-party diabetes mellitus risk prediction based on secure federated learning. Biomed. Signal Process. Control **85**, 104881 (2023). https://doi.org/10.1016/j.bspc.2023.104881

18. Wang, H., Yurochkin, M., Sun, Y., Papailiopoulos, D., Khazaeni, Y.: Federated learning with matched averaging (2020)

19. Yaqoob, M.M., Nazir, M., Khan, M.A., Qureshi, S., Al-Rasheed, A.: Hybrid classifier-based federated learning in health service providers for cardiovascular disease prediction. Appl. Sci. **13**(3) (2023). https://doi.org/10.3390/app13031911

20. Yaqoob, M.M., et al.: Modified artificial bee colony based feature optimized federated learning for heart disease diagnosis in healthcare. Appl. Sci. **12**(23) (2022). https://doi.org/10.3390/app122312080

21. Zhang, H., Cisse, M., Dauphin, Y.N., Lopez-Paz, D.: mixup: beyond empirical risk minimization. arXiv preprint arXiv:1710.09412 (2017)

22. Zhou, Z.H., Liu, X.Y.: Training cost-sensitive neural networks with methods addressing the class imbalance problem. IEEE Trans. Knowl. Data Eng. **18**(1), 63–77 (2005)

Intelligent Multi-document Summarisation for Extracting Insights on Racial Inequalities from Maternity Incident Investigation Reports

Georgina Cosma[1]([✉]), Mohit Kumar Singh[1], Patrick Waterson[2], Gyuchan Thomas Jun[2], and Jonathan Back[3]

[1] Department of Computer Science, School of Science, Loughborough University, Loughborough, UK
g.cosma@lboro.ac.uk
[2] School of Design and Creating Arts, Loughborough University, Loughborough, UK
[3] Health Services Safety Investigations Body (HSSIB), Poole, UK

Abstract. In healthcare, thousands of safety incidents occur every year, but learning from these incidents is not effectively aggregated. Analysing incident reports using AI could uncover critical insights to prevent harm by identifying recurring patterns and contributing factors. To aggregate and extract valuable information, natural language processing (NLP) and machine learning techniques can be employed to summarise and mine unstructured data, potentially surfacing systemic issues and priority areas for improvement. This paper presents I-SIRch:CS, a framework designed to facilitate the aggregation and analysis of safety incident reports while ensuring traceability throughout the process. The framework integrates concept annotation using the Safety Intelligence Research (SIRch) taxonomy with clustering, summarisation, and analysis capabilities. Utilising a dataset of 188 anonymised maternity investigation reports annotated with 27 SIRch human factors concepts, I-SIRch:CS groups the annotated sentences into clusters using sentence embeddings and k-means clustering, maintaining traceability via file and sentence IDs. Summaries are generated for each cluster using offline state-of-the-art abstractive summarisation models (BART, DistilBART, T5), which are evaluated and compared using metrics assessing summary quality attributes. The generated summaries are linked back to the original file and sentence IDs, ensuring traceability and allowing for verification of the summarised information. Results demonstrate BART's strengths in creating informative and concise summaries.

Keywords: Dynamic clustering · Abstractive summarisation · healthcare

1 Introduction

In recent years, deep learning (DL) and natural language processing (NLP) models have demonstrated immense potential for automatically analysing and summarising textual data across application areas. Within the healthcare domain,

© The Author(s), under exclusive license to Springer Nature Switzerland AG 2024
X. Xie et al. (Eds.): AIiH 2024, LNCS 14976, pp. 316–329, 2024.
https://doi.org/10.1007/978-3-031-67285-9_23

key use cases include generating concise summaries of electronic health records (EHRs) to accelerate access to patient histories, extracting key findings from the latest medical literature to keep professionals informed of advancements, and simplifying health education content into more readable materials for patient consumption. However, applying DL in sensitive domains like healthcare also introduces confidentiality, privacy, and ethical considerations which demand accurate yet traceable model behaviours that respect patient data sensitivity. To address the ethical considerations and data privacy requirements when applying deep learning models to sensitive healthcare data, it is crucial to ensure that any datasets used are fully anonymised before analysis or modelling, with all personally identifiable information removed from the outset.

Our prior work saw the development of the Intelligence-Safety Intelligence Research (I-SIRch) framework/tool [10], which utilises multi-label text annotation with the Safety Intelligence Research (SIRch) human factors taxonomy to systematically categorise contributing factors in adverse maternal care incidents. Trained on a corpus of real (anonymised) and tested on real and synthetically generated maternity investigation reports from UK cases, I-SIRch demonstrated robust performance across numerous evaluation metrics, including recall, precision, and balanced accuracy [10]. Our research represented an important step towards utilising advanced NLP techniques to enhance patient safety and address care quality gaps, especially within maternal health across different demographics. This paper aims to advance the I-SIRch framework [10] by proposing an extended I-SIRch:CS[1] system with robust multi-document summarisation capabilities to effectively analyse maternal incident investigation reports across various dimensions, including generating concise yet sufficiently informative summaries, ensuring complete traceability back to source data, and facilitating comparative equity evaluations by constructing separate summaries across ethnic groups to identify any care quality disparities underlying adverse incidents.

2   Related Work

Models including Long Short-Term Memory (LSTM) networks and Transformer-based architectures have been at the forefront, leveraging their ability to understand context and sequence in texts. Specifically, the use of pretrained models such as BERT (Bidirectional Encoder Representations from Transformers) and its adaptations in the medical domain (e.g., BioBERT, ClinicalBERT) have demonstrated promising results in improving the accuracy and relevance of summaries. For instance, LSTM and Transformer models have been applied to summarise patient Electronic Health Records (EHRs), extracting critical information that can aid in diagnosis, treatment planning, and patient monitoring [5,6,11,13,14]. These summaries provide a comprehensive view of a patient's medical history, current condition, and potential risks, distilled into a format that is easily accessible to healthcare providers. The introduction of models such as BERT (Bidirectional Encoder Representations from Transformers) [1] and

---

[1] https://github.com/gcosma/I-SIRchpapers.

GPT (Generative Pretrained Transformer) [7] marked a significant milestone in NLP. These models have shown remarkable success in various NLP tasks, including text summarisation. Their ability to capture deep contextual relationships within text makes them particularly suited for summarising complex healthcare documents. One notable advancement is the adaptation of these models for domain-specific tasks. For instance, BioBERT [3] and ClinicalBERT [2] have been fine-tuned from BERT for biomedical and clinical text processing, respectively, showing improved performance in tasks such as disease classification and patient information summarisation. Moreover, transformer-based models like BART (Bidirectional and Auto-Regressive Transformers) [4] and T5 (Text-to-Text Transfer Transformer) [8] have been utilised for both extractive and abstractive summarisation. BART, in particular, has been effective in generating coherent summaries of medical research articles by rephrasing and condensing the original text. While the effectiveness of these models is well-documented, their computational demands pose challenges, particularly in real-time healthcare applications. This has led to the development of more efficient variants, such as DistilBERT [9] and MiniLM [12], which maintain a balance between performance and computational efficiency. These models enable the deployment of advanced NLP techniques in resource-constrained environments, such as mobile health applications and low-resource organisations.

3   I-SIRch:CS Framework

We propose an automated system for summarising text data, capable of clustering sentences by similarity, determining the best number of clusters, and generating concise summaries and keywords for each cluster. This process transforms raw text into structured, actionable insights. We utilised offline generative models to ensure patient confidentiality by anonymising and synthesising data, preserving the integrity of insights while safeguarding personal information.

Algorithm (1) provides the text clustering and summarisation process. The algorithm takes as input a set of sentences, denoted mathematically as set S, along with an associated set of labels (a.k.a concepts) $\mathcal{L}$ that categorises the sentences. It also requires two machine learning models - a clustering model M_c and a pretrained summarisation model M_s. In the first stage, the algorithm groups the input sentences by their labels (i.e. concepts) in $\mathcal{L}$. For each label $l \in \mathcal{L}$, it extracts the subset of sentences S_l that have that label value l assigned. Next, it applies the clustering model M_c to embed the sentences in a vector space and determine an optimal number of clusters based on the elbow method. The sentences with the same label l are then clustered into these topics, denoted by $\{C_1, C_2, \ldots, C_k\}$. The second stage is a summary and evaluation loop over the clusters. For each cluster C_i covering a topic, the sentences are concatenated into a single text excerpt T_i. This is passed into the summarisation model M_s to generate a summary text S_i. Additional metadata including a heading H_i and the sentence IDs used are also extracted for summary S_i. Evaluation metrics are then calculated for summary S_i - including quantification of the diversity,

---

Algorithm 1. I-SIRch: CS Text clustering and summarisation

    Input:
      Set of sentences S with labels L
      Clustering model M_c
      Summarisation model M_s
1: **for** each label $l \in L$ **do**
2:     Filter S to get subset S_l with label l
3:     Embed sentences in S_l using M_c getting embeddings E_l
4:     Determine optimal clusters k using elbow method on E_l
5:     Cluster S_l into k clusters $\{C_1, \ldots, C_k\}$ using k-means on E_l
6: **end for**
7: **for** each cluster C_i **do**
8:     Concatenate sentences in C_i into text T_i
9:     Generate summary S_i by applying M_s to T_i
10:    Generate heading H_i by applying M_s to T_i
11:    Store sentence IDs used in S_i as ID_i
12: **end for**
13: **Outputs:**
14: Summaries S_i and corresponding Headings H_i for each summary
15: Sentence IDs ID_i used in each summary
16: Evaluation metrics for each summary

---

relevance, coverage, coherence, conciseness, and readability. These metrics are appended to a master output list. In the end, the full pipeline outputs: the set of summaries S_i for each topic cluster; the headings H_i; sentence IDs ID_i used; and evaluation metrics on the different quality attributes for each summary. The algorithm thus performs multi-document summarisation guided by data labels, with integrated quantitative assessment.

4 Methodology

4.1 Dataset of Maternity Incident Investigation Reports

The Healthcare Services Safety Investigation Branch (HSSIB) provided a random set of 188 anonymised investigation reports describing adverse maternity incidents. The reports were written between 2019 to 2022. The number of reports for each year is as follows: 4 reports in 2019, 115 reports in 2020, 42 reports in 2021, and 27 reports in 2022. Ethnicity was provided for 76 reports.

4.2 Experiment Methodology

The I-SIRch:CS framework is presented in Fig. 1 and its components are described as follows. **Healthcare reports repository:** The I-SIRch tool is used for loading, cleaning, and preparing reports. During processing, the tool generates a text file in CSV format that includes File IDs, Sentence IDs, sentences, and concepts derived from the SIRch taxonomy. This phase involves

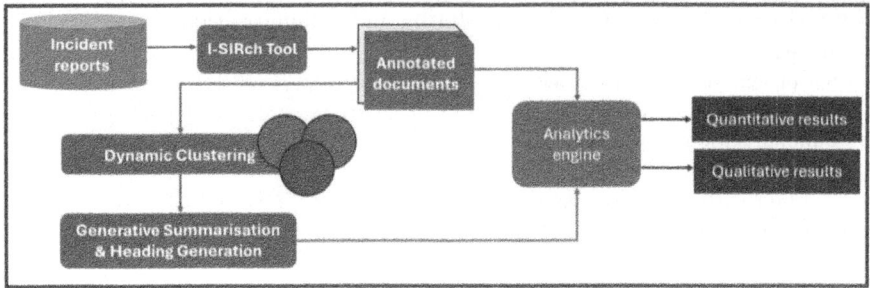

Fig. 1. I-SIRch:CS pipeline. Shows how the I-SIRch tool has been extended to include clustering and summarisation capabilities analysing intelligence from maternity incidence investigation reports.

cleaning the files by selecting particular sentences from each report, specifically targeting those with negative connotations, references to physical characteristics, and mentions of medication names associated with dispensing. These selected sentences are annotated according to the SIRch taxonomy and aggregated into a CSV file for subsequent clustering and summarisation tasks. Table 1 shows the list of SIRch concepts with the number of sentences per concept shown in brackets. **Dynamic clustering:** Employs the `all-MiniLM-L6-v2` Sentence-Transformer model for sentence embeddings and the elbow method with KMeans for clustering. This process groups text data into semantically similar clusters, maintaining traceability via file and sentence IDs. **Generative summarisation and heading generation:** Selects from predefined offline models (e.g., BART, T5, DistilBART) for summarisation. Keywords extracted by KeyBERT for headings ensure summaries are informative and traceable to original file and sentence IDs. **Analytics engine (Qualitative results):** Outputs include the textual summaries and their corresponding topic headings, where each summary is linked to each file and sentence ID. **Analytics engine (Quantitative results):** Outputs include a detailed CSV report with analysis on summarisation models, clustering, generated headings, summaries, and evaluation metrics, ensuring explainability through file and sentence ID traceability. **Batch processing and process automation:** The framework's scalable design allows for automated batch processing, enhancing the system's ability to handle large datasets efficiently, with a focus on traceability and organisation.

4.3   Methods

We employed the following transformer-based architectures that have been fine-tuned for summarisation, and which have demonstrated their capability to address complex NLP challenges, particularly in healthcare. **Sentence Transformers ('all-MiniLM-L6-v2'):** A compact model that generates semantically meaningful sentence embeddings suitable for semantic search, clustering and summarisation, balancing performance with computational efficiency. **BART**

Table 1. ID, concept and number of sentences per concept. Total sentences: 3760.

ID	Concept	Index	Label
1	Acuity (54)	2	Antenatal (69)
3	Assessment, investigation, testing, screening (381)	4	COVID (142)
5	Care Planning (132)	6	Communication factor (477)
7	Decision error (169)	8	Dispensing, administering (62)
9	Documentation (168)	10	Escalation/referral factor (158)
11	Guidance factor (42)	12	Interpretation (197)
13	Language barrier (30)	14	Local guidance (88)
15	Monitoring (118)	16	National and local guidance (80)
17	National guidance (169)	18	Obstetric review (147)
19	Physical characteristics (320)	20	Physical layout and Environment (35)
21	Psychological characteristics (54)	22	Risk assessment (94)
23	Situation awareness (77)	24	Slip or lapse (188)
25	Teamworking (530)	26	Technologies and Tools-issues (112)
27	Training and education (40)		

('**facebook/bart-large-cnn**'): A transformer model pretrained for generation tasks, including summarisation. The 'bart-large-cnn' variant excels at creating coherent and concise summaries, optimised for tasks requiring detailed summary outputs. **T5** ('**t5-small**'): Adapts the text-to-text approach, treating all NLP tasks as such. The 't5-small' version offers a balance between size, speed, and quality, ideal for diverse summarisation needs. **DistilBART** ('**sshleifer /distilbart-cnn-12-6**'): A lighter, faster distilled version of BART, maintaining robust summarisation capabilities. Optimised for efficiency, it provides a viable alternative to its parent model for summarisation tasks.

4.4 Evaluation Metrics

Several metrics have been used to assess different aspects of summarisation quality, including diversity, relevance, coverage, coherence, conciseness, and readability. Each metric provides insights into how well the summarisation process captures and conveys the essential information from the original text. Higher values across these metrics indicate better summarisation model performance in producing summaries that are diverse, relevant, comprehensive, logical, concise and readable.

Diversity measures the variety of vocabulary used in the summary. It is calculated as the ratio of unique words to the total number of words in the summary.

$$\text{Diversity} = \frac{\text{Number of Unique Words}}{\text{Total Number of Words}} \qquad (1)$$

Relevance assesses the similarity between the original text and its summary. Cosine similarity between the vector representations of the original text and the summary is often used for this purpose.

$$\text{Relevance} = \cos(\theta) = \frac{\mathbf{A} \cdot \mathbf{B}}{\|\mathbf{A}\| \|\mathbf{B}\|} \tag{2}$$

where $\mathbf{A}$ and $\mathbf{B}$ are the vector representations of the original text and the summary, respectively.

Coverage evaluates the extent to which the summary captures the key concepts of the original text. It can be quantified by the proportion of original text tokens (or concepts) that appear in the summary.

$$\text{Coverage} = \frac{\text{Number of Unique Tokens in Both Summary and Original Text}}{\text{Number of Unique Tokens in Original Text}} \tag{3}$$

Coherence measures the logical flow and connection between sentences within the summary. While more challenging to quantify, coherence can be assessed by evaluating sentence embeddings' similarity in sequence.

$$\text{Coherence} = \frac{1}{N-1} \sum_{i=1}^{N-1} \cos(\theta_{i,i+1}) \tag{4}$$

where N is the number of sentences in the summary, and $\cos(\theta_{i,i+1})$ is the cosine similarity between consecutive sentence embeddings.

Conciseness indicates the brevity of the summary. It can be inversely related to the summary's length, encouraging summaries that convey information efficiently.

$$\text{Conciseness} = \frac{1}{\text{Word Count of Summary}} \tag{5}$$

Readability measures how easy it is to understand the summary. The Flesch Reading Ease score is a common metric, calculated as follows:

$$\text{Readability} = 206.835 - 1.015 \left(\frac{\text{Total Words}}{\text{Total Sentences}} \right) - 84.6 \left(\frac{\text{Total Syllables}}{\text{Total Words}} \right) \tag{6}$$

5   Results

The IDs of sentences assigned to each cluster are tracked and used for generating the summary of that cluster. Hence, all sentences grouped into a specific cluster are considered in the summarisation process. However, the actual summary may not incorporate these sentences verbatim. Instead, the summary provides a condensed version that captures the main points from these sentences. An analysis of the summaries is presented below.

5.1 Performance Comparison of Summarisation Methods

Table 2 provides the results when comparing the summarisation models using the evaluation metrics defined in Sect. 4.4. Figure 2 provides an overview of the performance and variability of each model across concepts. Among the models, BART achieves the best overall performance and generalisation. BART creates relevant and coherent summaries that maximise vocabulary diversity, and it attains this reliable performance as evidenced by low standard deviations in key metrics like diversity, relevance, and coherence. Below is a summary of the results shown in Table 2. **Diversity:** BART's diversity score is 0.806±0.058 standard deviation, indicating its summaries incorporate the richest unique vocabulary with low variability run-to-run. **Relevance:** BART has highest relevance at 0.922 ± 0.015. This shows its summaries strongly preserve source semantics with minimal fluctuation. **Coverage:** All models exhibit low coverage of $\sim 0.07 \pm 0.03$ standard deviations because summaries significantly condense full text. **Coherence:** BART's scores 0.794 ± 0.022 coherence, meaning summary sentences interrelate accurately. This combination enables easy comprehension. **Conciseness:** The models achieve similar conciseness ($\sim 0.02 \pm 0.004$), quantifying the summary brevity. **Readability:** T5-small tops at 190.288 ± 5.799 in linguistic simplicity. But BART nearly matches at 189.148 ± 5.863.

Table 2. Evaluation metrics for summarisation models

Metric	BART	DistilBART	T5-small
Diversity Score	0.806 ± 0.058	0.770 ± 0.057	0.771 ± 0.059
Relevance	0.922 ± 0.015	0.709 ± 0.028	0.818 ± 0.035
Coverage	0.070 ± 0.034	0.072 ± 0.034	0.064 ± 0.032
Coherence	0.794 ± 0.022	0.674 ± 0.038	0.670 ± 0.030
Conciseness	0.021 ± 0.004	0.019 ± 0.003	0.022 ± 0.004
Readability	189.148 ± 5.863	186.896 ± 6.253	190.288 ± 5.799

5.2 BART's Summarisation Performance Across Concepts

Figure 3 depicts the performance of BART's summarisation model across each concept. The x-axes show the concept numbers, and these correspond to the IDs found in Table 1. Hence number 1 on the x-axis of Fig. 3(a) corresponds to the Acuity concept that has ID 1 in Table 1.

The areas of strength are: **Relevance:** Across all labels, the model consistently showed high relevance scores, with means above 0.9. This indicates that the model is adept at generating content that is closely related to the given topics. Low standard deviations in relevance scores, such as 0.012 for Acuity and 0.007 for Assessment, investigation, testing, screening, suggest that the model

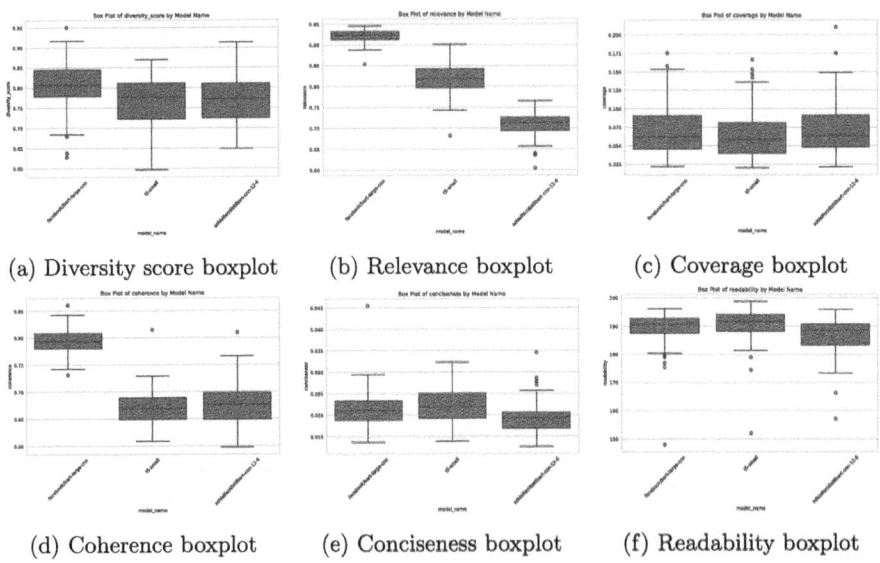

(a) Diversity score boxplot   (b) Relevance boxplot   (c) Coverage boxplot

(d) Coherence boxplot   (e) Conciseness boxplot   (f) Readability boxplot

Fig. 2. Overall comparison of evaluation metrics.

maintains this relevance across different instances reliably. **Coherence:** The model also performed well in terms of coherence, particularly for labels such as COVID, with a mean of 0.836 and Acuity with a mean of 0.809. These scores suggest that the generated text logically flows from one sentence to the next, making it easier for readers to follow the narrative.

The areas for improvement are: **Coverage:** The model struggled with coverage across several labels, notably so for Assessment, investigation, testing, screening, with a mean of 0.03 and a very low standard deviation, indicating consistently narrow topic coverage. This suggests that the model may not fully address all relevant aspects of a topic, possibly omitting important details. **Diversity:** While not as critical as coverage, diversity scores varied more widely across labels, with COVID showing a notably lower mean (0.702) and higher standard deviation (0.079). This indicates that the model's ability to generate varied text differs significantly across topics, which could limit its effectiveness in engaging readers with novel content or perspectives. **Readability:** The readability scores were consistently high across labels, with means around 187 to 192, suggesting the text may be complex and potentially challenging for a general audience to understand. While not a direct measure of performance like relevance or coherence, high readability scores indicate room for improvement in making the content more accessible to a broader audience.

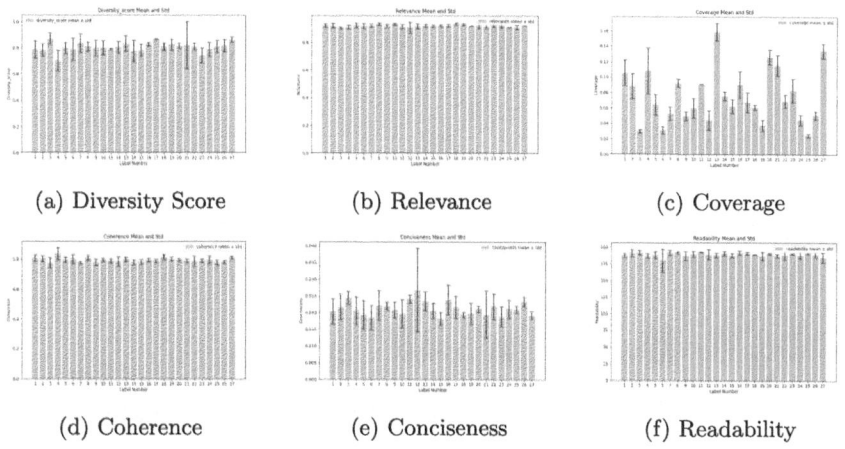

(a) Diversity Score   (b) Relevance   (c) Coverage

(d) Coherence   (e) Conciseness   (f) Readability

Fig. 3. Summary of model evaluation metrics for BART.

Table 3. Average and std. values of metrics by ethnicity when using BART

Metric	Asian	Black	DNR	MB	OW	WB
Diversity	0.67 ± 0.08	0.64 ± 0.07	0.67 ± 0.06	0.69 ± 0.08	0.65 ± 0.04	0.68 ± 0.04
Relevance	0.89 ± 0.18	0.87 ± 0.17	0.95 ± 0.09	0.97 ± 0.04	0.93 ± 0.10	0.40 ± 0.22
Coverage	0.89 ± 0.18	0.87 ± 0.17	0.95 ± 0.09	0.97 ± 0.04	0.93 ± 0.10	0.40 ± 0.22
Coherence	0.46 ± 0.32	0.54 ± 0.29	0.65 ± 0.26	0.63 ± 0.18	0.42 ± 0.27	0.18 ± 0.19
Conciseness	0.01 ± 0.00	0.01 ± 0.00	0.01 ± 0.00	0.01 ± 0.00	0.01 ± 0.00	0.01 ± 0.00
Readability	21.54 ± 5.12	17.53 ± 2.54	19.23 ± 3.37	16.08 ± 0.59	19.54 ± 3.63	19.62 ± 3.58

5.3   Evaluating Equity in Summaries of Investigation Reports

Table 3 and Fig. 4 present a summary of various evaluation metrics across different ethnic groups: Asian, Black, Data not received (DNR), Mixed Background (MB), Other White (OW), and White British (WB) when using BART.

Diversity: The diversity scores are relatively similar across all ethnicities, ranging from 0.64 to 0.69, with small standard deviations (0.04 to 0.08). This suggests that the BART model generates diverse outputs for all ethnicities. **Relevance and Coverage:** The relevance and coverage scores are identical for each ethnicity, indicating that these metrics are closely related. Asian, Black, DNR, MB, and OW have high scores (0.87 to 0.97) with small standard deviations (0.04 to 0.18), suggesting that the model generates relevant and comprehensive outputs for these ethnicities. However, WB has a lower score (0.40) with a larger standard deviation (0.22), indicating that the model's outputs for this ethnicity may be less relevant and comprehensive. **Coherence:** The coherence scores vary across ethnicities, with DNR and MB having the highest scores (0.65 and 0.63) and moderate standard deviations (0.26 and 0.18). Asian, Black, and OW have lower scores (0.42 to 0.54) with larger standard deviations (0.27 to 0.32), sug-

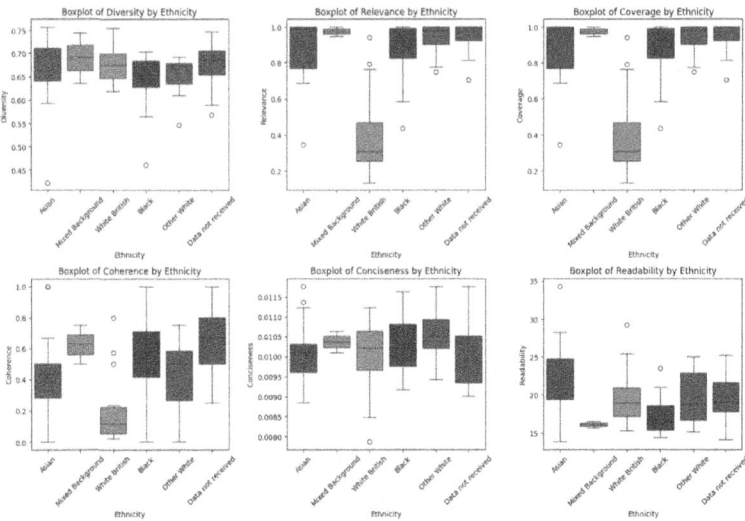

Fig. 4. Results per ethnic group when using BART

gesting that the model's outputs for these ethnicities may be less coherent. WB has the lowest coherence score (0.18) with a small standard deviation (0.19), indicating that the model's outputs for this ethnicity are the least coherent. **Conciseness:** All ethnicities have the same conciseness score (0.01) with no

standard deviation, suggesting that the model generates equally concise outputs for all ethnicities. **Readability:** The readability scores range from 16.08 to 21.54, with standard deviations ranging from 0.59 to 5.12. MB has the lowest

Table 4. Sample summaries from multiple reports for two ethnic groups. Ethnicities cannot be disclosed. Each summary is generated from multiple reports.

Concept	Summary
Communication	**Staff not heard.** Staff voiced their concerns about this decision to the senior obstetrician. They were left feeling that their concerns had not been heard. There was no formal debriefing afterwards, which staff would have valued. The opportunity to share reflections and learning was not completed with all staff involved. The incremental delays caused by finding and allocating staff to the concurrent theatre cases, and communication breakdown within the team further impacted on the DDI
Acuity	**Reviews with seniors did not occur.** The ambulance Trust was experiencing high volumes of 999 calls at the time of a Mother's call. Due to the high acuity on the labour ward the initial decisions were not discussed with the senior clinician. A senior face to face review did not occur until 16:05 h, 2 h and 50 min after the initial recognition of abnormalities of the Baby's heart rate. The abnormal CTG trace from the IOL suite was not reviewed by the senior obstetrician

readability score (16.08) with the smallest standard deviation (0.59), indicating that the model's outputs for this ethnicity are the most readable and consistent. Asian has the highest readability score (21.54) with the largest standard deviation (5.12), suggesting that the model's outputs for this ethnicity are the least readable and have the most variability. In summary, the BART model generates diverse, relevant, and concise outputs for most ethnicities, with some variations in coherence and readability. The model's performance appears to be the weakest for the WB ethnicity, with lower relevance, coverage, and coherence scores. These low scores could be attributed to the sample size and variability of the WB sentences. While the WB group has the most sentences, this does not guarantee better performance. A larger dataset can introduce more variability, making it harder for the model to learn consistent patterns. Table 4 presents two sample summaries (from reports of different ethnic groups) generated by the BART summarisation model.

6 Ethical Risks of Abstractive Summarisation Models

- **Risk of information hallucination and bias amplification:** Abstractive summarisation models like BART, T5, and DistilBART risk generating content not found in the original data and amplifying biases from their training data. **Mitigation:** Diversifying training datasets, implementing debiasing techniques, and cross-referencing with original texts. Regular bias audits and integrating ethical guidelines directly into the training process can enhance accuracy, transparency, and fairness.
- **Risk of inadequate control over content:** Unlike extractive methods, abstractive models generate summaries based on learnt patterns, which can result in misrepresentation or underrepresentation of certain groups or incidents. **Mitigation:** Developing more sophisticated models with embedded ethical and fairness constraints, and employing precise source mapping mechanisms like sentence IDs, can strengthen control and ensure verifiability and trustworthiness of the content generated.
- **Risk in processing sensitive data:** Utilising online LLMs for sensitive data can pose risks of data breaches and privacy violations. **Mitigation:** Switching to offline LLMs lessens these risks but may reduce performance, as it depends on local computing resources. Organisations need to balance security against performance to find an appropriate balance.
- **Sample Size and Variability:** Large datasets, whilst rich in information, present challenges due to variability and the potential inclusion of low-quality data. This complexity hinders a model's ability to learn consistent patterns, adversely affecting summarisation metrics. **Mitigation:** Explore robust data preprocessing techniques to enhance data quality. Utilising machine learning algorithms customised for high variability will enhance consistency and equity in summarisation outcomes across diverse groups.

7   Conclusion

The I-SIRch:CS framework automates the analysis and summarisation of textual data in maternity incident reports, holding significant potential for uncovering critical insights and contributing factors to preventable harm. Future work will prioritise enhancing the framework's traceability capabilities by implementing mechanisms to provide clear links between generated summaries and original reports, allowing for easy verification of accuracy and context. Explainable AI techniques will also be explored to offer insights into how models generate summaries. A key limitation of the I-SIRch:CS framework is the lack of Patient and Public Involvement (PPI) in assessing its outputs. PPI is crucial as it ensures solutions are relevant to patient needs and experiences, potentially improving the framework's summaries and their real-world applicability. Engaging with patients and the public could also increase the model's transparency and trustworthiness. Future development will aim to integrate PPI feedback, enhancing the framework's effectiveness and its contributions to patient safety and care quality.

Acknowledgments. This report is independent research funded by NHSX and The Health Foundation and it is managed by the National Institute for Health Research (AI_HI200006). The views expressed in this publication are those of the author(s) and not necessarily those of the NHSX, The Health Foundation, National Institute for Health Research, or the Department of Health and Social Care.

Disclosure of Interests. The authors have no competing interests to declare that are relevant to the content of this article.

References

1. Devlin, J., Chang, M., Lee, K., Toutanova, K.: BERT: pre-training of deep bidirectional transformers for language understanding. In: Burstein, J., Doran, C., Solorio, T. (eds.) Proceedings of the 2019 Conference of the North American Chapter of the Association for Computational Linguistics: Human Language Technologies, NAACL-HLT 2019, Minneapolis, MN, USA, June 2-7, 2019, Volume 1 (Long and Short Papers), pp. 4171–4186. Association for Computational Linguistics (2019)
2. Huang, K., Altosaar, J., Ranganath, R.: ClinicalBERT: modeling clinical notes and predicting hospital readmission. ArXiv arXiv:abs/1904.05342 (2019)
3. Lee, J., et al.: BioBERT: a pre-trained biomedical language representation model for biomedical text mining. Bioinformatics **36**(4), 1234–1240 (2019)
4. Lewis, M., et al.: BART: denoising sequence-to-sequence pre-training for natural language generation, translation, and comprehension. In: Annual Meeting of the Association for Computational Linguistics (2019)
5. Luo, Z., Ji, Y., Gupta, A., Li, Z., Frisch, A., He, D.: Towards accurate and clinically meaningful summarization of electronic health record notes: A guided approach. In: 2023 IEEE EMBS International Conference on Biomedical and Health Informatics (BHI), pp. 1–5 (2023)

6. Patil, S.S., Moorthy, V.: Extraction of unstructured electronic healthcare records using natural language processing. In: 2023 International Conference on Networking and Communications (ICNWC), pp. 1–6 (2023)
7. Radford, A., Narasimhan, K.: Improving Language Understanding by Generative Pre-Training (2018)
8. Raffel, C., et al.: Exploring the limits of transfer learning with a unified text-to-text transformer. J. Mach. Learn. Res. **21**(1) (Jan 2020)
9. Sanh, V., Debut, L., Chaumond, J., Wolf, T.: DistilBERT, a distilled version of BERT: smaller, faster, cheaper and lighter. ArXiv arXiv:abs/1910.01108 (2019)
10. Singh, M.K., Cosma, G., Waterson, P., Back, J., Jun, G.T.: I-SIRch: AI-powered concept annotation tool for equitable extraction and analysis of safety insights from maternity investigations. Under Review (2023). Preprint available: https:// github.com/gcosma/I-SIRchpapers
11. Tsai, H.Y., Huang, H.H., Chang, C.J., Tsai, J.S., Chen, H.H.: Patient history summarization on outpatient conversation. In: 2022 IEEE/WIC/ACM International Joint Conference on Web Intelligence and Intelligent Agent Technology (WI-IAT), pp. 364–370 (2022)
12. Wang, W., Wei, F., Dong, L., Bao, H., Yang, N., Zhou, M.: Minilm: deep self-attention distillation for task-agnostic compression of pre-trained transformers. In: Proceedings of the 34th International Conference on Neural Information Processing Systems. NIPS'20, Curran Associates Inc., Red Hook, NY, USA (2020)
13. Zelina, P., Halámková, J., Nováček, V.: Extraction, labeling, clustering, and semantic mapping of segments from clinical notes. IEEE Trans. Nanobiosci. **22**(4), 781–788 (2023)
14. Zhu, Y., Yang, X., Wu, Y., Zhang, W.: Leveraging summary guidance on medical report summarization. IEEE J. Biomed. Health Inform. **27**(10), 5066–5075 (2023)

Synthetic Patient Perspective Data for the Curation and Evaluation of Rare Disease Patient-Facing Technology

Emily Nielsen[(✉)] [ID], Tom Owen [ID], Matthew Roach [ID], and Alan Dix [ID]

Swansea University, Swansea, Wales
{e.e.nielsen,t.owen,m.j.roach,a.j.dix}@swansea.ac.uk

Abstract. Patient-facing technology to support rare disease patients seeking diagnosis has received comparatively little focus from the literature, despite the recognition of its importance. We hypothesise that this is due to the challenges presented when designing pre-diagnostic patient-facing technology within this area. A significant obstacle for research in this area is the lack of data which represents the patient's perspective. Existing data typically does not present the temporal aspects of diagnosis which are crucial to evaluate the diagnosis time of technology and consists of clinical terminology which is not representative of patients. This work aims to bridge this gap by creating open-source data which: (i) utilises patient-friendly terms and (ii) facilitates the sequencing of phenotypes to temporally recreate the informational journey of a rare disease patient. Therefore, this work facilitates evaluations on whether pre-diagnostic technology reduces the time to a rare disease diagnosis, thus providing more meaningful metrics for success.

Keywords: Rare disease · Patient-facing technology · Diagnosis · Health · Synthetic data · Data generation

1 Introduction

This paper looks at the generation of data for the evaluation of systems for rare disease diagnosis considering the need for (i) a temporal lens (importance of early diagnosis); and (ii) a patient-centred approach. Rare disease patients face a long and difficult journey to attain a diagnosis, resulting in severe, permanent and debilitating effects on their health [6]. This is often referred to as a diagnostic odyssey, with the average patient waiting four years, consulting with five clinicians, and receiving three misdiagnoses before they are correctly diagnosed [16]. Technologies to support rare disease diagnosis are almost always clinician-facing [7]. However, the role of the patient may be far more significant for rare conditions [4,6]. 94.6% of clinicians believe that they have insufficient or very poor knowledge of rare diseases [21] and lack time to research rare diseases. In contrast, it is common for patients to research their health, utilising resources such as ChatGPT, Google or Facebook [3,19]. It follows that patients may be able to contribute significantly to consultations with their healthcare providers. Indeed, The UK Strategy for Rare Diseases states that patients can play a significant role in diagnosis and treatment decisions *if given suitable resources* [4].

However, patients with rare diseases feel that they lack the support they need [5] which may be why patients resort to technology which is not specifically designed for health. In addition, applications designed with the common interest in mind will not cater for rare disease patients; information that is relevant to a rare condition is inevitably irrelevant for the majority. This suggests that patients do not have the resources required to play an active part in their health. Therefore, there exists a need for patient-facing pre-diagnostic technology which caters for the needs of people with undiagnosed rare diseases. Since this need has been established, we hypothesise that the limited focus in this area is due to the lack of data which is representative of the patient's perspective. Patient-facing works include Kühnle et al.'s [12] paper on the design of RarePairs, a peer-matched social media platform for rare disease patients. This required the use of an extensive 50-question survey to match patients based on their experiences through the healthcare system. The use of low-data approaches like this suggests that the lack of patient perspective data is a key barrier to data-driven approaches within this area.

Given that rare disease diagnosis is a long process where patients are unlikely to be diagnosed at the first consultation, a positive outcome for patients with rare conditions can be defined as the identification of a diagnosis as early in their journey as possible. As such, the performance of pre-diagnostic technology for rare disease patients needs to be evaluated throughout the diagnostic odyssey. Hence, test data must facilitate this temporal aspect of evaluation. However, as far as the authors are aware, there is only one paper [17] which evaluates the time taken for the proposed model to reach a correct diagnosis. Ronicke et al. evaluated their system, Ada DX, for each consultation that a patient has by manually removing data which would not be available for a given consultation. This revealed that only 33.3% of cases identified the correct condition in the top-5-fit disease list at the first consultation, however, Ada DX suggested the correct disease before clinical diagnosis for 53.8% of cases. This shows a non-trivial difference in the evaluation of this system since reducing the time to diagnosis for over half of the cases is highly significant in this context, however, to only show a single-point accuracy of 33.3% does not accurately portray the effectiveness of this system. Therefore, technology to support the diagnosis of rare diseases must be evaluated at multiple points to get an accurate impression of its effectiveness. While the evaluation approach presented by Ronicke et al. facilitates this, it may not be feasible in several research projects since the breakdown of cases into each of the clinical visits may not be possible (i.e., this information may not be present in the data, or it may be too time-consuming). Moreover, this approach aims to support evaluations of clinically-based technologies and thus is based on clinical data which does not represent the patient's perspective, so other methods may be required for patient-facing technologies. Therefore, there exists a need for approaches to evaluate pre-diagnostic technologies for rare diseases which can support the evaluation of patient-facing technology and does not require significant editing of data for each evaluation.

Hence, we identify two key barriers to accessing suitable data for the implementation and evaluation of rare disease patient-facing technology. Firstly, many sources of patient data are obtained from Electronic Health Records (EHR) [11,22] which consist of technical, clinical terminology. These data are not suitable for patient-facing technology as they do not use patient terminology for symptoms. Secondly, each of the numerous consultations involved in a rare diagnosis [6] presents an opportunity for diagnosis, so static performance metrics do not offer sufficient insight into the benefits of pre-diagnostic technology for rare diseases. Hence, a suitable test set must present different stages of the informational journey of each rare disease patient in order to assess the performance of pre-diagnostic technology over the stages of the diagnostic odyssey. Therefore, we need data which not only uses non-expert terminology, but that also sequences data in the order of a patient's information discovery. To address this gap, we present a data generation process to curate patient perspective data which we make freely available on GitHub[1]. This dataset provides a basis from which we generate: the Static User Profile Data which provides a static dataset for the curation of pre-diagnostic technology; and the Time-Series Persona Data which provides a suitable test set for evaluating pre-diagnostic technology for rare disease patients. These datasets aim to facilitate early-stage and proof-of-concept studies for rare disease pre-diagnostic technology.

2   Data Curation Process Overview

Figure 1 provides an overview of the processes to curate the datasets presented in this paper. The process begins with the established Orphanet rare diseases and phenotypes dataset, which contains phenotypes and the frequency of occurrence of each phenotype within each given disorder, and which is described in more detail later. We then augment Orphanet's data with patient perspective information (layman terminology and patient information discovery) to curate the Patient Perspective Dataset. This dataset provides a basis from which we generate the Time-Series Persona Data and the Static User Profile Data. We describe this process in more detail below.

2.1   Included Disorders

Creating a dataset for the estimated 10,000 types of rare diseases [13] presents a significant amount of work for proof of concept evaluations. Therefore, to establish a challenging but tractable basis on which to evaluate the potential of early-development pre-diagnostic technology, we adopt a subset of three

---

[1] https://github.com/902549/patient_perspective_data.

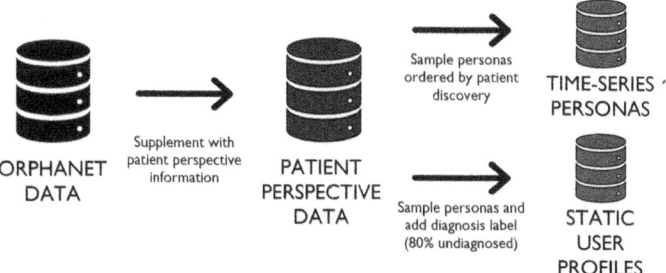

Fig. 1. Overview of the curation process for each of the three datasets

main rare diseases: Fabry Disease[2], Gaucher Disease[3], and hypermobile Ehlers-Danlos Syndrome (hEDS)[4] as the 'positive' classes for the test data. These were chosen because they are well documented, have varying diagnostic difficulties, and are easily misdiagnosed [2,9,15]. Thus, they provide a suitably challenging information-seeking task but also have sufficient documentation to scrape additional data. Clearly, for the purposes of evaluation, we need additional conditions in the databases to sufficiently assess their performance. The inclusion criteria were chosen to create a real-life distribution of the experimental context. That is, the three main rare diseases provided the basis for the Time-Series Persona Data (i.e., the positive classes), but prototypes should also include similar conditions (i.e., the negative classes - conditions that are most likely to be mistaken as the positive class).

The inclusion of misdiagnoses was guided by the relevant literature on the disease in question [1,10,14,15]. Psychological conditions were excluded and only specific named conditions were included. This resulted in a total of 16 rare disorders to provide the negative classes[5] (19 disorders including the three positive classes). Note that our data aims to facilitate comparative evaluations between completing systems, not aiming to give an absolute measure for any given system; therefore it is sufficient to have a range of conditions, but not match base-rate prevalence. In addition, our data aims to facilitate symptom-based patient matching systems which aim to cater for those facing a diagnostic odyssey, so people with common diseases would not have the need of this tool. The database

---

[2] https://rarediseases.org/rare-diseases/fabry-disease/   https://medlineplus.gov/genetics/condition/fabry-disease/   https://www.ninds.nih.gov/health-information/disorders/fabry-disease.

[3] wikipedia.org/wiki/Gaucher's_disease/   https://www.ncbi.nlm.nih.gov/books/NBK1269/.

[4] https://www.nhs.uk/conditions/ehlers-danlos-syndromes/   https://www.ncbi.nlm.nih.gov/books/NBK1279/   https://www.ehlers-danlos.com/what-is-eds/hypermobile-ehlers-danlos-syndrome-heds/.

[5] rheumatic fever, dermatomyositis, erythromelalgia, myelofibrosis, five rare forms of leukemia, two rare types of avascular necrosis, two rare forms of rheumatoid arthritis, vEDS, cEDS, cardiac-valvular EDS.

in a real-world context would be comprised of its users, so there would not typically be patients with common conditions in the database.

3   Curating the Patient Perspective Dataset

Both the Static User Profile Data and the Time-Series Persona Data require realistic patient data which represents the patient's perspective. However, many sources of patient data are obtained from Electronic Health Records (EHR) which consist of technical, clinical terminology [11,22]. These datasets show patients, their condition, and their phenotypic information, either stored as codes or in raw text. However, they are often difficult to access and do not represent a patient's perspective, since this would naturally consist of non-expert language. Some datasets exist which reflect the patient perspective, for example, a number of companies, such as Apple or Google, collect health data (e.g. symptom logging and sensor readings) from smart devices, but these datasets are considered proprietary information and as such are not publicly available. We therefore propose an approach to generate synthetic patient data consisting of non-expert terms for the phenotypes.

We need to create unique and realistic profiles to ensure both our Time-Series Persona Data and Static User Profile Data are as close to real data as possible, thus some form of real patient data must be used as a basis. Since data reflecting the patient perspective is not easily accessible, we use clinical patient data as a basis to create patient perspective profiles. Therefore, several aspects of the clinical patient data will need to be edited to make it representative of the patient's perspective. To ensure this process is efficient, we utilise a knowledge base to create the Patient Perspective Dataset (as opposed to data consisting of individual patient cases) to act as a base from which we can generate as many patient profiles we choose without creating additional work.

Orphanet has endeavoured to gather and improve knowledge on rare diseases since 1997, and as such has created several knowledge bases which provide insight into many different aspects of rare diseases. One knowledge base that Orphanet curated is their rare diseases and phenotypes knowledge base[6]. This contains phenotypes as well as the corresponding frequency of occurrence of each phenotype within each given disorder. In addition, it consists of standardised clinical terminology, is widely used for rare disease research, is frequently updated, multilingual, open source, and spans thousands of rare disorders. Moreover, it enables reproducibility and ensures that, if used in future development, it remains up to date and this process can be expanded to curate larger and more comprehensive datasets. Therefore, Orphanet's knowledge base provides a suitable starting point to create the Patient Perspective Dataset which provides the base from which we generate both the Time-Series Persona Data and the Static User Profile Data. Below we first describe the process used to create the Patient Perspective Dataset, then we present the remaining processes for the Static User Profile Data as well as the Time-Series Persona Data.

---

[6] https://www.orphadata.com/phenotypes.

Now that we have chosen the clinical data to base our patient profiles on, we need to alter this data to represent the perspective of rare disease patients. To create the Patient Perspective Dataset, we enrich the Orphanet data by augmenting the phenotype information for each disease with: HPO categories, layman terms, phenotype discovery group (i.e., development traits, symptoms, exploratory clinical findings, specific clinical findings), and probability of occurrence. Then we define a phenotype sampling process to dynamically generate a range of varied patient profiles from the Patient Perspective Data, using the probability of occurrence and some perturbation noise, each patient profile samples a proportional amount of phenotypes.

3.1   Identifying Patient Terminology for Phenotypes

For each phenotype associated with the 19 disorders, the knowledge base used standardised clinical terminology, namely Human Phenotype Ontology (HPO) terms [18]. HPO not only provides a standardised list of clinical terminology, but it also has synonyms and definitions and classifies phenotypes into categories of the human body (i.e., organ systems and parts of the body). All of this information is accessible on their website[7].

Using HPO's synonyms and definitions, we created initial patient terms. In particular, where synonyms were deemed to be patient- or non-expert-friendly, these were chosen. If there were no synonyms or only expert synonyms, the definitions were checked for short phrases which could be considered synonymous terms in themselves. Phenotypes that did not have clear patient-friendly terms from HPO were researched and discussed among multiple groups of two to four non-experts (people who were not healthcare professionals) until a term was unanimously agreed upon.

Once all terms were finalised by the non-experts, an experienced healthcare professional was shown the original HPO terms as well as the non-expert terms that we created for the three main disorders. They then checked that the patient phenotypes matched the original HPO term. The non-expert terms were then updated according to the suggestions made by the healthcare professional.

3.2   Labelling Phenotypes with Their Discovery Group and HPO Category

Now that we have finalised our layman phenotype terms, let us consider the order of discovery of the different types of patient data and group them accordingly. First, we define and categorise phenotypes into four different discovery groups: developmental traits, symptoms, exploratory clinical findings, and specific clinical findings. Second, we identify pre-requisites for specific clinical findings from existing phenotypes. Finally, we add additional pre-requisite symptoms for phenotypes which can be considered conditions in themselves identified by a clinician. These stages provide the crucial sequencing information which we later use to create the Time-Series Persona Data.

---

[7] https://hpo.jax.org/.

Define and Label Phenotypes by Discovery Group. We can consider each phenotype to either be symptoms (i.e., patient observable) or clinical findings (i.e., not observable by the patient). Since patients would clearly identify phenotypes they can observe themselves before those which require a clinical investigation, these phenotypes should come first. Some symptoms, such as *feeding difficulties in infancy*, would be observable from birth or a very young age. Therefore, it is important to distinguish these phenotypes, so the first two discovery groups are symptoms and developmental traits.

In addition, we can consider clinical findings to have two main types: exploratory clinical findings and specific clinical findings. We define exploratory clinical findings to be traits that are likely to be identified from routine investigations (e.g., blood tests, standard physical examinations). As such, many of these findings will be identified during or shortly after a patient visits their primary care physician.

We define specific clinical findings as traits which are likely to only be identified from specific investigations. It would be unrealistic for specific investigations to be conducted without the presence of symptoms to prompt these investigations. For example, the probability of discovering an *abnormal myocardium morphology* (abnormal heart wall muscle) is increased with the presence of cardiovascular symptoms, such as chest pain. Therefore, for each specific finding, we must ensure that the pre-requisite symptoms that are needed to prompt the necessary investigations are also sampled along with the specific finding.

Identify Pre-requisites for Specific Clinical Findings. This stage utilises HPO categories to identify pre-requisites for specific findings, namely the HPO category of a specific finding denotes the HPO category to identify required pre-requisites. That is, (i) we scrape HPO categories for each phenotype within the dataset, (ii) when a specific finding is sampled, 1-2 symptoms with the same HPO category are sampled.

First, we need to establish which symptoms should be considered pre-requisites for a given specific finding. To do this, we augment each phenotype in our data with its HPO category (i.e., organ systems and other physiological categories) as gathered from HPO's website. Then, for each sampled specific clinical finding, we additionally sample pre-requisite symptoms with the same HPO category as the finding. We generate one to two pre-requisite symptoms for each specific clinical finding using a random number generator to add perturbation noise. For example, if *abnormal myocardium morphology* was sampled, cardiovascular symptoms such as *heart palpitations* would also be sampled.

Add Clinician Identified Pre-requisites. In addition, some phenotypes, such as anaemia, may be considered conditions in of themselves. As such, there would naturally be symptoms associated with them, however, this was not present in the data. Since a clinician will know these conditions well, by denoting the presence of the condition, the associated symptoms may be implied. However, a patient will not necessarily recognise these associated symptoms. Therefore, we also add key symptoms associated with conditions that are present in the dataset. The underlying symptoms of phenotypes of this nature were identified by a healthcare professional and as such these symptoms were added and categorised into a new discovery group, pre-requisites. This ensured that they were only sampled if they are a pre-requisite of a phenotype that has been sampled, and otherwise cannot be sampled.

3.3   Probabilistic Sampling of Phenotypes

To generate a realistic range of phenotypes for each patient profile for a given disease we transformed unstructured frequency values from Orphanet's ontology into a probability density. The Orphanet ontology consisted of categorical values stored as strings (namely, always present: 100 %, very frequent: 99%-80% frequent: 79%-30%, occasional: 29%-5%, rare: 4%-1%, excluded: 0%). For values in a range, we took the mid-point of the percentage values and converted these to numbers between 0 and 1.

To generate unique patient profiles, we take a sample of phenotypes for a given disorder by randomly sampling from their defined frequency distribution using Numpy's random choice function[8]. Since the phenotypes in each discovery group are generated separately, we need to normalise our frequencies for each discovery group (this is a requirement of the sampling function). Since we sample within each discovery group, we lose the distribution of each group, so we set the number of phenotypes sampled to be representative of the weight of the discovery group's frequency. In addition, the proportion of phenotypes for each discovery group will vary from patient to patient, so we add some perturbation noise to the number of phenotypes sampled within the discovery group.

Now, let us formalise this as an equation for clarity. Given a disorder there is a set D of phenotypes for that disorder and a collection $G_1...G_5$ of the discovery groups for the disorder that have the properties: (i) $G_k \subset D$ – a disorder's discovery group only includes phenotypes for that disorder, (ii) $D = \bigcup(G_k)$ – every phenotype for the disorder is in a discovery group, (iii) $G_k \cap G_l = \emptyset$ for $k \neq l$ – no phenotype in more than one discovery group. So, we define the weight, w, of the discovery group as $w = \frac{\sum_{i \in G_k} F_i}{\sum_{i \in D} F_i}$, where F_i is the frequency of phenotype i. Therefore, given the total number of desired phenotypes per patient profile T, the size of phenotypes sampled within a specific discovery group is $T * w$ with some perturbation noise and then rounded to the nearest whole number.

4   Static User Profile and Time-Series Persona Data

Two separate processes follow now that we have created our Patient Perspective Data and defined our process for sampling phenotypes. For the Static User Profile Data, a diagnosis status and a name are assigned to the patient profile to create a user. For the Time-Series Persona Data, the phenotypes are sequenced based on their discovery group and divided into informational stages. We describe these steps in more detail in the following sections.

---

[8] https://numpy.org/doc/stable/reference/random/generated/numpy.random.choice.html.

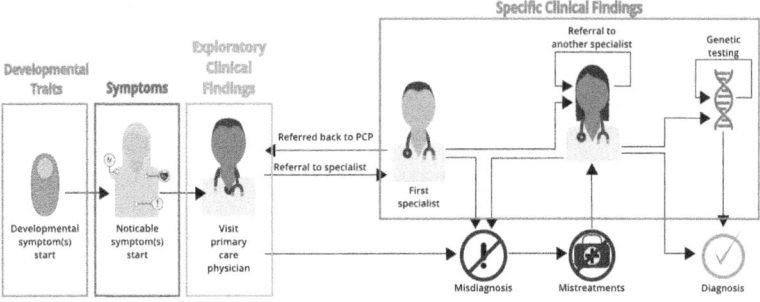

Fig. 2. Information discovery during a rare disease diagnostic odyssey

4.1 Creating the Static User Profile Data

Using the method described above, we sample patient personas from the Patient Perspective Dataset. The Static User Profile Data is intended to provide a user base for recommendation systems for symptom-based patient matching, so now we augment the data for this purpose. First, we set a diagnostic status for users. Let's consider a patient matching system that is predominantly aimed to be a pre-diagnostic application but not limited to pre-diagnosis. As such, we assume the majority of users are undiagnosed, so some people with diagnoses will be on the system. Therefore, we populate 80% of the users in the Static User Profile Data to be undiagnosed, the remaining users' diagnostic status displays the sampled disorder name. In addition, to ensure that the data presents humanistic users (as would be the case in a real-world context), we include randomly generated first names for each of the profiles. Therefore, the Static User Profile Data portrays a patient profile with a name, diagnosis status and a list of phenotypes.

4.2 Creating the Time-Series Persona Data

In this section, we outline our process to create the Time-Series Persona Data. The Patient Perspective Dataset that we generated above to provides a basis from which we can generate the Time-Series Persona Data. Given that the Patient Perspective Dataset was based on a rigorous knowledge base, it provides a realistic static basis for the Time-Series Persona Data. However, to simulate the informational journey of a rare disease patient, we need to augment the data with critical sequencing information which is representative of a patient's discovery of phenotypes. In particular, we use the sampling process described above to create patient personas. We then use the discovery groups to sequence phenotypes of each patient persona based on the patient information discovery of the phenotype group. These steps are described in more detail below.

First, we recreate the temporal aspect of information discovery from a patient's perspective. To do this, let us relate the phenotypes from our data to the diagnostic odyssey. In particular, as shown in Fig. 2, we can augment the patient journey diagram with the discovery groups, showing the order in which clinical discoveries are made and observed by the patient. The different types of data which we divided into the following discovery groups: developmental traits; symptoms; pre-requisite symptoms; exploratory clinical findings; specific clinical findings. This grouping can be utilised to provide the synthetic data with critical sequencing information to facilitate the revelation of phenotypes as each discovery group is perceived by the patient.

Patients discover the different types of phenotypes at different rounds of their diagnostic journey. Firstly, phenotypes which are observable by patients would be discovered first. Since developmental traits are present from an early age, it follows that these phenotypes should occur first, followed by non-developmental symptoms. Secondly, once the patient seeks medical help, clinicians will start providing them with information from tests or physical examinations. Routine investigations are often made on the first few visits, so exploratory findings will be identified first. Specific findings will occur latest in the diagnostic odyssey since these findings require specific investigations prompted by the phenotypes observed thus far. Therefore, to ensure that the Time-Series Persona Data is representative of a rare disease odyssey, we order the synthetic data so that developmental traits come first, followed by symptoms (including pre-requisites), exploratory findings, and finally specific findings.

Following this, we divided the phenotypes into different stages of information discovery by distributing the sorted phenotypes equally into the number of stages desired. In our case, we distributed the phenotypes equally to ensure that each stage was consistent in the amount of information that was revealed. Table 1 shows an example of the final generated Time-Series Persona Data for each of the three conditions included in the laboratory study.

Table 1. Time-Series Persona Data example for the three conditions

Condition	Early Stage	Middle Stage	Late Stage
hEDS	Sleep disturbance, Joint dislocation, Stretchy skin, Elbow dislocation, Muscle pain	Fatigue, Heartburn, Thin skin, Depressivity, Vertigo	Nausea and vomiting, Soft skin, Constipation, Gastrointestinal dysmotility, Extra bones in the cranium
Fabry Disease	Small dark-red spot, Poor appetite and weight loss, Lack of sweating, Nausea and vomiting	Joint pain, Blood in urine, Thickened skin, Vision loss	Kidney damage/Kidney disease, Cataract, Optic atrophy, Corneal dystrophy
Gaucher Disease	Squint, Corneal opacity, Joint pain, Abdominal pain, Recurrent fractures	Tremor, Falling, Delayed skeletal maturation, Recurrent fractures	Osteopenia: Decreased bone density, Enlarged liver, Cranial nerve paralysis, Enlarged spleen

5 Evaluating the Database

The steps above augmented a clinical knowledge base with patient terminology and sequencing information to create the Static User Profile Data and the

Time-Series Persona Data. These datasets provide data which represents the patient perspective for the curation of patient-facing technology. In addition, the Time-Series Persona data provides a temporal dataset to facilitate evaluations at different stages of the diagnostic odyssey. This provides more meaningful measures of the efficacy of technology by facilitating assessments on how quickly and consistently it suggests the correct diagnosis. However, before we use this data to perform evaluations, we must assess its suitability for purpose. In particular, we need to evaluate whether it provides a suitable representation of the informational journey of a real-world rare disease diagnosis.

Typical methods of evaluating synthetic data include comparing with other data using statistical methods or the performance of machine learning models. We do not have other data to compare our synthetic data to, so we could not use this evaluation method. Another method of validation is through feedback from domain experts, or by evaluating the utility of data for its intended application.

The Patient Perspective Dataset intends to represent patients, but is based on clinical data, so we can consider both healthcare professionals (HCPs) and non-HCPs to be domain experts in different ways. As non-HCPs would not know medical terminology, their input was important to provide terminology which was understandable to patients, whereas the HCPs knowledge of medical terminology verified that these terms were representative of the original HPO term. So, there was continual formative evaluation by domain experts throughout the process. As such, a subsequent expert evaluation of the Patient Perspective Data was not deemed necessary. Instead, we incorporate expert input to evaluate whether individual personas are realistic in the Time-Series Persona Data.

A healthcare practitioner with experience in primary care and rare diseases tested the Time-Series Persona Data by participating in a blinded simulation task, where the underlying condition of a given persona was only revealed at the end. They were presented three informational stages where new phenotypes were revealed and were asked to identify the condition using Google. Once the condition was revealed at the end of the three informational stages, they were asked about the realism of the task based on their clinical experience. They expressed that the patient persona made sense and was similar to their clinical experiences.

However, they discussed that when making diagnostic decisions, they would typically inquire about the patient's family history and duration of symptoms. Given that patients do not typically consider their family history until a genetic condition is suspected [8, 20], we did not consider this data feature to be necessary for the study. Moreover, we also deemed it could potentially lead participants to actively pursue genetic causes who would not have otherwise considered a genetic condition. The duration of symptoms, however, would be a relevant addition to the data, but as we did not have this information in the Orphanet dataset, we could not add this aspect. For future studies, we could explore methods to curate additional data features, such as the duration of symptoms. However, we deemed the current data to be sufficient for preliminary evaluations.

The Time-Series Persona Data may facilitate evaluations for a small number of conditions. In the context of proof of concept and early-stage evaluations, this provides a strong indication on potential. However, a larger dataset of patient phenotypes would be necessary to allow for evaluations on a greater scale. Large Language Models (LLMs) have shown significant promise in generating textual data based on a given input. Pre-trained transformer models, such as BART may be fine-tuned on the manually curated Patient Perspective Dataset, in addition to text scraped from HPO's website to provide a model which will translate clinical terminology to patient terminology. In addition, due to the variability of outputs from models like GPT 4, this may also provide multiple synonymous terms, thus adding to the realism of the patient data.

Future work may explore whether the Time-Series Patient Persona Dataset may be adapted to facilitate evaluations for clinician-facing technology. This may facilitate evaluation approaches that assess technology based on the time taken to diagnosis, rather than as a single-point accuracy. Ronicke et al. [17] performed a temporally-aware evaluation, however, it required significant manual edits to separate data based on the information that would be available at specific clinical visits. Researchers may not have sufficient time to perform these manual edits, so this dataset may provide a low-resource approach to facilitate temporal evaluations to support clinicians with rare diagnosis.

6   Conclusion

This paper presents a data generation approach for the curation of the Patient Perspective Dataset which aims to provide patient data which utilises (i) a temporal lens; and (ii) patient-centred language. We provide the Patient Perspective Dataset along with the code for sampling patient profiles on GitHub[9]. This data aims to bridge the gap where existing datasets were not suitable for patient-facing technology. Firstly, this data utilises non-expert terminology to represent the language used by patients. Secondly, this data is augmented with sequencing information to allow for temporal evaluations.

Clearly, the dataset presented in this paper provides a small sample of manually curated data. This provides a starting point from which a larger dataset could be curated with an automated pipeline. For example, a pre-trained transformer models may be fine-tuned on the Patient Perspective Dataset to provide a model which will translate clinical terminology to patient terminology. In addition, the HPO category, synonyms and definitions from HPO's website can easily be scraped using the phenotype's HPO ID and the disorder's Orphanet ID. Hence, this work can act as a basis from which an automatically generated patient perspective dataset may be curated. This would facilitate temporally aware evaluations to promote the design of pre-diagnostic technology which performs well throughout the stages of diagnosis. As such, this could open a new avenue of research to apply algorithms more suited to temporal contexts to this area which could prove more effective for this context of a lengthy diagnosis.

---

[9] https://github.com/902549/patient_perspective_data.

Considering temporal approaches for pre-diagnostic technology for rare diseases may increase the potential to support more challenging diagnoses where further investigations facilitate differentiation from common conditions.

Acknowledgments. The authors would like to thank Amicus Therapeutics for their support during this project. The main author is funded by the EPSRC Centre for Doctoral Training in Enhancing Human Interactions and Collaborations with Data and Intelligence Driven Systems (EP/S021892/1).

Disclosure of Interests. The authors have no competing interests to declare that are relevant to the content of this article.

References

1. Berglund, B., Nordström, G., Lützén, K.: Living a restricted life with ehlers-danlos syndrome (eds). Int. J. Nurs. Stud. **37**(2), 111–118 (Apr 2000). https://doi.org/10.1016/S0020-7489(99)00067-X, https://www.sciencedirect.com/science/article/pii/S002074899900067X
2. Colomba, P., et al.: Fabry disease and multiple sclerosis misdiagnosis: the role of family history and neurological signs. Oncotarget **9**, 7758–7762 (2018). https://doi.org/10.18632/oncotarget.23970
3. De Choudhury, M., Morris, M.R., White, R.W.: Seeking and sharing health information online: comparing search engines and social media. In: Proceedings of the SIGCHI Conference on Human Factors in Computing Systems, pp. 1365–1376. CHI '14, Association for Computing Machinery, New York, NY, USA (Apr 2014). https://doi.org/10.1145/2556288.2557214
4. Department of Health UK: The UK strategy for rare diseases (2013). https://assets.publishing.service.gov.uk/government/uploads/system/uploads/attachment_data/file/260562/UK_Strategy_for_Rare_Diseases.pdf
5. Depping, M.K., Uhlenbusch, N., von Kodolitsch, Y., Klose, H.F.E., Mautner, V.F., Löwe, B.: Supportive care needs of patients with rare chronic diseases: multi-method, cross-sectional study. Orphanet J. Rare Dis. **16**, 44 (2021). https://doi.org/10.1186/s13023-020-01660-w
6. Faurisson, F.: Survey of the delay in diagnosis for 8 rare diseases in Europe: Eurordiscare2 (2004). https://www.eurordis.org/wp-content/uploads/2009/12/EURORDISCARE_FULLBOOKr.pdf
7. Faviez, C., et al.: Diagnosis support systems for rare diseases: a scoping review. Orphanet J. Rare Dis. **15**(1), 94 (2020). https://doi.org/10.1186/s13023-020-01374-z
8. Genetic Alliance, The New York Mid-Atlantic Consortium for Genetic and Newborn Screening Services: Understanding Genetics: A New York, Mid-Atlantic Guide for Patients and Health Professionals. Genetic Alliance, Washington (DC) (Jul 2009). https://pubmed.ncbi.nlm.nih.gov/23304754/
9. Halverson, C.M.E., Cao, S., Perkins, S.M., Francomano, C.A.: Comorbidity, misdiagnoses, and the diagnostic odyssey in patients with hypermobile ehlers-danlos syndrome. Genetics Med. Open **1**(1), 100812 (Apr 2023). https://doi.org/10.1016/j.gimo.2023.100812, https://www.sciencedirect.com/science/article/pii/S294977442300821X

10. Hershenfeld, S.A., et al.: Psychiatric disorders in Ehlers-Danlos syndrome are frequent, diverse and strongly associated with pain. Rheumatol. Int. **36**(3), 341–348 (2016). https://doi.org/10.1007/s00296-015-3375-1

11. Kruse, C.S., Smith, B., Vanderlinden, H., Nealand, A.: Security techniques for the electronic health records. J. Med. Syst. **41**, 127 (2017). https://doi.org/10.1007/s10916-017-0778-4

12. Kühnle, L., Mücke, U., Lechner, W.M., Klawonn, F., Grigull, L.: Development of a social network for people without a diagnosis (rarepairs): Evaluation study. J. Med. Internet Res. **22**(9), e21849 (Sep 2020). https://doi.org/10.2196/21849, http://www.jmir.org/2020/9/e21849/

13. Haendel, M., et al.: How many rare diseases are there? Nat. Rev. Drug Discov. **19**(2), 77–78 (2020). https://doi.org/10.1038/d41573-019-00180-y, https://www.ncbi.nlm.nih.gov/pmc/articles/PMC7771654/

14. Mehta, A., et al.: Fabry disease defined: baseline clinical manifestations of 366 patients in the fabry outcome survey. Europ. J. Clin. Invest. **34**(3), 236–242 (2004). https://doi.org/10.1111/j.1365-2362.2004.01309.x

15. Mistry, P.K., et al.: A reappraisal of Gaucher disease-diagnosis and disease management algorithms. Am. J. Hematol. **86**(1), 110–115 (2011). https://doi.org/10.1002/ajh.21888

16. Muir, E.: The rare reality - an insight into the patient and family experience of rare disease (2016). https://www.raredisease.org.uk/media/1588/the-rare-reality-an-insight-into-the-patient-and-family-experience-of-rare-disease.pdf

17. Ronicke, S., Hirsch, M.C., Türk, E., Larionov, K., Tientcheu, D., Wagner, A.D.: Can a decision support system accelerate rare disease diagnosis? Evaluating the potential impact of Ada DX in a retrospective study. Orphanet J. Rare Dis. **14**(1), 69 (2019). https://doi.org/10.1186/s13023-019-1040-6

18. Köhler, S., et al.: The human phenotype ontology in 2021. Nucleic Acids Res. **49**(D1), D1207–D1217 (2021). https://doi.org/10.1093/nar/gkaa1043

19. Shahsavar, Y., Choudhury, A.: User intentions to use chatgpt for self-diagnosis and health-related purposes: Cross-sectional survey study. JMIR Hum Factors **10**, e47564 (May 2023). https://doi.org/10.2196/47564, http://www.ncbi.nlm.nih.gov/pubmed/37195756

20. Walker, H.K., Hall, W.D., Hurst, J.W.: Clinical Methods: The History, Physical, and Laboratory Examinations. Butterworth-Heinemann Ltd, Boston, 3rd edn. (Apr 1990), https://www.ncbi.nlm.nih.gov/books/NBK201/, chapter 215 The Family History

21. Walkowiak, D., Domaradzki, J.: Are rare diseases overlooked by medical education? awareness of rare diseases among physicians in Poland: an explanatory study. Orphanet J. Rare Dis. **16**, 400 (2021). https://doi.org/10.1186/s13023-021-02023-9

22. Wen, Q., Ouyang, Z., Zhang, J., Qian, Y., Ye, Y., Zhang, C.: Disentangled dynamic heterogeneous graph learning for opioid overdose prediction. In: Proceedings of the 28th ACM SIGKDD Conference on Knowledge Discovery and Data Mining. p. 2009-2019. KDD '22, Association for Computing Machinery, New York, NY, USA (2022). https://doi.org/10.1145/3534678.3539279

Author Index

GPSR Compliance

The European Union's (EU) General Product Safety Regulation (GPSR) is a set of rules that requires consumer products to be safe and our obligations to ensure this.

If you have any concerns about our products, you can contact us on ProductSafety@springernature.com

In case Publisher is established outside the EU, the EU authorized representative is:

Springer Nature Customer Service Center GmbH
Europaplatz 3
69115 Heidelberg, Germany

The manufacturer's authorised representative in the EU is Springer
Nature Customer Service Centre GmbH, Europaplatz 3, 69115 Heidelberg,
Germany. If you have any concerns regarding our products, please
contact ProductSafety@springernature.com

Printed and bound by CPI Group (UK) Ltd, Croydon, CR0 4YY
24/04/2026
02096351-0009